Aristotle on the Essence of Human Thought

OXFORD ARISTOTLE STUDIES

General Editor
Lindsay Judson

PUBLISHED VOLUMES INCLUDE

Aristotle on the Sources of the Ethical Life
Sylvia Berryman

Doing and Being
An Interpretation of Aristotle's Metaphysics Theta
Jonathan Beere

Aristotle on Knowledge and Learning
The Posterior Analytics
David Bronstein

The Undivided Self
Aristotle and the 'Mind-Body Problem'
David Charles

Time for Aristotle
Physics *IV. 10–14*
Ursula Coope

Aristotle and the Eleatic One
Timothy Clarke

Passions and Persuasion in Aristotle's *Rhetoric*
Jamie Dow

Teleology, First Principles, and Scientific Method in Aristotle's Biology
Allan Gotthelf

Aristotle on Shame and Learning to Be Good
Marta Jimenez

The Powers of Aristotle's Soul
Thomas Kjeller Johansen

Aristotle on Teleology
Monte Ransome Johnson

How Aristotle Gets by in *Metaphysics Zeta*
Frank A. Lewis

Aristotle on the Apparent Good
Perception, Phantasia, *Thought, and Desire*
Jessica Moss

Priority in Aristotle's Metaphysics
Michail Peramatzis

Aristotle's Theory of Bodies
Christian Pfeiffer

Aristotle on the Essence of Human Thought

KLAUS CORCILIUS
ANDREA FALCON
ROBERT ROREITNER

Funded by the European Union
European Research Council
Established by the European Commission

OXFORD
UNIVERSITY PRESS

OXFORD
UNIVERSITY PRESS

Great Clarendon Street, Oxford, OX2 6DP,
United Kingdom

Oxford University Press is a department of the University of Oxford.
It furthers the University's objective of excellence in research, scholarship,
and education by publishing worldwide. Oxford is a registered trade mark of
Oxford University Press in the UK and in certain other countries

Published in the United States of America by Oxford University Press
198 Madison Avenue, New York, NY 10016, United States of America

British Library Cataloguing in Publication Data
Data available

Library of Congress Control Number: 2024945854

ISBN 9780198921790

DOI: 10.1093/9780198921820.001.0001

The manufacturer's authorised representative in the EU for product safety is
Oxford University Press España S.A. of El Parque Empresarial San Fernando
de Henares, Avenida de Castilla, 2 – 28830 Madrid (www.oup.es/en or
product.safety@oup.com). OUP España S.A. also acts as importer into Spain
of products made by the manufacturer.

Contents

Figures

Note on the Text, Translations, and Transliteration

Abbreviations

The list of abbreviations for Aristotle is based on the one printed in the first volume of *Aristoteles Graecus* (Moraux et al. 1976).

Alexander of Aphrodisias

An.	*De anima*	*On the Soul*
De Int.	*De intellectu*	*On the Intellect*

Aristotle

An.	*De anima*	*On the Soul*
Cael.	*De caelo*	*On the Heavens*
EE	*Ethica Eudemia*	*Eudemian Ethics*
EN	*Ethica Nicomachea*	*Nicomachean Ethics*
Gener. An.	*De generatione animalium*	*Generation of Animals*
Gener. Corr.	*De generatione et corruptione*	*Generation and Corruption*
Hist. An.	*De historia animalium*	*History of Animals*
Inc. An.	*De incessu animalium*	*On the Progression of Animals*
Insomn.	*De insomniis*	*On Dreams*
Int.	*De interpretatione*	*On Interpretation*
Juv.	*De juventute et senectute*	*On Youth and Old Age*
Long.	*De longitudine et brevitate vitae*	*On the Length and Shortness of Life*
Mem.	*De memoria*	*On Memory*
Metaph.	*Metaphysica*	*Metaphysics*
Mete.	*Meteorologica*	*Meteorology*
Mot. An.	*De motu animalium*	*On the Motion of Animals*
Part. An.	*De partibus animalium*	*Parts of Animals*
Phys.	*Physica*	*Physics*
Poet.	*De arte poetica*	*Poetics*

Probl.	*Problemata*	*Problems*
Respir.	*De respiratione*	*On Respiration*
Rhet.	*Rhetorica*	*Rhetorics*
Sens.	*De sensu et sensato*	*On Sense-perception*
Soph.	*Sophistici Elenchi*	*Sophistical Refutations*
Somn.	*De somno et vigilia*	*On Sleep and Waking*
Top.	*Topica*	*Topics*

Philoponus

De Int.	*De intellectu*	*On the Intellect*
In An.	*In libros De anima commentaria*	*On Aristotle's On the Soul*

Plato

Phaed.	*Phaedo*	*Phaedo*
Phlb.	*Philebus*	*Philebus*
Soph.	*Sophista*	*Sophist*
Theaet.	*Theaetetus*	*Theaetetus*
Tim.	*Timaeus*	*Timaeus*

Sextus Empiricus

M	*Adversus mathematicos*	*Against the Professors*

Ps-Simplicius

In An.	*In Aristotelis De anima commentaria*	*On Aristotle's On the Soul*

Sophonias

In An.	*In Aristotelis De anima paraphrasis*	*On Aristotle's On the Soul*

Theophrastus

Sens.	*De sensibus*	*On Perception*

Themistius

In An.	*In Aristotelis De anima paraphrasis*	*On Aristotle's On the Soul*

Thucydides

Hist.	*Historiae*	*History of the Peloponnesian War*

Presocratics

DK *Die Fragmente der Vorsokratiker*. 3 vols. H. Diels and W. Kranz (eds.). Zürich 1951^{6}.

Convention

Square brackets, [ ], indicate that the enclosed words are added to improve the translation of the original Greek text.

Note on Translations

Unless otherwise indicated, all translations are ours.

Rules of Transliteration

α	*a*
β	*b*
γ	*g*
δ	*d*
ε	*e*
ζ	*z*
η	*ê*
θ	*th*
ι	*i*
κ	*k*
λ	*l*
μ	*m*
ν	*n*

ξ	*x*
ο	*o*
π	*p*
ρ	*r*
σ	*s*
τ	*t*
υ	*u*
φ	*ph*
χ	*ch*
ψ	*ps*
ω	*ô*
γγ	*ng*
γκ	*nk*

The iota subscript is transliterated by an *i* on the line.
Rough breathing at the beginning of a word is rendered by an *h*, while smooth breathing is ignored.

Foreword

This book offers a novel interpretation of Aristotle's treatment of the capacity for thought in *An.* III 4–8. The argument of the book differs from recent monographic studies of Aristotle's account of human thinking in more than one way. To begin with, (1) the book offers a reading of *An.* III 4–8 as firmly embedded in Aristotle's theory of the soul as the principle of the science of living beings and its methodology; (2) it argues that the stretch of text in *An.* III 4–8 contains a unitary and coherent definitory account of the essence of the human capacity for thinking; (3) it claims that Aristotle's account is capable of *explaining* important features of human thinking such as the ability to entertain a proposition or the universality and objectivity of human thought; (4) it accepts Aristotle's statements to the effect that the essence of human thinking is matterless (in a certain way); and last but not least, (5) it accepts Aristotle's description of human *nous* as a capacity (e.g., in *An.* III 4, 429a30).[1]

This is emphatically not a co-edited volume. Rather, it comes as close as possible to a co-authored book insofar as the three authors have come to agree on a large number of general points constituting an overall new approach to Aristotle's account of human thought (*nous*). They have, moreover, come to agree on how Aristotle's argument unfolds in *An.* III 4–8. This does not mean that the three authors necessarily agree on how to read every single detail of this exceedingly difficult stretch of text. But they believe that the remaining areas of disagreement are local and at no point undermine the overall coherence and novelty of the reading advanced in this book.

The book was written in the new and strange world into which we all were plunged with the outbreak of COVID-19 in February 2020. Unable to travel, the authors used the Zoom platform to meet and discuss drafts of their essays in long, and at times exhausting, work sessions. These meetings were instrumental in developing not only a coherent reading of *An.* III 4–8 but also a common language to describe what Aristotle is up to in this stretch of text. Each author remains fully

[1] Recent monographic treatments of human thought in Aristotle are Jiménez 2017 and Kelsey 2022. While Erick Jiménez agrees with none of the above claims, Sean Kelsey, following a very different method of interpretation that does not involve a close reading of *An.* III 4–8, seems to agree at least with (2), (4), and (5). In their recent books, respectively concerned with Aristotle's psychological hylomorphism and his account of the powers of the soul, David Charles (Charles 2021) and Thomas Johansen (Johansen 2012) argue that human theoretical *nous* depends existentially, but not essentially, on the human body. We agree with them. Johansen, who does not offer an in-depth interpretation of *An.* III 4–8, seems to agree with (1), even if the account of the methodology offered in his book is different from the one advanced here. He also agrees, with some important qualifications, with (2), (4), and (5).

responsible for the contents of his chapter (or chapters). Each chapter is the equivalent of a building block toward the development of a single argument in support of a single position. The first-person singular "I" is employed in each chapter to underscore that each author remains solely responsible for what is said at each step of the argument. By contrast, the conclusion of the book, which is also the conclusion of the argument, is jointly written by the three authors with the goal of highlighting some of the most important results reached in the book. By proceeding in this way, the authors want to preserve the co-authorship of the book while also allowing the reader to assign everything that is said at every step of the argument to a single author.

Klaus Corcilius wrote the Introduction (Chapter 1), Chapter 2 (on *An.* III 4–5), and Chapter 5 (on *An.* III 8); Robert Roreitner wrote Chapter 3 (on *An.* III 6) and Chapter 6 (Aristotle on *nous* and nature); Andrea Falcon wrote Chapter 4 (on *An.* III 7). The Glossary at the end of the volume was collectively written. This glossary is meant to serve as a point of reference for expert readers. It will also provide beginners with a first orientation to the contents of the book. In this respect, the authors' ambition was to write a book not only for historians of philosophy who are critically engaged with Aristotle but also for philosophers who are interested in what Aristotle has to say on the topic of human thought. For the reader's convenience, we attached, as an appendix to the book, the Greek text of *An.* III 4–8, along with a critical apparatus (taken from Aurelius Förster's edition) and an English translation (ours).

The origins of the book go back to a three-day seminar on *An.* III 4–5 led by Pavel Gregoric in the spring of 2018 at Charles University, Prague. It was during this seminar that Pavel Gregoric and Robert Roreitner conceived the idea of a workshop devoted to Aristotle's inquiry into *nous* in *De anima* beyond *An.* III 4–5. This second workshop was organized at the Warburg Institute, London, in November 2018. Robert Roreitner presented on *An.* III 6, Pavel Gregoric on *An.* III 7, and Klaus Corcilius on *An.* III 8. A follow-up workshop was organized in March 2019 at the University of Gothenburg. Leading up to and during this third meeting, some main points of the future Chapter 1 were sketched out, and a first version of the text and translation was prepared (Pavel Gregoric took a leading role in the latter). It was in Gothenburg that the group conceived the plan of co-authoring a book on the essence of human thought in Aristotle's *De anima* with an emphasis on how Aristotle's argument develops in *An.* III 6–8. The next workshop took place at the University of Tübingen, in November 2019, where *An.* III 4–8 was discussed in a larger context of related texts, such as *An.* III 3, *Mem.* 1, and *Posterior Analytics* II 19. In the meantime, regrettably, Pavel Gregoric had to withdraw due to other, more urgent commitments. But, fortunately for the project, Andrea Falcon agreed to join the group in October 2020. He wrote from scratch an essay on *An.* III 7 and assumed editorial tasks that helped to bring the project to its conclusion.

We would like to thank, above all, Pavel Gregoric, who gave the impetus to the project and contributed greatly to its initial phases, and Michel Crubellier, who participated in all the Zoom meetings and contributed to this book not only with his expert feedback but also by drafting one entry that is now incorporated in the Glossary (ACTUALITY, FIRST AND SECOND). Michel Crubellier also shared an unpublished article on the role of *An.* III 3 in Aristotle's argument. The seeds of the ideas on and around what is called "the grey zone" in Chapter 1 are to be found in that article.

Many thanks are due to the probing and encouraging audiences in London, Gothenburg, and Tübingen, and especially to Börje Biden, Peter Sjoerd Hasper, Sophia Connell, and Christina Thomsen Törnqvist.

We are also pleased to acknowledge the expert feedback received from two anonymous readers chosen by the Press and from Lindsay Judson in his capacity as General Editor of the series "Aristotle Studies." Their comments were helpful and always constructive in spirit. We have done our best to incorporate them into the final version of the book. We are grateful to Peter Momtchiloff for his expert editorial guidance in the early stages of the project.

Michael Arsenault read the final version of the manuscript. His sharp comments and helpful suggestions for improvement helped us produce a clearer and more readable book.

We acknowledge the generous support provided by the following institutions: the *Representation and Reality* project based at the University of Gothenburg, which provided the funds for the organization of the first two workshops, the Eberhard Karls University of Tübingen, and the Charles University of Prague. The bulk of the work for this book, including the drafting of its final version, was done under the aegis of ERC 2021 Advanced Grant: *Text and Idea of Aristotle's Science of Living Things* (acronym: TIDA).

The book is a gold Open Access publication with the generous support of the European Union (ERC, TIDA, grant agreement No. 101053296). The views and opinions expressed in the book are those of the three co-authors and do not necessarily reflect those of the European Union or of the European Research Council Executive Agency. Neither the European Union nor the granting authority can be held responsible for them.

Klaus Corcilius, Andrea Falcon, and Robert Roreitner

1
Introduction

1. What is *nous*?

The conception of *nous* lies at the heart of Aristotle's philosophy. On his conception, *nous* makes it possible that there is what we may call *objective knowledge*: that is, knowledge of how things really are, taken in themselves, and not how they might appear to different subjects at different times. *Nous* also explains why we can *know everything*, where "everything" is to be taken in a perfectly unqualified sense of "everything there is": that is, all things, including ourselves, *nous* itself, and even God. *Nous*, then, on Aristotle's understanding of it, somehow encompasses our subjective thinking as well as the objective being of things. It grounds the possibility of philosophical knowledge.

What is *nous*? As a term, *nous* is very hard, if not impossible, to translate. It is usually translated as "thought," "intellect," "understanding," or "reason." It is sometimes also rendered as "mind" or "spirit." But none of these translations seems to fully capture its meaning. One thing is clear, though: *nous*, along with perception (*aisthêsis*), is one of the two cognitive parts of the soul—namely, one of the two parts of the soul responsible for cognition in the wide sense of *gnôsis* (i.e., in the sense of the obtaining of information in a way such that something we may call "mental content" results). There are also other fields of application of the term *nous*, especially in Aristotle's theory of scientific explanation, his ethical theory, and his first philosophy (what we call metaphysics), but for the time being, and for reasons which will become apparent below, we will approach our question ("What is *nous*?") from the perspective of the human soul.

Nous and perception, then, are the two parts—and *capacities* (*dunameis*)—of the soul responsible for the fact that we can have "something in mind," whatever that may be—for instance, the sight of a landscape, a mathematical theorem, or the thoughts that pass through our minds when we are reading a poem.[1] If perception and *nous* together exhaust all kinds of cognition that perishable living beings are capable of,

I would like to thank Andrea Falcon, Michel Crubellier, and Robert Roreitner for their generous help and patience in discussing the contents of this chapter with me both in writing and orally.

[1] *Nous*, as defined in *De anima*, is a part of the soul (*meros tês psuchês*). See, e.g., *An.* III 4, 429a10–15 and 22–23; *Part. An.* I 1, 641a32–b10. Aristotle calls this part *to noētikon*. See *An.* II 4, 415a17; *An.* III 4, 429a30; *An.* III 7, 431b2). Parts of the soul, for Aristotle, are capacities of the soul (specifically for *nous*, see *An.* III 4, 430a8). For the conception of "parts of the soul" in Aristotle, I refer the reader to Corcilius and Gregoric 2010: 81–119 and Johansen 2012: 47–72. More on this in Chapters 2 and 4.

Aristotle on the Essence of Human Thought. Klaus Corcilius, Andrea Falcon, and Robert Roreitner, Oxford University Press.
 DOI: 10.1093/9780198921820.003.0001

that would leave us with *nous* as a capacity for the kind of cognition responsible for all mental content that is not due to perception. That, however, seems strange. Is it even *true* that perception and intellectual cognition comprise all forms of cognition? It certainly does not seem like that. After all, we can think of a variety of ways of having something "in mind"—imagining something, for instance, or whatever goes on in my mind when I am counting the stars in the sky or playing a board game. Does Aristotle, then, perhaps think of *nous* as an umbrella term encompassing other, perhaps more specific, kinds of cognition in a way similar to the way a class includes its members, or a genus includes its species? Not at all: Aristotle characterizes *nous* in a highly specific way: namely, as the capacity to "take in" the essences—the essential beings—of all things, including its own essence. This is no doubt a most wondrous and remarkable characterization. We will have a great deal more to say about it in this book. For the time being, let me stress that this characterization certainly does not give the impression of entailing in any way a *classificatory* conception of *nous*. On the contrary, cognizing essences is a very specific kind of cognition, which even seems to exclude most of the intellectual activities we are usually familiar with. Solving a mathematical problem, playing a board game, understanding a historical fact, designing a machine, thinking about what to do next summer, and many other such activities would seem to be intellectual activities; and yet, they could hardly count as cognizing, or "taking in," the essences of things. In which way, then, do we have to think of *nous* as extending over these other activities of our intellects?

To answer this question, and to begin approaching Aristotle's thinking about *nous* more systematically, it will be useful to take a step back and briefly survey the architecture of his thinking about what *nous* is supposed to be a part of: namely, the soul.

2. *Nous* in Aristotle's inquiry into the soul

Aristotle dedicates an entire treatise to the definition of the soul. This treatise is his book *On the Soul*, which is known by its Latin title *De anima*. The first thing to note about the treatise is that it is not, or at least not primarily, concerned with the definition of the soul in any of the senses that we today might take the word "soul" to have. Contrary to what a modern reader may expect, the soul is neither the seat of consciousness, nor the bearer of mental episodes, nor the self, nor the nucleus of personhood and moral sentiments. Aristotle, to be sure, nowhere denies that there are very important connections between the soul and these states or functions of the mind. Indeed, some of them are very important and arguably crucial ingredients of what he has to say on and around the soul in other parts of his work. But he does not talk about them in his treatise on the soul. His first and foremost concern in *De anima* is to arrive at a definition of the soul as the *principle of living things*. This is how he spells out his definitory aim in the second sentence of the treatise:

> The soul is like a sort of principle of living things (*zôiôn*). Our aim is to contemplate and understand its nature and its essence, and then all its accidental attributes. Some of the latter seem to be affections peculiar to the soul, whereas others belong to living beings (*zôiois*) as well on account of the soul.[2]

In his *De anima*, Aristotle wishes to arrive at a theoretical grasp of the soul as the principle of living things.[3] "Principle" here means that the soul is a "first thing" in the sense of the basic feature (or set of features) for which there is no further, more basic, ground or explanation, and which is (or jointly are) responsible for the facts that hold of living things insofar as they are alive. A further important issue, crucial to bear in mind in this context, is that Aristotle, in his *De anima*, wishes to define the soul not as the principle of your soul, or our own soul, or, indeed, anybody's soul in particular, but rather as the *general principle for the scientific explanation of the scientifically relevant facts about living things.* And as it turns out in the course of the argument of the treatise, and unlike what the above text may suggest to the uninitiated reader, the soul does not *have* a "nature and substance"; rather, it *is* the nature and common essence of all living things. A third important thing to note about the treatise is that Aristotle's science of living things, the principle of which *De anima* is trying to define, is an *Aristotelian science.*

The fact that the study of the soul offered in *De anima* contributes to an Aristotelian science has important consequences for us. They can be brought to light under two headings: (1) Aristotle's *explanatory essentialism* and (2) *the division of scientific labor* within Aristotelian sciences. Regarding the latter, we may say, in a nutshell, that all Aristotelian sciences divide into three basic components:

(i) *Explananda.* The things to be explained or demonstrated within a scientific domain, the so-called "that" (*to hoti*) of a science. These are the phenomena, facts, "*empeiria*," or data that constitute the *explananda.* They are the universal and necessary attributes that the items that constitute the respective scientific domain (a scientific 'genus' or subject kind) possess insofar as they are members of that domain.[4]

(ii) *Explanations.* The explanations, or, as Aristotle calls them, the "on account of which" (*to dioti*). They are the scientific accounts that explain or demonstrate the phenomena, facts, or *explananda* in (i).

[2] *An.* I 1, 402a6–10.

[3] *Zôia* in *An.* I 1, 402a7 and 10 at this very early stage in his inquiry most probably stands for living things quite generally—not only for non-human animals but also for plants and human beings. See Falcon 2024: 24–36.

[4] In the above quote Aristotle calls them, perhaps somewhat misleadingly, "all the accidental attributes" of the soul; what he means is the "*per se* accidents" in the second sense of the meaning of *per se* distinguished in *Posterior Analytics* I 4, 73a37–b4. He so calls them because the soul ought to provide their ultimate ground. See Corcilius 2017: xxii–xxvii, and footnote 7 below.

(iii) *Principles.* The starting points from which the explanations or demonstrations in (ii) are given. They are the ultimate *explanantia* of a science.[5]

Aristotle's explanatory essentialism does not just consist in the thesis that there *are* essences—that is, that there exist certain core features which things have, and which make it that they are the kinds of things they happen to be—but also in the thesis that these core features provide the grounds to explain why things have the other universal and necessary properties they possess insofar as they are bearers of their essences. What this means is that the ultimate *explanantia* of Aristotelian sciences—that is, the items to be found in (iii)—are typically the essences of their respective scientific domains or subject kinds. Thus, ultimately, all Aristotelian sciences explain the *explananda* of their given domains (their scientific data: i.e., their universal and necessary facts, or phenomena) with reference to the definition of the essence of that domain. For example, supposing that there is a science of animals, then that science consists of the collection of all the universal and necessary facts about animals insofar as they are animals, the scientific explanations of those facts, and the definition of the principle of the subject-kind "animal," which happens to be the essence of the subject kind: that is, *what it is to be* an animal. The essential being of the scientific subject-kind "animal" thus grounds the scientific facts or phenomena that are true of animals universally and necessarily and insofar as they are animals, as their fundamental principle.[6]

In compliance with explanatory essentialism, Aristotle's *De anima* is devoted to finding out about the definition of the essence of its domain, which is living things generally. In other words, this work is concerned with the definition of the ultimate *explanantia* of that science: that is, (iii). These *explanantia* will provide the ultimate ground for the scientific accounts or explanations of the *explananda* of that science, which are the universal and necessary attributes living things possess insofar as they are alive. The domain of the science of living things is humans, nonhuman (i.e., brute) animals, and plants: that is, perishable living things below the moon and to the exclusion of divine living things. The universal and necessary facts about all these living beings insofar as they are alive are the phenomena of that science. The ultimate *explanans* of these phenomena is the essence of these living things. This essence is the "soul in itself." (For the expression *psuchê kath'hautên*, see *Sens.* 1, 436a1.) The definition of that essence, as it will result from the discussion in *De anima*, will be at the very top, or at the foundation, of that science.[7]

[5] Aristotle distinguishes between different kinds of principles. See *Posterior Analytics* I 2, 72a14–24 and I 10. For the sake of simplicity, in this brief survey I take into consideration only principles that are specific to a given science.

[6] For an introduction to Aristotle's explanatory essentialism, see the Glossary (*s.v.* EXPLANATORY ESSENTIALISM) at the end of the volume.

[7] For Aristotle, all scientific *explananda* are "*per se* attributes" of the common essence of a science. Aristotle, we may say, is so much of an explanatory essentialist that he conceives of the structure of sciences as, so to speak, "built around" the essences of their respective scientific domains. Thus, since

So much for the general scientific framework in which Aristotle's *De anima* is to be situated. The definition of *nous*, as a part of the definition of the essence of living things, then, will range at the very top of that science too. It will provide the scientist of living things with the first, most basic, and therefore also most universal, propositions that are fundamental for the explanation of the phenomena related to human thinking: that is, of the universal and necessary attributes human beings possess in virtue of the fact that they are thinkers.[8]

It is hard to overestimate the extraordinarily high level of theoretical abstraction at which the definition of the soul offered in *De anima* operates. To illustrate what this means, it is instructive to look at Aristotle's general methodological principle of the so-called *commensurate universal explanations* (*prôton katholou*).[9] According to that principle, all explanations of a science ought to be given at a level of universality that is as general as possible and as specific as necessary so as to capture each phenomenon at its greatest extension, while at the same time excluding everything that does not pertain to it. Aristotle's stock example is the explanation of the proposition that the sum of the angles in a triangle is equal to two right angles (hereafter 2R). To demonstrate 2R for rectilinear figures without qualification would be false, since there are rectilinear figures such as squares for which 2R does not hold. Moreover, to demonstrate 2R for equilateral triangles would be true but unscientific, since it would not get the extension right, given that 2R holds of scalene and isosceles triangles as well. According to Aristotle, the scientist ought to demonstrate 2R at a level of universality *commensurate* with the extension of the phenomenon, which is triangles *simpliciter*. The same goes *mutatis mutandis* for all scientific explanations. The goal of this explanatory procedure is twofold: methodological economy—that is, minimizing explanatory work by way of avoiding repetitive explanations (*Part. An.* I 1, 639a15–b5; 5, 644a25–b15; cf. *Phys.* I 7, 189b31–32; *An.* I 1, 402b8–10)—and making sure that there is a proper hierarchical *sequence* of theorems. For Aristotle, more general (and therefore also more basic) facts ought to be dealt with first, not only because they are more fundamental, but also because they may serve as premises for other explanations to be offered "further down" in a given science: first things first.

Many important consequences follow from that methodological principle. For those who, like us, are interested in Aristotle's discussion of *nous* in *De anima*, the

the universal and necessary attributes of a given scientific domain are based on their common essence as their ultimate explanatory ground, Aristotle conceives of them as *per se* attributes *of that ultimate ground* as their subject. This is to say that he conceives of the *explananda* of a science—namely, the relevant facts, data, or phenomena—as attributes of their essence. This holds also for the soul and the phenomena of living things: the latter are *per se* attributes of the former. See *An.* I 1, 402a6–10, b16–403a2; *An.* I 5, 409b13–17; *Part. An.* I 1, 639a15–22, 641a21–31.

[8] Aristotle mentions "reasonings" (*logismous*) as *per se* accidents of the soul in *An.* I 5, 409b13–17. See previous footnote.

[9] *Posterior Analytics* I 4, 73b25–74a3; 74a32–b4.

most important consequence is this: the definition of the soul will operate at the highest level of explanatory abstraction that the science of living things allows for. But we must understand "highest level of abstraction" in a highly qualified sense here. In Aristotle's explanatory essentialism, the propositions that range at the top of a science are not just, or at least not primarily, the most general propositions that apply most universally; they are primarily the most *fundamental* propositions of that science, and it is only in virtue of their fundamentality that they are also the most general ones. The principle of commensurate universal accounts commits Aristotle to a strict *minimalism* regarding what may enter the accounts of scientific essences. For him, only and exclusively the most fundamental propositions of a science—namely, those that cannot be derived from another proposition (or from any combination of propositions)—may feature in the account of the essence. This means that mental phenomena, as for instance episodes of human thinking as we usually experience them, are most likely not what Aristotle is talking about in *De anima*, when he talks about *nous* as a principle, and certainly not in the first instance. In defining *nous*, Aristotle is not, or at least not primarily, concerned with mental acts as we know them, but with the fundamental capacity that constitutes merely the bare essence of our intellectual capabilities and the mental acts resulting from them.

It is possible to restate the last point by saying that the definition of *nous* in Aristotle's *De anima*, from a methodological point of view, though deeply connected to it, is *two steps removed from what we nowadays might expect a theory of the thinking mind to be concerned with.* We tend to think of such a theory as offering an account of the mind in the sense of an account of the corresponding mental phenomena. It should explain how the mind thinks. But, as I hope to have made clear, Aristotle's *De anima* is not—or at least not immediately—concerned with explanations of the phenomena of the mental (ii); rather, it is concerned with the definition of the principle on the basis of which scientists will be able to come up with such explanations: that is, with (iii). In Aristotle's way of thinking about the division of scientific labor, these should be carefully kept apart. The definition of *nous* we can extract from *De anima* neither states the phenomena (i), nor gives scientific explanations of episodes of human thinking, or of any other features that can be explained with reference to the essence and principle of human thought (ii); rather, it states only the fundamental principle from which such explanations should take their very first start.[10] This approach, to be sure, does not rule out that occasionally we find discussions, or even explanations, of such phenomena in the various thematic sections of Aristotle's *De anima*; but it *does* rule out that

[10] Hence, I cannot agree with Michael Frede's claim that Aristotle "clearly does not introduce reason to account for our ordinary thinking and reasoning" (Frede 1996a: 163, 162; likewise, Burnyeat 2008: 19, 32). Rather, it seems to me that Aristotle defines *nous* precisely in order to explain the phenomena of human thinking. He says explicitly that human *nous* is the capacity by virtue of which we engage in discursive thinking and suppositions (*hôi dianoeitai kai hupolambanein hê psuchê*, *An.* III 4, 429a22; cf. *An.* III 4, 429a10–13. More on these passages in due course).

rendering such explanations is the first and foremost, let alone the immediate, goal of the discussion of *nous* in that treatise.

Probably, what we tend to think of as our mental life will, from the perspective of Aristotle's science of living things, consist of different joint activities following from the exercise of various capacities and sub-capacities, which are likely to boil down to versions of "mixtures" of perception and *nous*. Full Aristotelian explanations of mental events as we know them are very likely to be much richer than what the definition of bare capacities advanced in Aristotle's *De anima* may suggest. In the case of episodes of human thinking, for instance, the explanations will most probably be causal. They will involve all the four Aristotelian causes and thus also include a story of how we come to think. This entails a reference to the moving causes of thinking, to thinking's material and organic conditions, and also to the representational and linguistic conditions for human thinking to take place. As we know from numerous passages inside and outside of *De anima*, Aristotle had many things to say about the material, causal, representational, and linguistic conditions of human thinking.[11] So he certainly was not naïve about what it takes for thinking to take place in human individuals. But he did not regard these material, causal, representational, and linguistic aspects of human thinking as pertaining to the *essence* of thought. By his lights, the essence of thought has much more to do with the intrinsic features of thinking and its content (what thought is *of*, or about).[12] So, even though Aristotle knew very well that humans would not be able to exercise their intellectual capacities without suitable bodily organs, highly developed perceptual apparatuses, linguistic abilities, and all sorts of other learning and acquired habits, his definition of *nous* in *De anima* does not concern itself with them; it focuses on the *essence* of human thinking, which is something different from the necessary enabling conditions of human thinking. That is why he scarcely mentions these conditions in his discussion in *De anima*. The reason for this, as I hope to have made clear, lies in Aristotle's views about the division of scientific labor.

Since Aristotle is self-consciously implementing the division of explanatory labor as outlined above, and since there can be no doubt that his *De anima* is an integral part of a scientific context, it is misleading to speak of the treatise as offering a "theory of the mind," and it is perhaps even more misleading to speak of the treatise as offering a "psychology," as many interpreters routinely describe it. An Aristotelian theory of the mind, or an Aristotelian psychology, would have to correspond to an *application* of the first explanatory principle to the explanation of the phenomena. It would have to fall under section (ii). But Aristotle's *De anima* offers us only the very first and basic steps toward such an explanation. It falls squarely

[11] On the bodily, causal, representational, and linguistic necessary conditions of human thinking in Aristotle, see Wedin 1993, Van der Eijk 1997, Labarrière 2004, Mingucci 2015, and Connell 2021.

[12] Cf. Charles Kahn's interesting discussion of Aristotle's tenet that *nous* is without matter in Kahn 1992: 376–379.

under (iii), which, as we have seen, pertains to a different, and more fundamental, *kind* of investigation. In virtue of Aristotle's explanatory essentialism, these first steps will be the crucial, and indeed explanatorily most powerful, steps because of their foundational status with respect to the relevant (mental or psychological) phenomena. But however that may be, the definition of the principle should not be identified with the explanations of the phenomena, which is why it is misleading to speak of *De anima* as offering a theory of the mind or a psychology.[13] As far as the latter are concerned, it seems that we do not possess scientific explanations of episodes of human thinking in Aristotle's works, at least not fully fledged ones.[14] But as we will see later, Aristotle does not strictly confine himself to simply defining the principles in *De anima*. There is also a certain tendency to go beyond them and to indicate, albeit very briefly, what their application to the explanation of the phenomena would look like.[15] The focus of the treatise, however, is clearly on (iii): that is, on the definition of the soul as the principle of the science of living things.

This, admittedly *very* short, overview of the project of Aristotle's *De anima* should allow us to answer the question of how *nous* as it is discussed in *De anima* relates to the corresponding mental phenomena of human thinking. It relates to them neither in the way in which an umbrella term relates to the terms it covers, nor in the way in which a class contains its members; rather, it relates to them in the way in which a first and essential explanatory principle relates to its *explananda*: namely, as their ultimate and fundamental ground. The various intellectual activities we engage in—from deciding what to eat for dinner to counting the stars in the sky—relate to *nous* as to the ultimate and essential ground of their being what they are. The fact that we can play a board game or solve a mathematical problem, for Aristotle, has its ultimate ground in our possession of a fundamental capacity to grasp essences. And this grounding relation holds irrespective of whether we are ever actually successful in grasping essences during our lifetimes. The essential core of all our thinking abilities is our capacity of *nous*. For Aristotle, *nous* is the principle of our intellectual activities even if this capacity should never fully actualize in us.[16]

[13] As is, unfortunately, often done in the literature. It would also be misleading to speak of a "science of the soul," as is done quite often in the literature as well, given that the soul is not the subject matter (i.e., the domain) of the science of living things as this locution suggests, but its principle.

[14] There is a very rough sketch of what such an explanation may look like in *An.* I 1, 403a3–b12, for the case of one member of a subclass of mental phenomena: namely, anger. From this rough sketch we can safely conclude that Aristotle asks for explanations that involve all his four causes (whenever this is possible). Aristotle's account of recollection in *Mem.* 2 (one of the works on topics "common to body and soul") does involve noetic features, and the theory of mental representation that we find in *Mem.* 1 would seem to be an important ingredient for accounts of the phenomena of human thinking.

[15] See, e.g., his discussions of different kinds of thinking advanced in *An.* III 6, which clearly go beyond the definition of the noetic capacity in *An.* III 4–5. For more on this issue, see Chapter 3. See also the brief offerings of models for the explanation of episodes of soul-involving activities that follow on the discussions of the corresponding capacities in *An.* II 4, 416b20–29, and in *An.* III 10, 433b13–27.

[16] Indeed, Aristotle thinks that most of us do not reach the full actualization of our capacity for thought. More on this point in Chapter 3.

It is important to bear in mind that when Aristotle talks about the soul in *De anima*, and in particular about *nous*, he is in the first instance talking about an explanatory principle and not about the soul as a subject of mental episodes, the seat of consciousness, and so on. The soul, as defined in *De anima*, is not a mind, nor does it have mental states.[17] It is not a mind or a living thing but a theoretical entity. Its definition expresses what all souls of living things share as their most fundamental and essential being. In this respect, the soul as defined in *De anima* may be compared to other entities that are hypothesized by Aristotelian sciences, such as the abstract zoological kinds "blooded" and "bloodless," which of course are not animals either but abstract common attributes of living things (see *Part. An.* I 1, 639a15–22, *Posterior Analytics* I 5, 74a20–25; II 14, 98a13–23). But this comparison must be taken with caution for at least two reasons. First, the soul is the *most fundamental* item in the domain of living things. This makes it in a way even more general than abstract kinds like "blooded" and "non-blooded animals," which are common features "further down" in the deductive hierarchy of the science of living things (namely, the branch of that science that we call zoology). Second, the soul, in Aristotle's thinking of it, is *not* an abstraction of a common feature that empirically existing living things happen to share; it is their *principle*. Unlike the abstract kinds "blooded" and "non-blooded," which are properties that empirically existing animals share, the soul is the essence that *makes* animals the kind of things they are in the first place: namely, perishable living things.

To sum up the main results reached so far. The soul in Aristotle's *De anima* is the first explanatory principle of the science of living things. It is not a mind or a bearer of mental states. *Nous* is a part of the soul and thus the principle of the *explananda* of the science of living things insofar as they regard human thinking. *Nous* relates to the phenomena of our intellectual lives as a principle relates to the things that depend on it: it is universally true of them in the way in which an ultimate explanatory ground is true of the things that depend on it. At this point we can see that *nous is*, as it were, *two methodological steps removed from the phenomena of our intellectual lives*. Aristotle's *De anima* is an inquiry centrally concerned with the definition of *nous* as such a principle. We should therefore not expect *De anima* to give explanations of the phenomena of our lives as thinkers, but only to give the very first—albeit crucial—steps toward such explanations. The scientific labor falling under sections (i) and (ii) is not within the purview of the investigation conducted in *De anima*. Those parts of the science of living things that regard mental episodes and that fall under (ii) are to be found in Aristotle's biological writings dedicated to "the actions and affections common to body and soul."[18] This is a description

[17] This does not prevent Aristotle from speaking, in and outside of *De anima*, of the soul as the place in which perceptions and other mental episodes take place. See, e.g., *Int.* 1, 16a3–13; *An.* III 8, 431b29. In these instances, Aristotle is simply following the common usage of the term "soul." He is not in these instances talking about the soul as the principle of the science of living things.

[18] *An.* III 10, 433b19–21. Cf. *Sens.* 1, 436a7–8.

that Aristotle uses to refer to the so-called *Parva naturalia* and *Mot. An.* When we turn to these writings, however, we do not find much about episodes of human thinking. As a result, we must conclude that Aristotle has not left us a full explanatory account of the phenomena of human thinking.

3. Methodology in Aristotle's *De anima*

Understanding the treatment of *nous* in Aristotle's *De anima* requires us to understand Aristotle's distinctive mode of inquiry in the relevant stretch of text (*An.* III 4–8). The problem with this, however, is that in *De anima* Aristotle adopts a method of inquiry that does not fall into any clearly circumscribed part of his methodology. Aristotle's *De anima*, as emphasized above, is concerned with the definition of the soul as the principle of the science of living things. But it seems that there is no general rule or mode of procedure that would tell us how to proceed in establishing such definitions of principles in the abstract *just like that.* Aristotle says so himself:

> However, it is wholly and in every respect one of the most difficult tasks to reach any kind of confidence concerning it [i.e., the soul]. For given that the inquiry is also common to many other subjects—I mean the inquiry into the essence and the what-it-is—*one might perhaps believe that there is a certain single method appropriate for all things whose essence we wish to find,* just as there is [one method of] demonstration of proper [*per se*] attributes, so that one ought to inquire about this method. *However, if there is no single common method for finding out the what-it-is, our work becomes even more difficult; for then one ought to grasp what [the right] procedure is in each particular case.* But even when it is evident whether it is demonstration or division or also some other method, there are still many further puzzles and [potential] errors about whence the inquiry ought to take its start. *For different things have different starting points,* just as in the case of numbers and planes.[19]

In this passage, Aristotle denies that there is a general mode of inquiry with respect to the definition of the essence of any subject kind. "General" here means *transgeneric.* In other words, there is no abstract, transgeneric method which is applicable across all scientific domains, and which gives us the essence of a given subject kind. In each case, there is no way around doing the hard work of deriving the accounts of the essence of subject kinds from the study of the particular facts that pertain to that subject kind. The essence of living things (i.e., the soul) is no exception to the rule. In our passage, Aristotle even goes so far as to make the following

[19] *An.* I 1, 402a10–22.

counterfactual claim: even if we *knew* which transgeneric method to apply—be it demonstration or division—this would still not give us what we are looking for: namely, the *starting points* for the application of such a method. Put otherwise, one must be an expert about a given subject kind before one can hope to successfully determine its essence.

In the immediate sequel to our passage, Aristotle comes up with a catalogue of questions that the inquirer into the soul must seek answers to. These questions are all very general (transgeneric) in character, but they surely do not add up to anything resembling a transgeneric *method*.[20] Aristotle, to be sure, will provide us with the conceptual resources to answer these questions in the course of *De anima*. Still, at this stage of the inquiry, it remains unclear what his overall method is: that is, what guiding principle (or principles) he will adopt in answering these questions. What matters most seems to be experience with relation to the relevant subject matter. One must already be an expert in it. Also, the generality and heterogeneity of the questions makes his catalogue very unlikely to be *the* method of defining the soul, especially since some of the answers involve the method of division (which is perfectly general), while others do not, but instead involve specific doctrines stemming from Aristotle's physics. In sum, it seems that, by Aristotle's lights, what is missing in the *idea* of a common and transgeneric method of finding essences is a positive reference to the specific phenomena whose essences they are supposed to be (cf. *An.* I 3, 407b13–26). But it is precisely our knowledge of the specific phenomena—in our case, our knowledge of the empirical facts about living things—that provides us with the information and the criteria we need to define their principles. And that is why there is no general mode of procedure in abstraction from the phenomena that will get us to their essence:

> It seems not only that knowing what a thing is (*to ti esti*) is useful toward the study of the attributes that belong to substances (just as in mathematics [it is useful to know] what the straight or the curved is, or what a line or a suface is toward seeing how many straight right angles a triangle's angles are equal to) but also, conversely, that the accidents contribute a great deal toward knowing what a thing is (*to ti esti*). Whenever we are able speak about the attributes according to their appearance (*kata tên phantasian*), then we will also be able to speak most finely about the substance. What a thing is (*to ti esti*) is in fact the starting point

[20] They concern the *category* of the soul (Is it a substance or one of the other categories?), its *modality* (Is it an actuality or a potentiality?), its *mereological structure* and the consequences this structure has with relation to the definition of the soul to be given (Does it have parts or not, and if it has parts, are these parts different in species or in genus? Moreover, if there is one common account, will each of the parts have to receive its own account as well?), and the mode of procedure in defining the soul (Should we first define the soul, or its functions or achievements? And, if the latter, should we perhaps define the objects that correspond to each of these achievements before we define the achievements themselves?). James G. Lennox refers to this set of questions as an "erotetic framework of inquiry into the soul" (Lennox 2021: 180–189).

> of every demonstration, so the definitions which do not result in knowedge of the accidents, or even in an easy conjecture about them, are all dialectical and empty.[21]

It is the knowledge of the phenomena—the *per se* attributes, data, and facts—of a science that will guide us in the process of finding their principles. And, as there is no general mode of procedure that allows the scientist to determine the essence of a scientific subject kind in abstraction from the specific data, there is a reciprocal dependency between coming to have knowledge of the facts and coming to have knowledge of the essence. The definition of the essence of a subject kind will only be as good as its value in the explanation of the phenomena.[22] In the production of a science, including the finding of its principles, there is no way around the study of the specific empirical facts, then, and, presumably, also no way around various testing stages of trial and error of hypotheses. There is, moreover, good reason to believe that the investigation of the definition of the principles of a given scientific subject kind, for Aristotle, strictly speaking, and in spite of its fundamental importance and the knowledge of the respective facts it involves, falls outside of that science.[23] The task of defining numbers—that is, of investigating and discovering the what-it-is (or the essence) of number—is not a part of arithmetic. It is the *philosopher* of mathematics who defines numbers, while mathematicians apply the concept of number in their theorems. The same holds for the definition of the soul as the principle of the science of living things. It will fall into the camp not of the biologist, but rather of what we nowadays would call the *philosopher* of biology, to find out that definition. In this sense we may say that *De anima* presents us, not with a science of living things, but with a *metaphysics* of living things. By defining the soul as the principle of living things, the philosopher offers an answer to the question "What is the basic common and explanatory essence of all living things?" or, putting it in slightly different terms, "What is, most fundamentally, biological life?" And there seems to be no ready-made procedure for answering these questions apart from being an expert in respect of the relevant facts about living things.

In the rest of this introduction, I will follow Aristotle's lead and observe the steps he takes in approaching the definition of *nous* in *De anima*, focusing only on the most important features of Aristotle's strategy. I begin with the discussion of his

21 *An.* I 1, 402b16–403a2.

22 Jason Carter (2019: 32–33) argues that the above passage *is* Aristotle's general method for the definition of principles. However, if that were the case, the general method would roughly consist in the arrangements of the facts of a science, as depicted in *Prior Analytics* I 30, plus the rule "find the right middle terms!" This is not so much a general method as a statement of the fact that, apart from almost trivially general precepts (like the ones mentioned above: determine the category, modality, and mereological structure of your subject kind!), there really is no sign of a general and *transgeneric* method for finding the essence of subject kinds in Aristotle's *De anima*. *That* the definition of the essence of a subject kind ought to be capable of explaining the *per se* accidents is, *pace* Carter, not a method, but merely a criterion for the success of, or a test for, a definition. A method, by contrast, would have to be a certain mode of procedure that tells us *how to get to* the definition of our target kind.

23 See *Metaph.* VI 1, 1025b5–13. Cf. *Phys.* I 2, 184b25–185a5.

predecessors on cognition and *nous* (Section 4), continue with his definition of the soul as a set of capacities of living things (Section 5), and end with his method in defining the capacity of perception, which later will serve him as a sort of blueprint for his method in defining *nous* (Section 6).[24]

4. Aristotle on his predecessors on cognition

In the second chapter of *De anima*, after the statement of the major questions, problems, and challenges facing the philosopher who wishes to define the soul, Aristotle starts out his investigation with a critical discussion of his predecessors and their views about the nature of the soul. This discussion is important for an adequate understanding of his own way of going about defining the soul in *An.* II–III.

Here is how Aristotle motivates this discussion.

> As we inquire into the soul, it is necessary [for us] (at the same time as we are going through the *aporiai* which we must solve as we progress [in our investigation]) to consult the opinions of the predecessors who have expressed views about the soul, so that we retain what has been said well; but if something has not been said well [by them], then we may stay away from that.[25]

On this description, Aristotle's discussion of the doctrines and opinions held by his predecessors pursues a twofold goal: (i) taking on whatever truths they stated about the soul, and (ii) avoiding their errors. This is certainly a terse description of what is going on in the chapters to come. Indeed, the description is so terse that the critical project pursued in *An.* I 2–5 might be underestimated. For one might take this project as merely consisting in sorting out the true propositions that his predecessors uttered about the soul from the false ones, as if what Aristotle was looking for was simply a list of true propositions to be integrated into his own account of the soul (and perhaps to create another list of false propositions to be avoided). But the discussion of the predecessors' doctrines in *An.* I, as we will see, certainly is not a mere sifting of true from false propositions about the nature of the soul. Rather, it prepares the ground for Aristotle's systematic treatment of the soul in *An.* II and *An.* III. It does so, chiefly, by securing two results: (i) it motivates the treatment of the soul as the *explanatory principle of the phenomena of living things* in the later books by sharpening our understanding of what this means, and (ii) it

[24] I leave out the famous hylomorphic discussion of the soul as the essential form of the living body advanced in *An.* II 1, as this discussion is limited to the soul as the form of a body, which does not apply to *nous*. *Nous* in human beings, even though it depends on the human body for its existence and operation, is not essentially something *of* the human body. This makes thinking different from nutrition and perception. More on this in Chapter 6.

[25] *An.* I 1, 403b20–25.

generates a *list of problems and questions* that any theory of living things, including Aristotle's own, will have to come to terms with. In this way, the discussion of the views held by his predecessors provides Aristotle with a general methodological outlook as to what to achieve: namely, a definition of the soul as a principle for the phenomena of living things that can actually explain the phenomena (something Aristotle claims most of his predecessors' theories have not been able to achieve). More specifically, the discussion provides Aristotle with criteria of failure and success for his own theory: namely, its ability to solve and explain the problems raised during the discussion of the predecessors' views. Now, clearly, neither (i) nor (ii) nor their conjunction can be explained starting from Aristotle's description that *An.* I simply collects true propositions about the soul from Aristotle's predecessors. What seems to be missing in this description is the *methodological* dimension of the discussion offered in *An.* I.

Whatever the reasons for Aristotle's apparent omission of the methodological dimension in the announcement of his discussion of his predecessors, his methodological interest is already implicit in his use of the Greek adverbial expression "*kalôs*" in the quoted passage, which translates as "fine" or "in a fine way." As we know from *Part. An.* I 1, judging whether something is or is not said *kalôs* does not only consist in knowing whether a given proposition is true or false, but can also consist in judging whether a certain *method* makes good sense in a given field of inquiry quite independently from any expert knowledge in that field.[26] And such a methodological focus would seem perfectly reasonable in the beginning of the *De anima*. For one might ask how the reader will be able to tell which of the predecessors' doctrines are true or false, as to be able to do that competently would require expertise in the field. But there is no reason to suppose that the beginning of *An.* I is addressing an expert audience.[27] Rather, Aristotle relies on a general competence for methodological matters in people who are generally educated, but lack expertise in the science of living beings. This general competence is sufficient for judging whether a given method of inquiry makes good sense or not. And Aristotle's criticisms of the previous theories are mostly situated at this general level. If this is correct, Aristotle's interest in his predecessors' methodological approaches in *An.* I 2–5 must be at least as strong as his interest in the contents of their doctrines.[28]

[26] The competence of judging what is said rightly in any given subject matter pertains to the generally educated person (*holôs pepaideumenos*, *Part. An.* I 1, 639a7, as opposed to the expert—see the extensive discussion in Kullmann 1974: 95–153).

[27] In fact, *An.* I 1 presupposes virtually no knowledge about the soul. Quite tellingly, *An.* I 1, 402a22–402b1 even asks in which category the soul belongs, and whether it is a potentiality or an actuality. *An.* I 1 starts from scratch, or least acts as if it did so; it presupposes no knowledge about the right method of procedure for the task at hand. We have already seen that, in *An.* I 1, 402a10–22, Aristotle browses through all sorts of methodological approaches without obviously favoring any of them, and he expresses puzzlement and even bewilderment as to the difficulty of figuring out how to proceed in defining the soul.

[28] See also the summary methodological judgment of the predecessors' views in *An.* II 2, 413a13–16.

This methodological interest shows already in the very first treatment of his predecessors in *An.* I. *An.* I 2 mainly enumerates the predecessors' doctrines, which then get their critical assessment in *An.* I 3–5, However, even before enumerating those views, Aristotle gives a methodological spin to the whole ensuing discussion:

> The starting point of this inquiry is to set out the things that seem most of all to belong to the soul by nature. Now, the ensouled seems to differ from what is deprived of soul most of all in two respects: motion and perception. These are also the two features we have taken over from our predecessors, or almost. For some of them say that the soul is most of all and primarily that which initiates motion; however, believing that what does not move itself cannot move something else, they assume that the soul is one of the things which are moved.[29]

Aristotle starts his review by setting out his own mode of procedure. He says that the natural beginning of his inquiry into the predecessors is a brief survey of the features that seem to belong to the soul most prominently: namely, motion (*kinêsis*) and perception (*aisthêsis*).[30] Now it is very interesting to observe Aristotle's strategy in presenting, and at the same time motivating, the survey of the views of his predecessors. For, in presenting their views, Aristotle moves from features of things that *have soul* (are "ensouled," *empsucha*) to the predecessors' doctrines about the features of the *soul* (*psuchê*). While it is things that have soul (ensouled things) that differ from inanimate things in exhibiting self-motion and cognition, Aristotle speaks as if his predecessors took these two prominent features of *animate things* to be features of the *soul*. Thus, to explain the phenomenon of self-motion, they conceived of the soul as a self-moved thing. While their explanation of cognition is more complicated (see Chapter 3 and especially Chapter 6), the theories of the largest group among them basically consist in a conception of the soul as of a *cognizing thing* that, moreover, very much behaves like the things it cognizes. Aristotle's wording in the above passage leaves little doubt, then, that he thinks his predecessors inferred from the effects that the possession of the soul has on living things to the nature of the soul itself. This, to be clear, is a fallacious inference from the phenomena (the *explanandum*) to their principle (the *explanans*). From the fact that a given phenomenon is such-and-such it does not follow that the cause of that phenomenon is such-and-such as well. So, the fact that living

[29] *An.* I 2, 403b24–404a1.

[30] Aristotle's talk of motion (*aisthêsis*) and perception (*kinêsis*) as the two most prominent features of living things should not (at least not at this early stage of the argument) be interpreted as if they were established terms of Aristotle's terminology. The latter will only emerge from his discussions later in the book. Therefore, we should understand *aisthêsis* as equivalent to cognition generally (as he hasn't yet argued for the existence of different modes of cognition), and we should perhaps think of *kinêsis* as self-motion rather than motion generally (or perhaps we should think of it *primarily* as self-motion, since this is one of the most obvious things that we observe living things doing). When it comes to cognition, in *An.* I, Aristotle generally oscillates between *ginôskein*, *krinein*, and *gnôrizein*.

things move about and cognize does not license the inference that their cause and principle—the soul—moves and cognizes as well. Indeed, as it turns out, Aristotle will largely deny that these features pertain to the soul.[31] What one could perhaps more legitimately infer from the prominent facts to be observed in living things is that the soul, whatever it may turn out to be, should be able to *explain* self-motion and cognition. That, however, is not what his predecessors seemed to have inferred; or, rather, they seemed to have inferred *more* than they were licensed to do from the facts. What Aristotle is doing here, then, is charging his predecessors, or most of them, with having fallen prey to some sort of *fallacy of isomorphism between cause and effect.* To his eyes, the methodological effect of the fallacy is this: the predecessors were supposed to *explain* the phenomena of living things with reference to the soul (*An.* I 1, 402a4–10, 402b22–403a2); instead, due to their conception of the soul as a moving or cognizing thing, far from explaining the facts in a satisfactory way, they ended up only adding to the number of *explananda.*[32] To say that the *soul* moves or cognizes may to some extent even explain the movement and cognition of living things, but it does so in a less than satisfactory way. Recall that for Aristotle the soul is a *principle.* So the way in which it explains phenomena of living things such as motion and cognition should be ultimate in the sense that, once the soul is given in reply to the question "why" (*dia ti*), there should be no further question to be asked.[33] But postulating a moving or a cognizing soul, as Aristotle's predecessors did, unavoidably raises the further question of *why* the soul can engage in motion and cognition. In this sense, their explanations are less than satisfactory because they are not ultimate.

Aristotle also offers explanations as to how and why his predecessors arrived at their theses. In the case of motion, he says that it was their unthinking assumption that motion can only be caused by other motion. Given this assumption, it was natural for them to think of the soul as a subject of motion as well.[34] His explanation of their views on the cause of cognition is slightly more complicated as it involves a further set of assumptions. Aristotle says that those who took cognition to be a

[31] He argues at length against the thesis that the soul is moved (*An.* I 3, 405b31–407b11) and strongly suggests that the soul is not a subject of any of the body-involving mental episodes ("affections of the soul," *An.* I 4, 408b1–30), saying that "discursive thinking, loving, and hating are not affections of the soul, but of that which possesses it, in so far as it possesses it" (*An.* I 4, 408b25–26). This excludes the soul from being a subject of mental episodes. The only possible exception is a certain kind of theoretical thinking, about which more in Chapter 2, which offers a full discussion of *An.* III 5. In other places, most prominently perhaps in *Metaph.* XII 3, Aristotle seems to advocate the so-called synonymy conception of causation, according to which a thing of kind *X* comes to be from some other thing of that same kind. That, however, is a theory restricted to the causation of substances (*ousia*) in substantial generation and does not apply across the board to all processes.

[32] He says that this is "roughly" (*schedon*) the features that his predecessors have attributed to the soul presumably because the *harmonia* theory of the soul (discussed in the first half of *An.* I 4 *in extenso*) seems to be an exception to the fallacy of isomorphism between *cause* and *effect.*

[33] See, e.g., *Posterior Analytics* I 24, 85b27–38.

[34] *An.* I 5, 411a24–26; see *An.* I 2, 403b29–31, and the survey of different views of the soul as a moved thing up until 404b8.

prominent feature of living things conceived of the soul as composed of the same elements as the things it cognizes. As for their reasons for thinking this, Aristotle invokes the fact that his predecessors were almost all committed to the like-is-known-by-like principle, which, in conjunction with their conviction that the soul cognizes all things, made them agree on the doctrine that the soul consists of as many elements as they happened to have posited in their various cosmologies, to the effect that like can be cognized by like with the soul as the subject of cognition (405b12–19).[35] As a result, the theories of his predecessors made the soul behave pretty much like an *ensouled thing*. In other words, these theories *reified* the soul. The importance of this point for Aristotle's own thinking about his predecessors can hardly be overestimated. It is a standing concern in Aristotle's criticisms in *An.* I 3–5 that his predecessors, by modeling their conception of the soul after things that have soul, have come to results which both are untenable in themselves and fail to explain the phenomena in a satisfactory manner.

Here is the summary statement made at the very end of those criticisms:

> Therefore, from what has been said it is clear that it is not because the soul is composed of the elements that cognition belongs to it, nor is it well said or true to say that the soul is moved.[36]

In sum, we may say that Aristotle organizes the discussion of almost all his predecessors on the soul along a single, albeit crucial, *methodological* point, which moreover seems to correspond to a basic motivation for Aristotle's own systematic treatment of the soul. By Aristotle's lights, all his predecessors (with few exceptions) jumped from the nature of the main *explananda* of the soul, which are self-motion and cognition, to substantive claims about the nature of the soul as *having* both of these features as well. That inference, however, is fallacious (for Aristotle, the cause of φ-ing need not itself be φ-ing; the cause of cognition need not be cognizing, and the cause of motion need not be moving) and results in unwarranted, reifying, and basically homuncular conceptions of the soul. The methodological lesson to be drawn from this is that the soul—whatever it should turn out to be—must be able to *explain* the phenomena. This lesson is stated implicitly in *An.* II 1, where Aristotle says that the soul (instead of being a thing that moves and cognizes) is not a thing in the sense of an (often bodily conceived) subject of motion and cognition at all, but rather the substantial *form* of the living body. And the lesson is drawn explicitly in *An.* II 2, where he gives a general job description of the soul as the explanatory principle (*archê*) of the phenomena of living things—that is,

[35] More on the like-is-known-by-like principle below. Among his predecessors, the only exception to the rule is Anaxagoras and the so-called *harmonia* theory of the soul. Aristotle will give them a separate treatment.

[36] *An.* I 5, 411a24–26.

thinking, perceiving, nutrition, and self-motion (413b10–13)—albeit without yet saying what this principle consists in.[37] Both statements are well motivated from a methodological point of view by Aristotle's description of his predecessors' fallacy of isomorphism between *cause* and *effect*.

But how does Aristotle criticize the views of the predecessors on *nous* more specifically? Aristotle's discussion in *An.* I 3–5 does not separate the treatment of perception from the treatment of thinking but deals with his predecessors' views on cognition in a summary fashion. The discussion can be organized under two headings. One type of criticism leveled against the predecessors is internal to their views. It takes its lead from what they had to say about the soul and attacks the internal consistency of their views. The other type of criticism is systematic: it attacks their views from the perspective of the explanation of the phenomena. Here, I concentrate on the latter type of criticism, since it works on the basis of criteria that should apply to Aristotle's own theory as well.

I focus on the basic structure of the discussion:

> They all define the soul by means of three features, so to speak: motion, cognition, and incorporeality. Each of these features is traced back to the principles (*archai*). This is why those who define the soul by means of cognition make it an element (*stoicheion*) or out of the elements (*ek tôn stoicheiôn*), thus offering similar accounts, with the exception of one of them. For they say that like is cognized by like, and since the soul cognizes everything, they put it together from all the principles. As a result, those who say that there is one cause and one element also hold that the soul is one thing (e.g., fire or air). But those who maintain that there is more than one principle also make the soul more than one thing. Anaxagoras alone says that *nous* is unaffected and that it has nothing in common with any of the other things. But he does not say how *nous*, being such a thing, cognizes and on account of what cause it does so; nor is it obvious at all from what he says.[38]

Aristotle arranges all the previous theories into two camps: those who follow the principle according to which "like is known by like" and those who don't. While the overwhelming majority of his predecessors endorsed, in one way or another, the like-is-known-by-like principle (hereafter LKL), Anaxagoras appears to be the sole thinker in the other camp.[39]

[37] In light of the hylomorphic analysis of natural substances into form and matter, which is to say into the principle and the bearer of that principle, we can safely say that Aristotle has the conceptual resources to offer a non-reifying, non-homuncular account of the soul which makes the latter something "of" a subject (hence making the *commonality—koinonia*—of soul and body in the compound all-important for the theory; see *An.* I 3, 407b14–26). That seems an important part of the point Aristotle wishes to get across in the introduction of the hylomorphic framework in *An.* II 1.

[38] *An.* I 2, 405b10–23.

[39] Unlike the classification by Theophrastus, who also names Heraclitus and Alcmaeon as members of that camp. I leave out the *harmonia* theory of the soul as Aristotle does not discuss it critically in relation to cognition.

The basic idea of LKL consists in the thesis that cognition is some sort of "match" between the object of cognition and some constituent part of the cognitive agent which is "like" that object. Since the holders of LKL are committed to the thesis that the soul cognizes all things (*An.* I 2, 405b15–16), that would have to imply that the soul *is* all things. In Aristotle's narrative, his predecessors were able to evade that conclusion by combining LKL with a further, reductive, thesis about the constitution of things, which is the thesis that all things in the world consist of elements: that is, basic constituent parts (*An.* I 2, 405b12: *toutôn d' hekaston anagetai pros tas archas*). On that basis, the holders of LKL established a much more economical way of making the soul a subject of the cognition of all things based on their reductive thesis. For they seem to have thought that if things can be reduced to basic constituents, then the soul, to cognize them, does not have to *literally be* all things; it only has to consist of the same basic constituent parts as things do. The most famous proponent of LKL is Empedocles (see DK 31 B 109), but Aristotle leaves no doubt that *all* his predecessors were committed to it, with Anaxagoras as the only exception, about which more in a moment.

LKL, therefore, must be understood on a high level of abstraction, greatly varying in accordance with the different basic constituents adopted by the different philosophers. Thus, Empedocles is said to have thought of the items that constitute the cognition relation on both sides as the elementary physical bodies (earth, water, air, and fire) and Love and Strife, and Plato in the *Timaeus* seems to have postulated conceptual elements—namely, the reflexive conceptions of sameness and otherness (cf. *Tim.* 35A–37C)—while other philosophers have argued for other elements (*diapherontai peri tôn archôn*: *An.* I 2, 404b31). What is important is that LKL is a substantive thesis about the *nature* of cognition: cognition is explained as *being* the matching of the two "like" parts on both sides of the cognition relation,[40] while that matching is brought about by way of an affection: the cognitive agent acts on the cognitive patient (*An.* I 2, 410a24–25). Somehow, the resulting identity is supposed to constitute the act of cognition. So, all holders of LKL agree that cognition takes place by way of affection and that it consists in the matching of like things on either side of the cognition relation.

The other camp is harder to pin down. Aristotle only says that Anaxagoras thought that *nous* cognizes while being unaffected (*apathês*) and having absolutely nothing in common with the things in the world. But he also says that Anaxagoras did not explain how *nous* cognizes, and for what reason, and that his answers to these questions are not apparent from what he has said either. So, as we lack any

[40] This, at any rate, is how Aristotle seems to see it, since he charges Anaxagoras, and not the holders of LKL, with having not explained to us, either explicitly or explicitly, "how the soul cognizes and an account of what" (*An.* I 2, 405b21–23). I use the term "cognition relation" here in a non-committal sense. I do not want to thereby presume or presuppose a certain understanding of relations, nor do I want to thereby claim that all kinds of cognitions *are* relations. In *Cat.* 7 Aristotle makes clear that he at least thinks that perception and knowledge are relata that correlate with their respective objects.

account of the workings of cognition in Anaxagoras, we cannot say whether his thesis amounts to a substantive theory of cognition or not. But we can say the following. Unlike LKL, Anaxagoras' basic intuition seems to have been that cognizing things requires being different from, and not being like or even a part of, them. We can call this position "Cognition by Unlike" or "Separatism," which—however vague the statement of it may be—conceives of cognition as involving some sort of *contrast* between the knower and the known. But it is not at all clear how this is supposed to work in the case of Anaxagoras' theory.[41]

As we will see in more detail below, Aristotle's own theory of cognition, both perception and intellectual cognition, exhibits elements from both camps—that is, LKL and Separatism—and combines them in new, interesting ways. At the most basic level, for both modes of cognition, the corresponding acts of cognition consist in some sort of (highly qualified) identity between the knower and the known thing, whereas the processes that lead to cognition in both instances are driven by the interaction between knower and known thing as qualified others. It also seems that two of the core conceptions of his theory of cognition—namely, the concepts of assimilation and discrimination—have their roots in these two earlier theory-types of cognition. Note also that Aristotle agrees with virtually all his predecessors that somehow "all things" are (or at least in principle can be) cognized (*An.* I 2, 405b15–16).

Aristotle's criticism of the previous theories of cognition focuses on the LKL camp, for lack of sufficient evidence for Anaxagoras' theory. He levels three arguments against the thesis, the first of which is found in this passage:

> It remains to be investigated how it is said that the soul is made out of the elements. For they say this for the soul to be able to perceive and cognize each of the things that exist. But this thesis must lead to many impossible consequences. For they assume that the like cognizes the like, as if they were assuming that the soul is the things. But there exist not only these things but also many other things (in fact, perhaps an infinite number), which are made out of them. So let us grant that the soul cognizes and perceives the components out of which each thing is. By means of what will the soul perceive or cognize the whole? [I mean to perceive and cognize,] for instance, what god, human, flesh, or bone is, and likewise for any other composite thing. Each composite thing is not the elements irrespective of the way in which they are arranged, but it is identical to them in a certain proportion or combination, as even Empedocles says.... It is no good, therefore, for the elements to be in the soul unless the proportions and combinations will also be present [in the soul]. Each [element] cognizes its like but nothing will cognize

[41] See the discussion of his views in Theophrastus' *Sens.* 507.7–510.4. Cf. also the instructive discussions of the relation between Theophrastus' *Sens.* and Aristotle's discussion in *De anima* offered in Laks 2020 and Johansen 2020.

> either bone or the human being unless they too are present [in the soul]. But this, needless to say, is impossible. Who in the world would wonder whether a stone or a human being is present in the soul? The same goes for what is good and what is not good, and likewise for the other things.[42]

After blaming his predecessors explicitly for reifying the soul—that is, for making it "the things" (*pragmata*)—Aristotle here argues that LKL fails to explain what it purports to explain: namely, the cognition of all things. His argument is based on the non-reductive assumption that things do not consist of their constituents alone but also of the arrangement, combination, or proportion of those constituents. Things are, accordingly, compounds (*sunhola*) of their constituent parts plus the modes of their combination: that is, their arrangement in the sense of the specific ways in which they are put together.[43] With this Aristotle basically denies the legitimacy of the reductive move his predecessors made when they reduced things to their elementary constituents. Given his non-reductive thesis, the fact that the soul consists of the same elementary constituents as things in the world is of no use for the explanation of the cognition of things other than the elementary constituents themselves, as the soul will fail to cognize the modes of combination of the constituent parts of things. Cognizing things like bones or humans, therefore, will either not take place at all, or require that the combinations and proportions of the elementary parts of things will be present in the soul as well. Otherwise, LKL won't work and won't explain the cognition of all things.[44] Now, quite interestingly, Aristotle adds: "needless to say, this is impossible. Who would be puzzled over whether there is a stone or a human being in the soul?" Famously, this is something that Aristotle himself will be claiming later in the treatise, although in a strongly modified version. More directly, in *An.* III 8, he says that not just all things, but *all beings* are in the soul, albeit with the qualification that only their *forms* are in the soul and even this only *potentially*.[45] This first line of criticism makes it a

[42] *An.* I 5, 409b23–410a3.

[43] This corresponds to familiar anti-reductivist arguments Aristotle makes in various places. See, e.g., *Metaph.* VII 17; *Phys.* II 1).

[44] Apparently, the idea of the holders of LKL was that those features of cognized things other than their elementary constituents would reach cognition, as it were, for free: an object consisting of elementary parts *X* and *Y* would be matched by the soul's constituent parts *X'* and *Y'*, where the arrangement of the object's *X* and *Y* would not require a separate receptor or act of cognition but would be somehow included in the matching story. Now, this may very well be an anachronistic, and perhaps even unfair, way of describing LKL, as Aristotle's predecessors probably did not explicitly distinguish between formal and material features of things, or they did not do so as sharply as Aristotle did. Aristotle appears to have thought that Empedocles and Democritus came close to some such distinction in *Phys.* II 2, 194a20–21; see *An.* I 4, 408a18–22; *An.* I 5, 410a3–8; *Metaph.* I 4, 985b4–22; *Metaph.* VIII 2, 1042b11–15. We forgo such complications. What we are concerned with here is making transparent Aristotle's way of thinking about the theories of his predecessors. It is striking that Aristotle, in using the terminology of "proportion" and "combination" of elementary constituents, seems to be deliberately avoiding the language of matter and form (in this respect, his discussion is reminiscent of *Metaph.* VIII 2).

[45] See my discussion of *An.* III 8 (in Chapter 5) for more on this point.

requirement for any theory of cognition, including Aristotle's own, that it must be able to explain the cognition of all things and in such a way that their formal, relational, and abstract features are taken into due consideration as well. As LKL in combination with the elementary reduction of things can only make a claim toward explaining the cognition of the basic material constituents of things, and not of their formal features, it does not meet that requirement.

The second objection to LKL follows immediately. It is similar to the above argument, except that this time it is based on Aristotle's doctrine of categories of being. The basic structure of the argument may be represented as follows:[46]

(1) Cognition happens by way of LKL.
(2) Things pertain to the different categories of being.
(3) The soul cognizes all things.
(4) There are no common elements for the different categories ("being is not a genus").
(5) Therefore, the soul will pertain to all categories.

The argument has the form of a *reductio*. That the soul, or any other item, consists of all categories is taken to be an absurdity. In a further step, Aristotle discusses an attempt to save the theory:

> Or will they say that there are elements (*stoicheia*) and principles (*archai*) proper to each kind (*genos*) and say that the soul is composed out of them? If so, the soul will then be quantity, quality, and substance. But it is impossible to obtain a substance, and not a quantity, out of principles of quantity.[47]

Only to reject it as well, on the (implicit) grounds that

(6) Nothing falls essentially into more than one category,

and, therefore, that it is impossible for any object to be composed of elementary constituent principles that fall into different categories while still being one unitary thing. This argument is particularly interesting from the point of view of the criteria for an adequate theory that it implies. For Aristotle, any theory of cognition must be able to account for the alleged fact that at least in principle everything can be cognized. As the objects of cognition fall into different categories of being, cognition will then have to somehow be trans-categorical: that is, to be in some way receptive of things that fall into different categories. The argument is particularly

[46] This is a *very* simplified representation of the argument. For a full reconstruction, see Shields 2016: 154–158.

[47] *An.* I 5, 410a18–21.

interesting because it seems to pose a serious challenge for Aristotle's own theory. Premise (4) says that there are no common elements for the different categories, while (6) denies the possibility that any object pertains essentially to a plurality of categories. Now add to this Aristotle's own commitment to the thesis, made later in the treatise, that the soul is the essence of the living body (a substance, and thus not pertaining to any other category). How will cognition of items of different categories be possible on that basis? As it turns out, Aristotle relegates perceptual cognition, in the most basic form that it takes, to just one category, the category of quality. Whatever the details of his theory of perception (we can leave them aside for now), this leaves the cognition of all other categories to intellectual cognition. But how can the intellect cognize things that pertain to different categories at once, if the LKL principle is involved, while there are no common elements for the different categories, there being no single item whose essence pertains to more than one category? Aristotle's theory of *nous*, as we will see, manages to avoid at least part of the challenge by conceiving of the capacity for thinking as being nothing, and hence also nothing categorial, at all: that is, nothing categorial in actuality (*An.* III 4, 429a21–27). But this is supposed to be the case only *before it thinks*. Once it is engaged in actual thinking, thought would seem to have to pertain to the category of the object it cognizes (given the principle according to which the essence of *X* pertains to the same category as *X*), so to that extent Aristotle remains committed to LKL. It would follow (non-trivially) that each thought can only be of objects in one category of being. However, in Chapter 5 I will show that at least as far as typical instances of human thinking are concerned, Aristotle sticks to the idea that not only perception but also thinking is—in a specific sense to be discussed—qualitative.

The third objection reduces LKL to panpsychism. If LKL is true, and it holds of all the elementary constituents of things, then there is no reason why all things should not have their own share in cognition (*An.* I 5, 410b7–10). The conclusion of this argument may not be philosophically as unacceptable as Aristotle apparently took it to be.[48] But however that may be, what is important is that Aristotle here seems to apply his doctrine of commensurately universal explanations. Explanations should be coextensive with the phenomena they purport to explain; cognition is something only animals, and neither their material components nor inanimate things, can do by themselves; therefore . . .

These three, then, are the main "systematic" objections against his predecessors' theories of cognition insofar as they were proponents of LKL. Aristotle agrees with his predecessors that cognition is of everything there is. The criteria (or demands)

[48] See his rhetorical question in *An.* I 5, 410b7: "In general, why is it not that everything that exists has a soul . . . ?" This question presupposes that it is not the case that everything has a soul. Parmenides seems to have allowed for panpsychism (Theophrastus, *Sens.* 5).

for an adequate theory of cognition that his criticisms appeal to either explicitly or implicitly may be summarized as follows:

(1) "Explain the cognition not only of the material but also of the formal features of things!"
(2) "Explain the cognition of beings in all of the different categories of being!"
(3) "Explain cognition on a commensurate universal level!"

5. The soul as a set of capacities and how to define capacities of the soul

After the discussion of Aristotle's predecessors and the famous definition of the soul as the form of the living body in *An.* II 1, which situates the science of living things within the metaphysical framework of hylomorphism (thus allowing Aristotle to stay clear of the reifying moves of his predecessors), *An.* II 2 makes a new start with a job description of the soul within his science of living things. According to that job description, the soul is the explanatory principle of the phenomena pertaining to living things:

> We say, therefore, taking up the beginning of the inquiry, that the ensouled (*empsuchon*) is distinguished from what is deprived of soul (*apsuchon*) by being alive (*zên*). But being alive is said in more than one way, and should even one of them be present, then we say that the thing is alive. I mean *nous*, perception, motion and rest with respect to place, and also motion with respect to nutrition, decay, and growth.[49]

Aristotle here moves from the *definiendum* to the *definiens* in a purely formal way. The *definiendum* is (trivially) the soul, and the soul, according to the common understanding, is responsible for making living beings "alive," which is to say that the soul is responsible for making it that living things are endowed with soul (i.e., that they are "ensouled beings," *empsucha*) and do the things living things do. That global result of the possession of a soul by living beings—namely, their "being alive"—is divided into four different sections in accordance with the four different ways in which we say about living things that they are alive and live (*zên*). Each of these four ways of being alive corresponds to a certain life-activity, and each life-activity is *sufficient* for the attribution of life:[50]

[49] *An.* II 2, 413a20–25.
[50] Aristotle seems to think that these four candidates are both: good candidates for *basic* life-activities, and together sufficient for generating an exhaustive account of the soul.

(i) *nous*;
(ii) perception (*aisthêsis*);
(iii) motion and rest with respect to place (*kinêsis kai stasis kata topon*);
(iv) motion in relation to nourishment, decay, and growth (*kinêsis kata trophên kai phthisis te kai auxêsis*).

Aristotle now moves from the division of the life-activities to the division of the soul as their *explanans* or principle:

> For now, let just this much be said: the soul is the principle of the things mentioned and is delimited by them—namely, capacity of nourishment, capacity of perception, capacity of thinking, and motion.[51]

The relevant capacities listed in the passage are:

(i′) capacity for nourishment (*threptikon*);
(ii′) capacity for perception (*aisthêtikon*);
(iii′) capacity for thinking (*dianoêtikon*);
(iv′) (local) motion (*kinêsis*).

This second list matches exactly the preceding list of life-activities. The crucial difference is the addition of the Greek -*ikos* ending in each case, indicating that now we are turning to the *capacities* (or faculties) that correspond to each of the activities as their principles and thus their *explanantia*.[52] This, then, is a preliminary definition of the soul as the *explanans* of the life-activities as the corresponding set of capacities. These life-capacities are the candidates for being the explanatory subprinciples of living things that together constitute the soul as the first explanatory principle of the science of living things. At this very early stage of the investigation, these basic capacities (or "parts" of the soul, as Aristotle will call them) are, to be sure, no more than mere placeholders for the items that are going to be jointly necessary and sufficient to fulfill the function of the first and basic principles of the phenomena of living things. This is all we know at this point. The soul is going to be the set of capacities that are jointly necessary and sufficient for the explanation of the phenomena of living beings; but we do not hear more than that. In this sense the definition of the soul in *An*. II 2 is merely formal and preliminary. Aristotle says

[51] *An*. II 2, 413b10–13.

[52] Leaving aside the case of locomotion, which does not seem to correspond to a basic *capacity* or "part" of the soul. Quite tellingly, Aristotle does not speak of locomotion as a capacity in the above list. He does not say "capacity for locomotion" but "motion." In this connection, the following passage is also relevant: "But is each of these a soul or a part of a soul, and if a part, is it separable only in account or also in place? Where some of them are concerned the answer is not difficult to see, whereas others involve an *aporia*" (*An*. II 2, 413b13–16).

that the soul to be defined is the *explanans* of the phenomena of living things as the set of their basic life-capacities, but he does not say by virtue of which features the soul can play that role. What these basic life-capacities will turn out to be can only be revealed by the philosophical inquiry into the what-it-is (i.e., the definition) of each of them. And this is also roughly what happens in the rest of the treatise. Aristotle discusses and defines each of these capacities, and he does so in the same sequence as in (i′)–(iv′). The list of capacities (i′)–(iv′), therefore, may be regarded as Aristotle's to-do list in the *De anima*. If this is correct, then the task that Aristotle sets for himself in *De anima* is, first and foremost, a *definitory* one. It consists in searching for definitions: namely, searching for answers to the question "What is it?" (*ti esti*) for each of the four life-capacities. This is exactly what one would expect from a foundational text such as *De anima*, which is concerned with the search for the principles from which explanations about living beings ought to be given.

The definitions that result from these discussions, Aristotle adds, will at the same time provide the most adequate definition of the soul (*An.* II 4, 415a12–13). This is because, on Aristotle's conception, the soul is the principle of the science of living things *by* being the basic capacities that explain the phenomena of living bodies as enumerated in (i)–(iv) as their ultimate and fundamental ground. Defining the soul's basic capacities, therefore, is equivalent to defining the soul itself (*An.* II 3, 415a12–13). There is, in other words, no underlying subject that would be the psychological bearer of these capacities. The soul as the principle of the science of living things *is* a set of capacities.

The claim that the soul is a set of basic capacities raises the question of the unity of the soul of *living things as they exist in nature*. For unlike the soul as the principle of the science of living things, for which the definitional separability of the parts is not a problem, our souls are not going to be "sets of definitionally separate capacities" but rather unitary souls which, moreover, are the principles of the unity of our bodies and lives (see *An.* I 5, 411a26–b14). So, in this case a stronger unity of the parts of the soul is required than merely forming a set of capacities. Aristotle deals with the question in *An.* II 3. His answer is that the lower parts of the soul of an individual living being as it occurs in nature (e.g., the soul of a dog) are not actual *parts* of the dog's soul, which is just one: namely, the dog's soul (a kind of perceptual soul). Rather, they are only *potentially contained* in them. Thus, the vegetative part of the dog's soul is not separate or separable from the dog's highest (perceptual) part as an independent module but is *operationally fused* with it. It will not act as a module separate from the perceptual part, but rather will reproduce and preserve the *dog* (and not just the dog's vegetative system). Indeed, it will exert its function in the service of the higher parts of the soul (*Gener. An.* II 3, 736a35-b8). That is to say that the lower parts of the soul are also *teleologically subordinated* to the higher ones. Teleological subordination and operational fusion, I think, allow Aristotle to conceive of the souls of actually existing living beings as strong *natural unities* capable of grounding the unity of the corresponding animals' lives and bodies.[53] In Chapter 2, we will see how teleological subordination cashes out in the case of some of the operations of the human intellect. In the rest of the book, we will refer to the teleologically and operationally unified soul of human beings insofar as it is responsible for cognition as the *cognitive soul*.[54] But for now we are first and foremost interested in the definition of the parts of the soul themselves, and not so much in the question of their unity in living things.

In *An.* II 4, Aristotle, responding to his last general question raised in *An.* I, 402b10–16, moves on and offers a methodology for the definition of the capacities of the soul. As they are capacities, they must be defined with reference to their manifestations, as for instance a runner—a person with the capacity to run—is defined with reference to its manifestation, which is the activity of running. But capacities of the soul behave in ways that are more complex than running. They are capacities of a more complex kind because they have not only corresponding manifestations but also corresponding objects.

> If one ought to say what each of them is—I mean what the capacity for thinking (*to noetikon*), the capacity for perception (*to aisthêtikon*), and the capacity for nutrition (*to threptikon*) are—one ought to say, still prior to that, what it is to think (*noein*), and what it is to perceive (*aisthanesthai*). The reason is that activities (*energeiai*) and actions (*praxeis*) are prior in account to capacities (*dunameis*). But if this is the case, and the corresponding objects should have been studied even prior to these things, one would have to make distinctions about these objects—I mean about nourishment (*trophê*), about the object of perception (*aisthêton*), and the object of thought (*noêton*)—and for the same reason.[55]

Like all capacities, the capacities of the soul have their corresponding manifestations. These manifestations are the activities of the soul (*hai energeiai kai hai praxeis*). They are prior in account (*logôi*) to the corresponding capacities, and they must therefore be determined before them. But the basic activities of the soul, unlike running or other ordinary activities, are themselves by definition object-related. This is an important fact about life and living things. Therefore, understanding the capacities of the soul, and thus being able to define them, requires an

[53] The dog's soul is one *by nature* (*phusei*). Teleological subordination and operational fusion of soul-parts allow Aristotle to explain how the soul-parts can be natural (*phusei*) unities while remaining separate in their definitions (cf. *EE* II 1, 1219b34–36). See Chapter 2, footnote 52.

[54] The term has already been used by Ron Polansky (2007: 494). See the Glossary (*s.v.* COGNITIVE SOUL) for our attempt at a definition of the concept of a cognitive soul.

[55] *An.* II 4, 415a16–22. Note, however, that it is also true that, as one anonymous referee writes, these manifestations also cannot be fully understood with reference to the objects at which these manifestations are directed.

understanding not only of their manifestations but also of the objects that correspond to these manifestations.[56] These objects need to be determined prior to the definition of their manifestations "for the same reason": that is, because they are prior in account to the corresponding activities. To define the capacity of perception, for instance, we need to know what perceiving is, and before we can know that we need to know what the object of perception is. This methodological insight will determine Aristotle's mode of procedure in defining the main capacities of the soul in the rest of the treatise. He starts from the definition of the objects of each of the activities of living things to approach the definition of the corresponding activities (i.e., the manifestation of each capacity), from there to arrive at the definition of the corresponding capacity.

So much for the general method which Aristotle adopts in defining the capacities of the soul in *De anima*. His discussion of the nutritive capacity follows that method and the same goes for the perceptual capacity, even if there are certain additions, as for instance in *An.* III 1, where Aristotle discusses the completeness of the five senses, or when he gives introductory explanations, as for instance in *An.* II 5, where he distinguishes perceptual affection from change. Having arrived at this point, before turning to the thinking capacity, however, I still need to direct attention to some of the basic features of Aristotle's definition of the perceptual capacity (Section 6), since his account of the essence of human thinking will to some extent depend on it. I will also have to turn to Aristotle's somewhat complicated discussion in the chapter that immediately precedes the chapters on the thinking capacity: namely, *An.* III 3 (Section 7). I will do this only to the extent that it is immediately relevant for the discussion of the thinking capacity. Unavoidably, I will say many things that are going to be controversial without being able to take the—extremely rich—secondary literature into account. I hope the results will justify this mode of procedure.[57]

[56] Even in the philosophers' stock example of a capacity defined by reference to its manifestation only, brittleness (the capacity to break easily), there are constraints on the range of objects that may bring about the relevant manifestation. But this is an incomparably weaker sense of object-relatedness than in the case of life-activities.

[57] The past few decades have seen a veritable explosion of major publications on and around perception in Aristotle. This is largely a result of the intense debate between two interpretative camps: spiritualists and literalists. This is a debate about the particular way in which the perceptual capacity is said to become "like" its object, as Aristotle says it does (*An.* II 5, 418a3–4). While literalists claim that perception involves the 'literal' assimilation of the sense organ to the sensory quality it receives, spiritualists maintain that perception for Aristotle is a *sui generis* kind of change consisting in perceptual awareness and that it essentially involves no 'ordinary' change. A highly informative summary and philosophical analysis of this debate (including a new suggestion) can be found in Caston 2005. It is not my purpose here to contribute to this debate. I deal with Aristotle's account of perception in *De anima* only to the extent that it helps us understand the account of human thinking in *De anima*. What I wish to bring out is the way in which Aristotle conceives of perception as an *essentially embodied* (or physically implemented) capacity, since, as we will see below, his account of the essence of human thinking is based on the explicit denial of such essential embodiment for the human *nous*.

6. Before thinking (1): the perceptual capacity

In *An.* II Aristotle defines the capacity of perception by its corresponding objects as the methodology of *An.* II 4 requires him to do. He defines it in a *causal* way and without saying much about its content. He can do this because, in Aristotle's theory, the object of perception is both: it is the object of the act of perceiving (what perception is "of" or what it is "about") *and* it is the efficient (moving) cause of the change (process) leading to the act of perception. The causal impact of the external object of perception brings about its own being perceived by the perceiver: cause and object of perception coincide.[58] Perception is in this sense *of* what causes it. Now it is important to realize that, in his account of perception in *De anima*, Aristotle largely focuses on the causal ancestry of perception—namely, on the change that the object of perception causes in its environment (in the medium) so as to produce a perceptual stimulus in a perceiver—whereas he remains relatively silent with respect to what perception is "of" or what it is "about," beyond some rather schematic claims. He focuses on the object of perception *qua* its causal powers to affect the perceptual apparatus, and he avoids statements about the phenomenal content (or the qualitative features) of perception as they result from the soul's actuality in perceiving objects. Thus, he says, for instance, that the object of sight is color, and that color has the causal power to affect a perceiver so as to result in its being perceived, but he does not say what color, as we see it, is. The reason for proceeding in this way most probably has to do with methodological concerns Aristotle has regarding the division of explanatory labor I have discussed above in Section 2. Since the phenomenal content of perception is the *result* of the soul's activity *as it operates in a living body* (i.e., the cognitive soul)—the soul *does* something so that the living body can receive the perceptual object—the definition of the perceptual soul should not presuppose the result of its own activity in a living body, on pain of definitional circularity. So, Aristotle has reason to avoid doing the work of the scientific explanation of episodes or acts of perception in a treatise that is still devoted to finding the principle for such explanations. The scientific explanation of episodes of perception, including their phenomenal content, should, from an architectonic point of view, fall into the camp of the works dedicated to the actions and affections common to body and soul.[59]

This methodological concern may well be the main reason why Aristotle remains largely silent concerning the analysis of the phenomenal content of perception and the inner bodily workings of the perceptual apparatus in *De anima*,

[58] See Caston 2009: 323. This holds of the causally basic cases of perception (which for Aristotle also have explanatory priority). More complex kinds of perception, e.g. incidental perception, are different in this respect.

[59] Perceptions (*aisthêseis*), which I take to be a generic expression for occurring episodes of perception, are explicitly mentioned as *explananda* of the definition of the soul in *An.* I 5, 409b13–17, and as *explananda* of the soul that are "common to body and soul" in *Sens.* 1, 436a1–6.

apart from generic statements (hearing is of sound, seeing is of color, and so on, all objects of perception consist in certain proportions of the extreme positions on qualitative scales). But, presumably, Aristotle's mode of inquiry in *An.* II 5–11 also has to do with the specific method he adopts for the definition of the perceptual capacity. Perception is, as we have seen, to a large extent explicable in terms of its causal ancestry. However, in his introductory discussion of the relation between perception and change in *An.* II 5, Aristotle emphasizes that the act of perception is not to be identified with change. He classifies perception as an actuality (*energeia*) and a having (*hexis*) of a psychic state: namely, as the actuality of one's soul as one's nature. That requires a causal affection by the external object of perception, but that affection is importantly different from *being changed by that object*. It rather is, he says, the preservation of a natural capacity: namely, the *exercise* of our natural capacity to perceive external things (*An.* II 5, 417b3). To perceive external things, therefore, is to be affected by them but not so as to be changed by them.

Aristotle then proceeds to define the capacity of perception. He starts by introducing the different ways in which the object of perception (*to aisthêton*) is said: namely, exclusive, common, and incidental objects of perception (*An.* II 6). From there onward, Aristotle concentrates on exclusive objects of perception. Exclusive objects of perception are the modally specific objects of perception. They are exclusive to each sense modality: color to seeing, sound to hearing, smell to the sense of smell, taste to the sense of taste, and the qualities of bodies *qua* bodies to the sense of touch. Aristotle concentrates on them because in their case cause and phenomenal content coincide most strictly, so that the perception of the exclusive objects of perception is (almost always) veridical. A color, for instance, is a quality in an external object that has the causal power to affect its environment in such a way as to bring about its own being perceived in perceivers, and the analogue holds for the exclusive objects of the other sense modalities. This makes the exclusive objects of perception an ideal starting point for his account of perception (*An.* II 6, 418a14–16).

In the chapters that follow (*An.* II 7–11), Aristotle discusses each of the five sense modalities by defining their corresponding objects, and by showing how these objects in each case causally affect their environment in such a way as to convey perceptual stimuli to the corresponding peripheral sense organs. Once Aristotle has gone through each sense modality individually, he defines the common underlying capacity of perception as the "capacity to take on perceptual form without the matter" and as the capacity "to be affected according to the proportion" (*An.* II 12, 424a17–24). Saying that perception is the capacity to take on perceptual forms of external objects without their matter, and saying that perceiving is to be affected by them according to the proportion (more on both notions below) avoids saying much by way of a positive description of what the objects of perception consist in *as they are perceived*.[60]

[60] But note that Aristotle's definition of the perceptual capacity as the capacity to take on *perceptual* forms without their matter is not *vacuous* (or circular); "perceptual" here stands in for the various

However, saying that much seems to suffice for the purposes of finding the principle of the science responsible for the explanation of the phenomena of living things.[61] This reservation with respect to a positive description of the achievements of perception, as we have seen, follows from Aristotle's general methodology. Aristotle's *De anima* is devoted to the definition of the soul. Describing the results of the operations of the soul, such as the achievements of the operation of the perceptual soul, is a task to be pursued not in *De anima* (at least not primarily) but in other parts of Aristotle's science of living things, such as in *De sensu*. So much for the method of definition of the perceptual capacity in *De anima*.

For an adequate understanding of the discussion of *nous* it is necessary to provide a few additional details about the way in which Aristotle goes about discussing the causal ancestry of perception in *An.* II 7–11. This is important because in *An.* III 4 he will rely on his account of the perceptual capacity as a template for the discussion of the thinking capacity (*nous*). Although in the end Aristotle will leave behind perception as a model for the thinking capacity, as we will see, it is crucial for an adequate understanding of his argument to be aware of *what* it is that he is leaving behind. What he is leaving behind is, in a word, the *physical model* of the explanation of perceptual episodes. This model has two relevant aspects: (1) the aspect of a physical affection by a corresponding perceptual object (perceptual stimulus), and (2) the aspect of sensory discrimination.

The explanatory model on which Aristotle's discussion of perception is based is the causal model of *assimilation*, which is largely prefigured in Aristotle's general hylomorphic account of change in his *Gener. Corr.* I 7 and *Phys.* III 1–3; however, in *De anima*, this causal model is adapted to the special circumstances of perception. The resulting account of perception, as we will see, combines elements from LKL and Separatism. Let me first give the main lines of the general account of physical change before looking at the way it is adapted to perception.

The general account of physical change. According to the general hylomorphic account of physical change advanced in *Gener. Corr.* I 7 and *Phys.* III 1–3, a physical change is *a process of property exchange*. It consists in the *process of assimilation of properties in things*. Substance x is the bearer of the active relatum of change, the property F; the other substance y is the bearer of the passive relatum of change, G. Upon contact between the two substances, the two relata become actual: x assimilates y in respect of F, while y, in being assimilated, loses its property G and

objects of the five senses (color for sight, sound for the sense of hearing, and so on, and presumably generally for all the *per se* objects of perception).

[61] This can be seen, e.g., in Aristotle's arguments in his *Part An.* II 1, which scientifically account for parts of the physical structure of the heart from the general definition of perception as it is given in *An.* II 12. It follows, trivially, that *An.* II 12 gives the definition of the capacity of perception and that this definition is explanatorily powerful despite the relative silence about the qualitative and phenomenal features of acts of perception.

acquires *F* instead. The change itself is the process of *transition* from *F* to *G*: that is, the process of becoming assimilated. *F* and *G*, to qualify as relata of change, must be *contraries*. That means that they must stand in a relation of *qualified otherness*. They have to be unlike each other because, if they weren't, they would be the same, and nothing can *change* from being *F* toward being *F*.[62] At the same time, *F* and *G* have to be the same in that they must pertain to the same "genus" as Aristotle says: that is, they have to be the same *sort* of property, since otherwise no interaction between them would be possible—for instance, a color cannot change into a sound; change can only occur from one kind of color toward another kind of color. The process takes place in the bearer of the passive relatum of change *G*, which is the substance *y*. Also, the properties *F* and *G* must be *positive and existing physical qualities* (e.g., cold, warm, blue, green, small or large, here or there), otherwise change is not going to happen. All change necessarily requires *physical contact* between the bearer of the active and the bearer of the passive relatum of change ("contact requirement" in what follows). Change unfolds in time; it is continuous and linear in structure. That means that any individual process of change is infinitely divisible and is structured by a starting point and an endpoint. *G* is the *starting point* of change (*terminus a quo*), while *F* the endpoint (*terminus ad quem*), which is to say that during the process of change *y*'s *G* disappears to the degree in which *x* assimilates *y* to itself in respect of *F*. At the end of the process (everything going well), *y* will be identical to *x* in respect of *F*. Change *per se* occurs only in the categories of place, quality, and quantity. In sum, physical change is the assimilation of properties in things, which are contrary to each other: that is, unlike in a qualified way. So much for physical change in general.

The account of perceptual change. In his account of *perceptual* change, Aristotle sticks to the general hylomorphic account of physical change, modifying it in one, albeit crucial, respect. Perceptual change, unlike ordinary change, is *not exactly* a property exchange in things and it is also not the acquisition of a new hylomorphic property by the perceiver. While perceivers are assimilated to perceptual objects in a certain way, they are not assimilated to them in such a way as to receive them *as their properties*. When we perceive a red tomato, we do not thereby become either a red tomato or red. We do not take on the redness in a way that makes the red quality a constitutive part or property of us as hylomorphic compounds. Perceiving qualities such as red does not require that we embody these qualities. Rather, perceivers take on the perceptual qualities, yes, but they take them on "without the matter" and "according to the proportion" (*An.* II 12, 424a17–24; the latter qualification is added because Aristotle thinks of perceptual qualities as proportions of qualitative

[62] *Metaph.* X 8, 1058a16–19 makes the point that any difference on a scale (i.e., non-identity of *F* and *G* on a qualitative scale) counts as contrariety. Since every point on such a scale can serve as a starting point or an endpoint of a given process of change, different positions on the scale are functionally equivalent to the extreme positions.

values on scales of qualitative values, about which more in a moment). But it is important to see that this modification of the general account of change does not result in a completely different kind of account. It is a *modification* of the general physical account. This is to say that Aristotle does take on board the rest of the general account of physical change. There are two modifications Aristotle inserts into his general account to adapt it to the special circumstances of perception. They are *mediation* and *discrimination*.

Mediation is a modification of the *contact requirement* of change. Supposing that *x* is the external perceptual object and *y* the perceiver, mediation makes it possible that there is causal affection and hence contact without there also being an immediate interaction between *x* and *y*; the contact will be mediated by a physical body that lies in-between *x* and *y*. This body is the so-called medium (*metaxu*). That mediating body, however, will not embody the property that it conveys to the perceiver. Colors, for instance, affect us not by traveling through the air in-between the perceiver and the perceived thing *as colors*. The air in-between the perceiver and the perceived thing will not become colored but remain transparent. What the medium conveys is a *sensory stimulus*. It conveys an affection, not with color, but with causal properties carried by the medium and having the power to affect the perceiver in such a way as to make the latter see the color of the external objects. Aristotle argues that direct contact between perceiver and perceived thing would make perception impossible. He thinks that mediation is a necessary feature of a perceptual affection.[63]

Perceptual discrimination. Media convey sensory stimuli to the perceiver. Perceptual stimuli are not sufficient for perception on their own, even if they reach the peripheral sense organs. The stimuli must reach the perceptual center located in the heart where they are *discriminated*. The result of perceptual discrimination is the perception of the external object. This is why Aristotle classifies perception, and later also thinking, as *discriminatory capacities* (*kritikai dunameis*).[64] Aristotle offers a brief discussion of how perceptual discrimination works. The details of the account are obscure, and it is likely that he operates with a simplified model. However, the basic framework of how Aristotle wishes to explain perceptual discrimination is reasonably clear.[65] This is what he says:

[63] This holds even in the case of the so-called contact senses; see *An.* II 11, 422b34–423b26.

[64] *An.* III 3, 427a17–21; *An.* III 4, 429b12–18; *An.* III 9, 432a15–16; *Mot. An.* 6, 700b20; *Posterior Analytics* II 19, 99b35. However, this classification is very likely to be an *a posteriori* commonality between these two capacities; their respective modes of discrimination seem to be very different from each other, so that it would not be justified to speak of the discriminatory capacity as the common genus of perception and thinking. More on this front below.

[65] Interpreters often restrict the scope of Aristotle's account of perceptual discrimination only to the sense of touch. Corcilius 2014 and 2022 argue that interpreters assume this without good reason and that the scope of the passage is perfectly general and unspecific, concerning all kinds of perceptual discrimination, even if he does not spell out how things are supposed to work in all sense modalities (and to be sure it is not entirely clear how it could work in all sense modalities). But not much hangs on this. For even if we suppose that the above account applies to haptic discrimination only, it is still the only Aristotelian account of sensory discrimination we possess, and there is no reason to suppose that he

> Perceiving is a sort of being affected (*paschein ti*), hence that which acts makes that which is potentially as it is, such as it is itself actually. This is why we do not perceive what is equally as hot or cold, or [equally] hard or soft, but their excesses, perception (*hê aisthêsis*) being a kind of mean (*mesotês*) of the opposition present in the objects of perception.[66]

Aristotle here says that perception is a sort of being affected, which, as we have seen above, requires the *qualified otherness* of the agent and the patient of change, which in our case is the perceptual object and the perceiver. So the *capacity* for perception must be different from the perceptual object (a perceptual quality) but it must be of the same genus, which is to say that it must somehow be on the same scale; in other words, the capacity for perception, in order to receive qualities, must be qualitative as well. Aristotle here presupposes his general theory of perceptual qualities.[67] According to this theory, perceptual qualities are defined as positions on qualitative spectra or scales, the extremes of which are maximally different from each other. Qualities on the same scale that are maximally different from each other are *contraries*.[68] To be a certain perceptual quality, a color for instance, on this theory, is nothing but to be a certain *proportion* (*logos*) of the extreme values on the relevant scale (*akra*). For instance, red—the quality red itself—is nothing but a certain proportion of light and dark, the extreme contrary qualities on the relevant qualitative spectrum: namely, a certain portion of bright (say, 2) plus a certain portion of dark (say, 7) (see Fig. 1.1).[69]

The perceptual capacity, to be receptive of a perceptual quality, as we have seen, has to be potentially like it. We have just seen that this means that the perceptual capacity has to be on that same qualitative scale as the quality that it is going to receive and that it has to be "qualifiedly other": that is, different from it. Now, on

thought about the workings of discrimination in the other sense modalities in radically different ways. Hence, even if the following offers an account of haptic discrimination only, discrimination in the other sense modalities will be *mutatis mutandis* the same.

66 *An.* II 11, 423b31–424a5.

67 For what follows, see *An.* II 12, 424a17–24; *An.* III 2, 426b3–8; *Sens.* 3, 440b18–25 (cf. 6, 445b20 ff.); *Metaph.* X 7. An anonymous reader sees a tension between the qualitative nature of the capacity for perception on the one hand and its ontological role as the form of the body on the other. I do not see why qualitative forms could not be structuring principles for a bodily structure.

68 See *Metaph.* X 3, 1054b23–26.

69 How good this is as a theory of colors is a difficult matter that need not interest us here. The answer depends, crucially, on how exactly we conceive of the extreme values and the character of their "mixture." Sean Kelsey (in Kelsey 2022: 95) criticizes the theory, arguing that qualitative contraries (the "extremes") are not possible candidates for quantitative ingredients because they are not divisible into parts. But the character of the mixture need not be physical in the way in which a paint color is produced by the mixing of other paint colors. It is open to Aristotle to conceive of the "mixtures" in-between the extremes of a given qualitative spectrum as proportions of fractions of the full *possession* of the extreme qualities. All that needs to be divisible is the *extension of the relevant qualitative spectrum*, not the contraries that make up its "extremes."

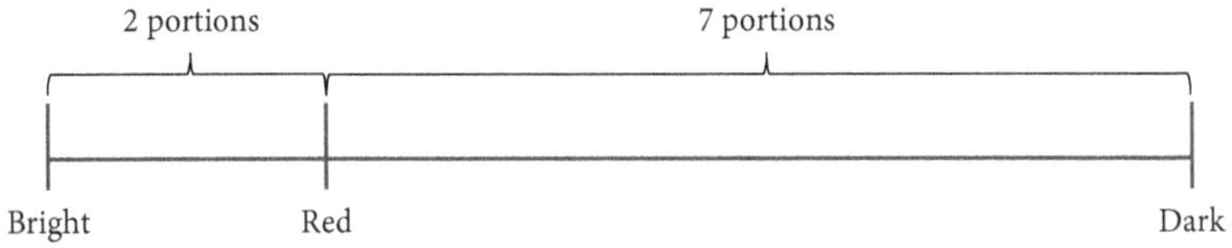

Fig. 1.1 The color red according to Aristotle's metaphysics of qualities

Aristotle's account, the capacity for perception is a mean proportion on the relevant qualitative scale. In the case of the sense of sight, this should mean that the proportion of the perceptual mean (*aisthêtikê mesotês*) is neither bright nor dark—it is the exact mean between the extreme values. Based on this account of perceptual qualities and the perceptual capacity as proportions (*logoi*), Aristotle now moves on to explain *perceptual discrimination*.[70] He says:

> And that is why it [i.e., the mean] discriminates (*krinei*) the objects of perception. For the mean is capable of discriminating (*to gar meson kritikon*); because it becomes (*ginetai*), relative to each extreme, in turn the other extreme (*akron*).[71]

Given that the perceptual capacity is situated in the middle position on the qualitative scale, as Aristotle here says that it is, discrimination happens whenever there is a *contrast* between the mean position of the perceptual capacity and the qualitative value of an incoming perceptual affection. The perceptual mean, says Aristotle, can bring about sensory discrimination in virtue of becoming relative to the incoming value, "the other extreme." What this suggests is that when the sensory stimulus, which carries a value on the same qualitative scale as, but different from, the perceptual mean, has contact with the perceptual mean (capacity) located in the heart, there will be a juxtaposition of two positions on the scale. Since these positions will not be identical with each other but will be "extremes" that are different from each other, there will again be a proportion of values, which is just what a perceptual quality is by its definition. In that scenario, the reception of the *per se* features of that incoming perceptual value will be veridical because the contrast that the two positions on the scale generate has the neutral middle value as one of its "extremes;" it will therefore produce a quality that matches the quality of the external object (provided that neither the medium and its causal property to affect

[70] I cut a long story short here. It looks as though Aristotle does not think that the mean value of the perceptual capacity, which does the sensory discrimination, is divided into (or distributed over) the values of the five special senses; rather, there is only one perceptual mean which stands in an analogous proportion to the qualitative proportions of the different sense modalities and that, in virtue of this analogous proportion, is capable of receiving them all. More on this in Chapter 4.

[71] *An.* II 11, 424a5–7.

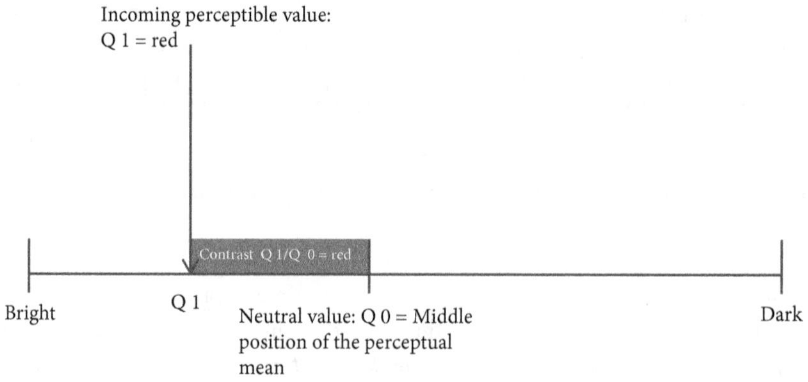

Fig. 1.2 How the senses work: perceptual discrimination of red

perceivers nor the perceptual mean is distorted). The result is a quality without matter in the perceiver: that is, a contrast between two qualitative values—namely, the incoming value, say, *Q* 1, and *Q* 0, which is the value of the neutral perceptual mean (see Fig. 1.2).

In effect, Aristotle's account of basic acts of perception as the reception of perceptual qualities in the perceiver without the matter (i.e., the reception of the quality without proximate matter in the perceiver) can *explain* the sensory awareness of the perceptual qualities of external objects. For, in that scenario, Aristotle can explain how the received qualities will be received as *of* the external objects. This is because the matter of these objects remains outside in the external objects.[72] But be that as it may, what is important for Aristotle's account of the thinking capacity is that his account of perceptual discrimination is a *physical* account: the perceptual object assimilates the perceiver to its perceptual quality via the causal effect that it exerts on the medium. And even though perceptual change does not amount to full property exchange—the received perceptual quality does not become a hylomorphic property of the perceiver (but continues to be a property of the external object) —it still requires that the perceptual capacity itself occupy a certain *position* on the relevant scale of perceptual qualities.

> And just as that which is about to perceive white and black must be neither of them in actuality, but both of them in potentiality—and similarly also in the other senses—so must also in the case of touch [that which is about to perceive hot or cold must be] neither hot nor cold.[73]

[72] As argued in Corcilius 2022: 150–154.
[73] *An.* II 11, 424a7–10.

To be receptive of perceptual qualities is thus to be relatively unaffected by the corresponding extremes: that is, it is to be neither the one nor the other extreme. To be neither white nor black here does not mean to be something categorically different from being a color; it means to be neither white nor black *while occupying a position on the color spectrum* (namely, the neutral position of being neither bright nor dark, given that the colors are "mixtures" of bright and dark).[74] Otherwise, the perceiver would not be a possible object of affection by color (this is the qualified otherness that any kind of affection requires according to Aristotle). Similarly, to be neither warm nor cold means not to have no temperature at all but to be of *neutral temperature*. The neutral values on perceptual scales are *qualitative*. For Aristotle that means that they are physical because he is a realist about qualities (for Aristotle, as we have seen, qualitative alteration is a straightforward, intrinsic, and irreducible kind of physical change). However, that very same feature of the perceptual capacity that enables it to be receptive of perceptual qualities—its perceptual mean—makes it the case that there are "blind spots" in every sense modality, as Aristotle says in the above passage. Affections by perceptual qualities that are in the same positions as the middle position of the perceptual mean will *not* be perceived. That too follows from the qualified difference thesis. A wet hand will not be able to discriminate the wetness of the water that it touches etc. Likewise, perceptual stimuli that exceed the limits of the receptivity of the perceptual capacity of the perceiver will either fail to be perceived (because they fail to meet the minimal threshold of perceptibility) or destroy the corresponding organ. A sound that is too loud will destroy the eardrum and so on.[75]

In sum, perception is a *physical* system for the discrimination of (likewise physical) qualities. To be sure, the capacity of perception itself is a non-bodily proportion (*logos*); however, it is a proportion *of* physical (qualitative) values, which also occur as ingredients of physical properties of external physical bodies.[76] Without body, perception would be not only impossible but also *inconceivable*. Perception, for Aristotle, is *essentially* bodily. And it is so on both ends of the cognition relation, on the side of the perceiver and on the side of the perceived object. As we will see, in this respect perception is different from thinking, which also requires that the corresponding capacity be impassive or unaffected (*apatheia*); however, in the case of thinking, the impassivity is not neutrality in the sense of a physical and embodied kind of impassivity, but an altogether non-physical kind of impassivity. This will change everything.

[74] There are thus two ways of being transparent. One is the condition of bodies to be receptive of colors; the other is a neutral qualitative value on the color spectrum.

[75] See *An.* III 2, 426a27–b12, including for what follows.

[76] *An.* II 5, 417b19.

7. Before thinking (2): the "grey zone"

After his discussion of perception,[77] Aristotle does not immediately move to the definition of the next basic capacity of the soul, as one might expect him to do based on his announcement in his to-do list in *An.* II 2. Instead of discussing the next part of the soul, the thinking capacity, Aristotle discusses something else.[78]

An. III 3 is often regarded as a chapter concerned with the definition of *phantasia*, a capacity that is not even mentioned in the programmatic list of basic capacities of the soul in *An.* II 2. (It is only briefly mentioned as an object of inquiry in *An.* II 3, 414b16). Now, it is certainly true that the chapter contains a discussion of *phantasia*, and it is also true that this discussion results in a definition of that capacity. To be sure, this is in line with the definitory goals of *De anima*. And yet, there are good reasons to think that *phantasia* is not the chapter's main topic; the discussion of *phantasia* is more likely to be merely a component, albeit an important one, of its main topics. The main purpose of the chapter rather is to distinguish perception and perception-involving mental states from what Aristotle regards as thinking proper.[79] This is how the chapter begins:

> Since they [i.e., philosophers] define the soul most of all by way of two differences—namely, by way of motion with respect to place, and by way of discriminating (*krinein*) and thinking (*noein*) and perceiving (*aisthanesthai*)—it seems that both thinking (*noein*) and understanding (*phronein*) are just like some sort of perceiving; for in both cases the soul discriminates something and cognizes what there is. And the ancient thinkers anyway say that understanding and perceiving are the same, as Empedocles did say as well, "For the wisdom of human beings grows with respect to what is present to them," and elsewhere, "Whence the understanding presents to them different things in each moment." And this is also what the Homeric expression, "For such is the mind," wants to convey. For they all suppose that thinking is corporeal, just like perceiving, and [all suppose] that both perceiving and understanding is of like by like, just as we have set down at the outset of our treatise.[80]

[77] The chapters that immediately follow the definition of the perceptual capacity in *An.* II 12 discuss the completeness of our perceptual receptivity by the five sense modalities (*An.* III 1), and other important issues related to perception (*An.* III 2), such as the awareness of acts of perception, the factors of perceptual affection (agent and patient, their actuality, and their potentiality), the proportion-character of perception, and the principle responsible for the simultaneous discrimination of sensory input from different sense modalities. These topics, despite their intrinsic importance, do not have an immediate bearing on Aristotle's discussion of the thinking capacity.

[78] I would like to thank Michel Crubellier for sharing an unpublished article on the role of *An.* III 3 in the argument of the *De anima*. I also adopted his suggestion of referring to the area between perceiving and thinking as the "grey zone."

[79] Which also explains why the treatment of *phantasia* is not mentioned in Aristotle's to-do list in *An.* II 2. See above (Section 4).

[80] *An.* III 3, 427a17–29, taking the *de* in 427a19 as apodotic. This is not how the above sentence is usually construed (and consequently translated).

Aristotle here makes two observations. First, he notes that the majority of his predecessors, when they identified self-motion and cognition as the distinguishing marks of the soul, did not properly distinguish between perceiving and thinking.[81] His second observation is that the ancient predecessors' practice of treating perceiving and thinking as the same kind of thing—namely, as some sort of bodily discriminating and cognizing, in which like is cognized by like—creates the impression that perceiving and thinking are fundamentally the same sort of thing. So, to judge from the first sentence of the chapter, the beginning of *An.* III 3 is about that very question: how to distinguish perceiving from thinking, and more specifically whether the ancient predecessors are right in claiming that thinking is, like perception, a bodily kind of discrimination and a cognition of like by like. The ensuing discussion in *An.* III 3 can, and indeed should, be interpreted as contributing to settling this very question, and not so much, let alone primarily, as devoted to the definition of an additional capacity of the soul: namely, *phantasia*.[82] For obvious reasons, I cannot offer more than a rather sketchy discussion of this difficult and demanding chapter. But I should say something about the basic outline of its argument insofar as it prepares the ground for the study of human thinking offered in *An.* III 4–8.

An. III 3 is devoted to the question of where to draw the boundary between what Aristotle regards as thinking proper and other, at least on the face of it, similar cognitive states that in one way or the other involve perception.[83] Aristotle answers that question in three steps.

First, he attacks the claim that thinking is, like perception, a bodily kind of cognition and discrimination. He does agree with his predecessors that thinking is discriminative (all genuine cognition is discriminative for Aristotle). But, as it will turn out, he does not think that thinking is a *bodily* sort of discrimination. His argument to that effect, however, is negative; it does not offer a positive view of what sort of cognition or discrimination thinking is. For this the reader will have to wait until *An.* III 4.

Second, Aristotle introduces *phantasia* and distinguishes it from thinking, and, indeed, from all cognitive and discriminative states. As will eventually become clear, *phantasia* is a bodily change (*kinêsis*) serving as an enabling condition for

[81] Aristotle here uses the same two words for the activity of thinking, *noein* and *phronein*, that he will use at the outset of *An.* III 4 (429a10–11). It is very difficult to determine what exactly the difference between these two words is. It might also be that Aristotle uses *phronein* to limit, or to explicate, the meaning of *noein*. For a survey of different possible interpretations, see Gregoric 2007: 93–96.

[82] *Phantasia* is a capacity of the living body and not a capacity of the *soul* in the sense of a part of the soul as defined above. Unlike proper soul capacities, *phantasia* is purely passive (see Wedin 1988: 45–53) and causally and definitionally dependent on other capacities of the soul, see Corcilius and Gregoric 2010). More on this front momentarily.

[83] For a much more detailed and, in its effects, similar interpretation of *An.* III 3, see Polansky 2007: 403–433 ("Distinguishing Sense and Thought"). Unlike Polansky, however, I do not regard *phantasia* as a faculty of representation, but only of providing "the material" for mental representation.

all kinds of representative, cognitive, and other related states that go beyond mere sense perception.[84]

Third, Aristotle offers a causal account of *phantasia*. As a result, the discussion of *phantasia* serves Aristotle to distinguish mental representation and other *phantasia*-involving states, which he conceives of as bodily, from thinking, and hence to achieve the main purpose of the chapter, which is to distinguish thinking from bodily cognition.

First step (*An.* III 3, 427a29–b14). Aristotle raises the following points against the identification of thinking and perceiving:

(i) *Against the ancient version of LKL.* If perception is of like by like, and thinking is like perception, why can we go wrong and think and perceive falsely (427a29–b6)? This is an argument against the plausibility of the old version of LKL. On this pre-Aristotelian version of the theory, the explanation of misrepresentation and error seems impossible.

(ii) *The extensions of thinking and perceiving are not the same.* Since all animals (both human and nonhuman animals) can perceive but only a few can engage in propositional thought (which can be true or false), thinking and perceiving seem not to be the same; also their extensions are not the same in respect of veridicality: while the perception of modally specific objects can be exercised by all animals and is always true, propositional thinking (*dianoia*) can be false as well and can only be exercised by animals that possess speech (*logos*) (427b6–14).

This strongly suggests that thinking and perceiving are not the same thing, and Aristotle will draw that conclusion explicitly a little later in the text.

Second step (*An.* III 3, 427b14–428b10). Aristotle brings in *phantasia*. He says:

> For *phantasia* is different from both perception (*aisthêsis*) and propositional thinking (*dianoia*); and it itself does not come about without perception and without it there is no taking something to be the case (*hupolêpsis*).[85]

[84] Often *phantasia* is translated as "representation." That, however, seems wrong. *Phantasia* just by itself does not represent anything (see also the discussion of *An.* III 8, 432a12–14). *Phantasia* is functionally incomplete for Aristotle, as Wedin 1988, 45–57, rightly insisted. That means that its products, the *phantasmata*, require cognitive capacities to use them for their representational purposes. *Phantasia* itself is no more than a perceptual stimulus which is stored in the organism. It can, however, be retrieved, reconfigured, and used for representational purposes and also in other contexts, such as imagination, dreams, and illusions. These contexts can, but need not be, intentional. More on this in Chapter 5, and in the Glossary (*s.v.* PHANTASIA and PHANTASMA).

[85] *An.* III 3, 427b14–16.

This sentence introduces *phantasia* as something in-between perception and propositional thinking ("taking something to be the case").[86] *Phantasia*, Aristotle says, requires perception as a necessary condition, which would make it something bodily, while it is itself a necessary condition for *hupolêpsis* (propositional doxastic and epistemic states generally, hence "taking something to be the case"). In the immediate sequel, Aristotle first argues that *phantasia* is not *hupolêpsis* (427b16–27), and then he makes a point he has already established in the first step: namely, that perception and thinking are not the same thing. This seems to rule out the identification both of perception and of *phantasia* with the thinking capacity. However, contrary to what one might expect him to do after having established that thinking and sense perception are not the same and that *phantasia* is not propositional thinking, Aristotle does *not* immediately move on to discuss the thinking capacity; instead, he turns to a discussion of what he has just claimed to be somehow in-between perception and thinking: namely, *phantasia*. This is how he justifies his mode of procedure.

> But regarding thinking (*noein*), since it is different from perceiving, and [since] one part of it seems to be *phantasia*, and another *hupolêpsis*, we must, after having made our determinations concerning *phantasia*, in this way speak about the other [i.e., thinking].[87]

Interestingly, Aristotle here justifies the ensuing discussion of *phantasia* with the claim that thinking partly *consists* of *phantasia*. Since he has just claimed that *phantasia* neither is propositional thinking (*dianoia*) nor consists in taking something to be the case (*hupolêpsis*), this is a puzzling claim. But it could well be that Aristotle is not speaking in his own voice here; perhaps he is only reporting other people's beliefs. If this is correct, he justifies his discussion of *phantasia* with the observation that certain people have the impression that thinking is constituted partly by *phantasia* and partly by *hupolêpsis*.[88] On that assumption, the reason why

[86] This means all mental states that accept something to be the case: understanding, opinion, and, as he says, "their contraries" (*An.* III 3, 427b24–27). "Supposition" is a possible English translation. Aristotle there says that the treatment of the differences of *hupolêpsis* pertains to a different account (*heteros estô logos*). This seems to confirm our thesis from above that Aristotle, in *De anima*, is not so much interested in the account of the phenomena of living things as in the definition of the principle of such an account.

[87] *An.* III 3, 427b27–29.

[88] As Plato seems to have implied in the *Sophist*, where he argued that *phantasia* (in the sense of perceptual belief) is a mixing together of perception and belief. (See the next footnote.) Ronald Polansky takes Aristotle to endorse the claim that *phantasia* is somehow part of thinking (not implausibly from a textual point of view). He then removes the contradiction by claiming that Aristotle here uses the term "*noein*" (thinking) in a wide sense that includes animal cognition (as he does in *An.* III 10, 433a10, and *Mot. An.* 6, 700b18; Polansky 2007: 413). I find this unlikely as in both cases in which Aristotle applies the wider use of *nous* or *noesis*, he explicitly says that he is using that term in an extended sense. This is not the case here in *An.* III 3.

Aristotle discusses *phantasia* here rather than elsewhere is to dispel that impression and to show that *phantasia* is not a constitutive part of thinking. But Aristotle may also simply be looking forward to his own account of the phenomena of human thinking, according to which human thinking "involves" *phantasia* as a necessary enabling condition. In both cases we would have to stress the fact that he says that *phantasia* merely *seems* to be a part of thinking.

The ensuing discussion confirms the above assumption. It has the structure of an argument by elimination. Aristotle asks whether *phantasia* is one of the discriminative states by which we grasp what is true and what is false. They are perception (*aisthêsis*), infallible knowledge and awareness of principles (*epistêmê*, *nous*), fallible opinion (*doxa*), and any combination of perception and opinion (*doxa met'aisthêseôs*).[89] The result is that *phantasia* is none of them.[90] This eliminative procedure, even though it appears to be purely negative in character, turns out to be an important part of the investigation. For the elimination of all the cognitive-discriminative states serves not only to distinguish *phantasia* from thought, but also to contrast *phantasia* with those states; it thus reveals the non-cognitive and non-discriminatory character *of phantasia*.

A further upshot of the elimination procedure is a collection of facts about *phantasia* and its products, which Aristotle calls *phantasmata*.[91] His ensuing account of *phantasia* should be able to *explain* these facts. Roughly, these *explananda* are:

(1) *Phantasia* is the capacity in virtue of which we are capable of having *phantasmata*: that is, internal appearances (in all sense modalities).
(2) *Phantasia* is not necessarily of things that are externally present (like perception is).
(3) Not all animals have *phantasia*; in fact, many non-rational animals do not have it.
(4) The *phantasia* of some given thing can be true or false, but for the most part it is false.[92] Indeed, we can have *phantasmata* of a certain state of affairs, while simultaneously having the rational conviction that that state of affairs does not obtain.
(5) Having *phantasmata* depends at least in part on us and not so much on our environment. It is, to some extent, spontaneous and under our control.

[89] This goes against Plato's discussion of *phantasia* in *Soph.* 264 A (see also *Phlb.* 39 B).

[90] For roughly the same list of discriminative cognitive capacities, see *An.* I 3, 404b25–27. *Phantasia* is subsumed under the discriminative capacities in *Mot. An.* 6, 700b20–22. That, however, need not be taken as contradicting the discussion in *De anima*. For a discussion, see Corcilius 2020b: 314–327.

[91] The suffix *-ma* indicates the *result* of the activity of *phantasia*: that which this capacity brings about or produces.

[92] The meaning of "true" and "false" here is to be understood as follows. A *phantasma* is true whenever what appears in it is also externally present, whereas it is false if that which appears in it is not externally present.

(6) *Phantasmata* can also be present to us in a way that is not under our control (e.g., during sleep when we are dreaming).

Third step (428b10–429a8). Aristotle's causal account of *phantasia* serves him to explain the above features (1)–(6) in a rather minimalistic way. Aristotle defines *phantasmata* neither as intentional states nor as conscious mental events but as causal remnants of the affections that occur during episodes of sense-perception. They are remnants of perceptual stimuli. This means that they are bodily changes (*kinêsis*). More specifically, *phantasmata* are qualitative changes persisting in the body even after the event of perception.[93] They persist in the body, in the blood both in the region around the heart, which is the seat of the cognitive center of the animal (the perceptual soul), and in the peripheral sense organs. Their causal history as stored perceptual stimuli determines in a certain way what *phantasmata* can be taken to be "of"; taken *per se*, *phantasmata* preserve the causal power of the perceptual stimuli to affect perceivers with these same qualitative features as they are possessed by the external objects that originally brought them about. But Aristotle does not think that the being "of" is quite the same in the case of *phantasmata* as in perception. More directly, *phantasmata* do not have the same content as perception; indeed, Aristotle does not think that *phantasmata* taken *per se* have any mental content at all (similar to pictures or books). A *phantasma* is a stored perceptual stimulus; given the right circumstances, it has the power to affect the cognitive center of the animal in such a way as to result in a perception-like discriminative act (*Insomn.* 2, 460a32–b3). That perception-like act then will result in, as it were, the second-hand mental presence of the external perceptual object that brought the *phantasma* about when the object was originally perceived. Aristotle compares the way in which *phantasmata* are present in the body to the way in which a signet ring leaves its imprint in wax (*Mem.* 1, 450a31 ff.). It is only in such a second-hand way that a *phantasma* has the "power of the objects that bring it about;" it can act as a *causal substitute* of external things (*Mot. An.* 6, 701b18–23). This is important for Aristotle's theory of animal self-motion in *An.* III 9–11 and *Mot. An.*, as it gives him the resources to explain the seemingly radically spontaneous movements of animals (*Phys.* VIII 6, 259b1–6) as basically delayed responses to sense-impressions. This causal substitute function of *phantasia* implies an important role for it in representational contexts (even if a *phantasma* by itself is not sufficient for the mental act of representing an object). The internal presence of a *phantasma* as a causal substitute for an external object implies that it can also stand in for, or be taken as *representing*, that object, since otherwise the animal would not (as it in fact does) respond to it in a way that is similar to the way it responds to the perception of that same object. But apart from

[93] In this, they are like Sigmund Freud's *Tagesreste*.

their role in representational contexts, when they stand in for currently absent external objects to the animal, *phantasmata* also exert other functions during cognitive episodes, about which more below.

But, for all the causal powers *phantasmata* have, it merits emphasis that *phantasmata* by themselves, from a causal point of view, are entirely passive.[94] They require external moving sources to bring them back to the cognitive center of the animal (to make them "resurface" again) before they can make their impact on the animal's cognition and behavior. They are stored qualitative changes (*alloiôseis*; *Mot. An.* 7, 701b17–23; *Insomn.* 2, 459b1 ff.), which are said to somehow subsist in the blood (we do not know in which way; *Insomn.* 3, 460b28 ff.). Now, the moving causes of *phantasmata* (or sequences of *phantasmata*) that bring them back into an animal's cognitive life can be intentional, as in the case of an animal's desires which are teleologically guided (see *An.* III 7), or they can be non-intentional and occur without a teleological dimension: for example, when a person who sleeps next to a hot stove dreams of a fire, in which case it would be the unconscious sensation of the heat of the stove that stirs up *phantasmata* of hot things. The principle of the association of *phantasmata* would in that case not depend on a person's desires but be entirely dependent on the causal properties of the *phantasmata* themselves (association by physical similarity, in this instance).

Phantasia, as it is defined in *An.* III 3, is the capacity of a cognitive agent's body to store the remnants of perceptual stimuli. And this is all it is. It has no correlated object; nor does it have a second actuality that would correspond to a specific mental act.[95] As such, *phantasia* is not itself a cognitive capacity but an *enabling condition* for all cognitive and other mental states that go beyond the mere perceptual presentation of what is externally present. It is a provider of the, as it were, "material" of mental representation, but it is not itself *doing* the mental representation. Mental representation is a mental act that involves cognition. And that requires the activity of one of the genuine cognitive capacities, which takes us back to perception and thinking. Both perception and thinking can be *agents* of mental representation.[96] Perceptual representation, as for instance in memory and perceptual association, just like the mental representation in thinking contexts, certainly depend on the presence of *phantasmata* to be able to engage in their representations. Aristotle claims a number of times that human thinking cannot occur without a

[94] See Loening 1903: 95, and especially Wedin 1988: 57. The causal passivity and functional incompleteness of *phantasia* which Aristotle emphasizes in *An.* III 3 and *Insomn.* 2 is doubted by a number of scholars. For a survey of some of the more recent views on this, see the discussion by Jessica Moss (who herself assigns a necessary role to *phantasia* for animal motivation; Moss 2012: 51–66).

[95] In other words, *phantasia* is functionally incomplete. See Wedin 1988: 45–57. Of course, "having a *phantasma*" *can* refer to an occurrent mental episode: namely, to "having an appearance" (it is used in that way, e.g., in *An.* III 3, 428a1–2). That, however, does not make *phantasia* a cognitive capacity; the cognitive agent (mover) of such an episode will always be a perceiver or a human thinker. See the next footnote.

[96] For perception and thinking as the cognitive agents of *phantasia*, see *An.* III 11, 434a5–10.

phantasma.[97] But it is *them*, namely perception, memory and thinking, that are the movers and agents of the mental acts of representation.

This dependence on *phantasmata* as the material for representation makes it all the more important for Aristotle's project of defining the thinking capacity to distinguish *phantasia* from thought as clearly as possible. Such a clear distinction is certainly one of the upshots of the discussion in *An.* III 3. The chapter shows that *phantasmata* fall short of *being* thoughts (see also *An.* III 7 and *An.* III 8 with our discussion in Chapters 4 and 5), or indeed any properly cognitive state or proper *per se* object of cognition; they *enable* mental representation and as such will turn out to be necessary conditions of human thinking. They can do this in virtue of the fact that they, when stirred up properly by an external moving cause, can bring perception-like affections to the cognitive center of cognitive agents. The latter can then discriminate them anew and make use of them. Regarding their usage, the possibilities of variation and combination are almost unlimited. Since *phantasmata* are stored perceptual stimuli, the limits of their reconfigurability and recombinability, sequencing and resequencing, focusing, and so on, are determined by the causal properties of the qualitative changes that they are. All of this makes *phantasmata* an indispensable aid for higher forms of cognition and all kinds of animal behavior. The reconfigurability of *phantasmata*, as it were, emancipates cognitive agents from the influences of their immediate environment, as it broadens the scope of objects and scenarios that are available to them beyond what is immediately available to sense perception. In this way, *phantasmata* can determine the behavior of cognitive agents, which is also what Aristotle says at the end of his discussion of that capacity.

> And since they remain in the body and are similar to the perceptions, the animals do many things due to them [i.e., *phantasmata*]; partly because they do not have the capacity for thought (*nous*), as in the case of nonhuman animals, and partly because their thinking capacity (*nous*) is eclipsed at times either through emotion or illness or sleep, as in the case of human beings.[98]

Despite being an indispensable aid to thought, Aristotle points out that whenever *phantasmata determine* the behavior of cognitive agents (when they "do many things due to them," *kat' autas*), this is because thinking *fails* to do this. *Phantasmata* determine behavior of cognitive agents either because these agents do not have the capacity of thinking in the first place or because their thinking capacity is temporarily eclipsed. Thinking and *phantasmata* thus turn out to be very different: They mutually exclude each other as determinants of an agent's behavior. It follows that

[97] *Mem.* 1, 449b31–450a1; *An.* I 1, 403a8–10; *An.* III 3, 427b14–16; *An.* III 7, 431a16–17, 431b2; *An.* III 8, 432a8–10.

[98] *An.* III 3, 429a4–8.

when thinking agents make use of *phantasmata*, it will not be the *phantasmata* that determine their behavior but these agents themselves. Unlike Plato in the *Sophist*, Aristotle in *An.* III 3 sharply distinguishes thinking from *phantasia*.

In which way, then, are *phantasmata* enabling conditions of human thinking? This is a difficult question; a partial answer will be given in the course of the argument in the chapters on thinking in *An.* III 4–8, where Aristotle says that *phantasmata* are to human thought as percepts are to perception (*aisthêmata*; 431a14–17), and that human thinking thinks the intelligible forms "in the *phantasmata*" (431b2). This latter formulation presumably means that *phantasmata* serve as necessary means for mental representations that supply material for human thinking. Aristotle gives one example that may help to see how he might have thought about the way *phantasmata* contribute to the representation of intelligible content: that is, how the mental representation of the objects of thought works in one particular case. The example is unique in the Aristotelian corpus. It occurs in a passage in which Aristotle offers an account of the distinction between two different kinds of *phantasia*, which he calls perceptual and deliberative *phantasia*.[99]

> Well, then, perceptual *phantasia*, as has been said already, occurs in the other animals as well, deliberative *phantasia*, by contrast, in those that are capable of calculating; for, [to determine] whether one should do this or that already is the work of calculation, and it is necessary to measure by one [common] standard. For one pursues the greater. It follows (*hôste*) that [the calculating agent] is capable of making one *phantasma* out of a plurality of *phantasmata*.[100]

Here, Aristotle distinguishes intellectual calculation and perception by way of the former's minimum achievement:[101] namely, a minimal preference calculus resulting in a judgment about the relative preferability of one thing over the other (of the form "*A* is greater than *B*"). Doing this, he argues, requires measuring *A* and *B* by a common standard. And this in turn requires the capacity to *fuse* a plurality of *phantasmata* into one ("making one *phantasma* out of a plurality"). Why? Because whoever can compare two separate things by way of a common standard must be able to perform both: imagining two separate things or courses of action, *A* and *B*, simultaneously, *and* subjecting *A* and *B* to a common standard. The result of that complex operation is, or corresponds to, the judgment "*A* is greater than *B*." That

[99] *An.* III 10, 433b29–30. These names indicate the *sources* of the respective kinds of *phantasmata* (i.e., the agents that are responsible for their appearance). Perceptual *phantasia* is the kind of mental representation that occurs in perceptual contexts, or in contexts in which perception is the origin and driving force of the *phantasmata*, while deliberative *phantasia* is the kind of *phantasmata* as they come up in episodes of practical deliberation, which are driven by a rational desire (*boulêsis*).

[100] *An.* III 11, 434a5–10.

[101] Cf. Burnyeat 1980: 91n29 ("simplest achievement").

judgment is the expression of a relation in which *A* stands to *B* ("greater than"). However, as there cannot be a perception of relations, Aristotle infers that the calculating agent must be capable of *fusing* a plurality of *phantasmata* into one, to represent the imperceptible content of their judgment. If we suppose that Aristotle is committed to the thesis that the contents of human thinking require mental representation (he does not bother to spell out this hidden premise of his reasoning here, but he has argued for it previously in *An.* III 7, 431a14–17[102]), the underlying argument seems to run as follows.

(i) All human thinking requires mental representation of the objects of thinking.
(ii) *Phantasmata* are remnants of perceptual stimuli and thus are naturally capable of serving as material for the representation of perceptible objects.
(iii) There is human deliberative thinking.
(iv) Minimally, the content of the result of a deliberative episode is of the form "*A* is greater than *B*," which is the expression of a relation that obtains between two perceptible things *A* and *B*.
(v) Relations, unlike the relata *A* and *B*, are not perceptible.
(vi) Therefore, the material for the mental representation of relations as they figure in human deliberative thinking must result from a certain manipulation of *phantasmata* (which otherwise, originally and naturally, would serve to represent perceptual objects): namely, their fusion.

The conclusion in (vi) follows because *phantasmata* are the only available source from which cognitive agents can derive the material for their mental representations, and because without such fused *phantasmata*, all *phantasmata* would, in one way or the other, stand in for objects and their perceptual features. In other words, given his commitment to (i), what Aristotle needs is an account of *symbolic representation*.[103] Symbolic representation is representation of content that does not *picture* that content. Rather, the qualitative features of the mental representation itself (the *phantasma*) will stand in a more or less contingent relation to the content it represents. This is the difference to perceptual *phantasia*, where the *phantasmata* literally resemble ("picture") the (perceptual) objects they represent. And since there is no material for such representations other than perceptual *phantasmata*, the fusion of a plurality of the latter will be a natural source. As the passage in *An.* III 11 describes deliberative thinking by way of its minimum achievement, there is reason to think that symbolic representation as it is displayed in *phantasia bouleutikê*, or something like it, is required for the representation of all the specific (non-perceptual) content of human thought.

[102] Chapter 5 in this volume offers a more comprehensive justification for this same claim.
[103] Martha Nussbaum discusses the symbolic role of *phantasmata* in Nussbaum 1985^2: 266–267.

In sum, *An.* III 3 prepares the ground for the discussion and definition of the thinking capacity. The chapter distinguishes perception from thought, and it distinguishes *phantasia* from thought. It also offers an account of *phantasia*. By so doing, Aristotle makes it clear that *phantasia* is neither discriminative nor a mental state in its own right (cognitive or representative); rather, it is a causal and bodily enabling condition for such states. With this conclusion, Aristotle isolates the physical enabling conditions of thinking from what he regards to be thinking proper. The section on *phantasia* is thus only a part, albeit an important one, of the general argumentative line of *An.* III 3 to distinguish thinking from bodily discrimination. This is the main achievement of the chapter with relation to the ensuing chapters on thinking. With this conclusion in place, we are ready to turn to the stretch of text that contains the treatment of what Aristotle regards as the principle of thinking proper, *nous*.

2

Aristotle's account of the human capacity for thinking

1. Introduction

In *An.* III 4–5 Aristotle is centrally concerned with the definition of the human capacity for thinking. This follows directly from his announcement at the outset of *An.* III 4:

> Regarding the part of the soul by which the soul knows and understands—be it separate or separate not in extension but only in account—we must examine what distinguishes it and how thinking may ever come about.[1]

At this point of his argument, Aristotle takes it for granted that the thinking capacity is a part of the soul. What he is looking for is the definition of that capacity. As we have seen in the previous chapter, the investigation in *De anima* is concerned with the definition of the basic capacities of the soul ("the soul itself," *Sens.* 1, 436a1). Aristotle's ultimate goal is to provide his science of living things with a principle from which to derive explanations of the phenomena of living things. Thinking ("reasonings," *logismous*) is one of these phenomena (see *An.* I 5, 409b16). Hence, what Aristotle is looking for is the definition of the principle by reference to which he can scientifically explain the phenomena related to human thinking.

This principle is the part of the soul called "the thinking capacity" (*to noêtikon*; *An.* III 4, 429a30), "the thinking part of the soul" (*to noêtikon meros tês psuchês*; *Phys.* VII 3, 247b1), "thinking soul" (*noêtikê psuchê*; *An.* III 4, 429a28), or simply "thought" (*nous*; *An.* II 3, 414b18). *That* the thinking capacity is a part of the soul for Aristotle is clear from the fact that in the above text he brackets the question whether the thinking part of the soul is separate in account only or perhaps also separate in

I would like to express my gratitude to Michel Crubellier, Andrea Falcon, and Robert Roreitner for their comments and corrections in both oral and written communication. They have saved me from many errors. Some of the basic ideas of this chapter go back to my research published in Corcilius 2011b. I would also like to thank the audiences at the Universities of Tübingen, Vienna, Potsdam, and Frankfurt, where I had occasion to present parts of this chapter, for their remarks and questions, especially George Karamanolis, Johannes Haag, Luz Christopher Seiberth, and Markus Willascheck. I owe special thanks to Michel Crubellier for making available to me his unpublished manuscript on *An.* III 4–5.

[1] *An.* III 4, 429a10–13.

Aristotle on the Essence of Human Thought. Klaus Corcilius, Andrea Falcon, and Robert Roreitner, Oxford University Press.
 DOI: 10.1093/9780198921820.003.0002

extension. For, on either option, the corresponding capacity will turn out to be separate in account and hence be a part of the soul. This is because, as we have seen in the previous chapter, Aristotle conceives of each part of the soul as separate in account from the others and vice versa. As separation in extension, which I understand as spatial independence, implies separability in account—for Aristotle, the being of things has to be *in* the things whose being it is[2]—on either option the thinking soul will be separate in account and hence be a part of the soul. Seeking for a definition of that part of the soul and principle of the phenomena of human thinking, as we have seen, is to engage in an investigation that is *two methodological steps removed* from the scientific explanation of episodes of human thinking. With these goals and methods, Aristotle's investigation in *An.* III 4–5 does not offer what we today call a theory of the human mind; rather, it is a study devoted to finding the principles of a general science of living things, and in particular of that part of it which provides the ultimate ground for the phenomena of the mental *qua* intellectual.

From his to-do list, and the method of defining the fundamental capacities (i.e., parts) of the soul recommended in *An.* II 4, Aristotle's mode of procedure is clear.[3] First, we should expect him to determine the *object* of human thinking. Then, we should expect him to go on with a characterization of the corresponding *activity*, and to finish up his investigation with a definition of the *capacity* of human thinking, as he has already done in the case of the nutritive and perceptual parts of the soul. And, very roughly, this is also how Aristotle will proceed in the case of the thinking part of the soul, albeit with some important modifications. One modification is the emphasis on the difficulty of finding the "distinguishing mark" of thinking. Apparently, Aristotle does not seem to know even where to start with the identification of thinking. Another modification, for which there seems to be no parallel in the previous discussion of the nutritive and perceptive parts of the soul, is the focus on the question of how thinking "may ever come about."

A natural way of explaining the need for these modifications of the general program outlined in *An.* II 4 is to recall the result reached in *An.* III 3, where Aristotle has taken care to distinguish human thinking from bodily affection and mental representation.[4] For if thinking is neither bodily affection nor mental representation, it seems a perfectly natural question to ask what *else* thinking could be. After all, these are powerful intuitions about the nature of thinking that many philosophers had at the time, as Aristotle tells us in *An.* III 3, and many still have today. It is, then, an unavoidable side-effect of Aristotle's isolation of thinking proper from bodily

[2] See *Metaph.* I 9, 991a12–14, and XIII 5, 1079b15–18. That the non-rational functions of the soul are spatially inseparable from each other is one of the upshots of Aristotle's experiments with divided insects. On divided insects, see Lefebvre 2002.

[3] For more on the to-do list and the methodology it implies see Chapter 1 (Section 5).

[4] Under "mental representation" I understand the *act* of having of a *phantasma* in the soul as a representation (i.e., a "picture" or *eikôn*) of something else. See *Mem.* 1, 450b20–451a19. For more, see Chapter 1 (Section 7).

affection and mental representation in *An.* III 3 that at this point—namely, at the beginning of *An.* III 4—it should be utterly unclear to anyone not already familiar with Aristotle's conception of thinking what thinking is supposed to be in the first place. And if that is the case, and we do not even know the "distinguishing mark" of thinking with relation to the other parts of the soul, then *a fortiori* we are not in a position to know how thinking "may ever come about." This, I suggest, prompts Aristotle to ask these additional questions at the outset of his investigation.

The difficulty is seriously aggravated by the fact that in *An.* III 4–5 Aristotle is speaking not about just any kind of thinking, and not even about just any kind of theoretical thinking, but about a highly specific kind of theoretical thinking: namely, the thinking of essences (about which more shortly). And this kind of thinking, apart from the bodily and representational preconditions that it has, also has linguistic, educational, and further necessary conditions in terms of scientific research skills that the account of the thinking capacity in *An.* III 4–5 presupposes without discussion. We know this because in *An.* III 4, 429b5–10, Aristotle says what he takes the capacity for thinking essences to be like. He says that it is like the person who already is a knower (*epistêmôn*)—that is, a fully educated and able epistemic agent who possesses all the relevant scientific research skills and concepts—and who is able to engage in the thinking of essences, albeit without doing so currently:

> When it [i.e., the capacity for thinking] becomes each [object of knowledge] in such a way as the actual knower is said to be—this is the case when he is capable of being active by his own effort; and then it is still in potentiality in a way, not however in the same way as it was before learning or discovering; and then it is also capable of thinking itself. (*An.* III 4, 429b5–10)

The capacity for thinking Aristotle is concerned with in *An.* III 4 corresponds to the capacity for thinking as it is possessed by a *skilled researcher.* This is a person who has learned and has successfully engaged in research ("discovering") and only needs to activate and employ their knowledge (cf. *An.* II 5, 417a27–28). In other words, Aristotle' s account of thinking in *An.* III 4, even if supposedly fundamental for thinking more broadly speaking, is concerned with a highly specific kind of thinking, which presupposes a great deal of preparatory skills and knowledge. And that kind of thinking is unlikely to be familiar to most of his readers.[5]

Furthermore, there are also the volitional enabling conditions of thinking that the account of thinking in *An.* III 4 presupposes without discussion. Aristotle

[5] To be as clear as possible: in *An.* III 4–5 Aristotle is not concerned with "concept acquisition," because he seems to presuppose the possession of the relevant concepts on the side of the epistemic agent; nor is he concerned with "concept use," because he is not interested in concepts at all in *An.* III 4–5. Rather, Aristotle is interested in the thinking of essences, and essences are not "concepts" because the application of concepts can be adequate or not while the thinking of essences is supposed by Aristotle to be always true. On concepts in Greek philosophy see now: Betegh and Tsouna 2024.

mentions them briefly in *An.* II 5, where he says that we human thinkers are autonomous agents insofar as we are able to initiate episodes of thinking *when we so wish* (*boulêtheis*).[6] Our wishing to think is no doubt a necessary precondition of our thinking for Aristotle;[7] at the same time, it, no less than our bodily and representational apparatus, is something that pertains to us insofar as we are cognitive souls: embodied agents, that is, who act in the natural world. To be sure, saying "because I wished to" *is* an acceptable answer to the question why one is thinking. And Aristotle does at least mention the volitional conditions of thinking in his search for the principle of thinking (*An.* III 4, 429b7–8); however, it is important that for him these conditions, though necessary, are, strictly speaking, external to the act of thinking proper. Our wishing to think is something that precedes thinking and that can be separated from the proper act of thinking. This is why Aristotle does not discuss these necessary conditions in his account of the human capacity for thinking in the *De anima*.

Aristotle, then, at the beginning of *An.* III 4, faces the task of having to define a capacity of the soul whose primary manifestations, unlike those of nutrition, perception, and mental representation, are probably not immediately clear or familiar to most of his readers. Unlike the capacity for perception, of which we all know in one way or another that it comes about by way of an affection,[8] thinking, at this point in the argument, lacks even the most basic and preliminary description. As a result, since it supposedly is neither bodily affection nor mental representation, Aristotle must describe the very phenomenon of human thinking in a new and revisionary way. This is why he, in the first part of the chapter, engages in a piece of hypothetical reasoning to compensate for our lack of familiarity with the phenomenon of human thinking. His strategy consists in generating a preliminary and hypothetical account of our thinking capacity on the basis of an adaption of the account of perception advanced in *An.* II 5–12 to the special circumstances of thinking.[9] In that adaption Aristotle makes two basic assumptions about thinking which he takes for granted and which will shape his entire account—these are that thinking is some kind of reception of its cognitive object, and that thinking can think everything (including itself). The result will be an account of the thinking capacity as an entirely immaterial receptivity for the objects of thinking. I will refer to this adaption as the *transformative modification of the account of perception*. Aristotle then, after having presented his preliminary and hypothetical account of

[6] *An.* II 5, 418a27–28.

[7] With some exceptions. Corcilius 2009: 14 discusses scenarios in which a rational desire (wish) to engage in an episode of thinking is not a necessary condition for thinking to occur in Aristotle's theory. In what follows I shall speak, for the sake of simplicity, in a summary fashion of "necessary volitional conditions of thinking." It is important to note in this context that habitual thinking routines also have their origin in volitional thinking.

[8] *An.* II 5, 416b32–417a2.

[9] One may also describe it as a thought experiment.

the human capacity for thinking, seeks to confirm it by way of independent empirical observations.

It turns out that this new account conceives of thinking in a very narrow sense: namely, only as the *thinking of essences*. But for Aristotle, this form of thinking grounds the possibility of all the other, more familiar, kinds of thinking.[10] Essences, however, are not objects that most of us would be familiar with. Thus Aristotle, in a second step, introduces *the objects* of thinking in the narrow sense—the different kinds of essences—and discusses, briefly, how we cognize them. Finally, he returns to his account of the thinking capacity as the immaterial receptivity of the objects of thinking and confronts it with two difficulties (*aporiai*). These difficulties cast serious doubt on the consistency of the account Aristotle has just offered. They motivate the discussion in the rest of the chapter, which is devoted to finding a solution to these difficulties. As we will see, the solution Aristotle offers in the rest of *An.* III 4 does not fully answer the difficulties. Indeed, his discussion even raises an additional, and no less pressing, question. This question is treated in *An.* III 5.

In my view, therefore, *An.* III 4 and *An.* III 5 form a single argumentative unity. The text can be broken down into five sections.

(1) A preliminary account of the thinking capacity: the analogy between thinking and perception; the limits and the consequences of the analogy (*An.* III 4, 429a13–b9).
(2) The objects of thinking and the capacities with which we cognize them (*An.* III 4, 429b10–22).
(3) Two difficulties (*An.* III 4, 429b22–29).
(4) Solutions: the writing tablet and the cognitive transparency of thinking (*An.* III 4, 429b29–430a9).
(5) Two kinds of thinking, and the intrinsic nature of the active cause of thinking (*An.* III 5, 430a10–25).

In these five sections Aristotle offers a highly revisionary and bold account of human thinking. The account is based on his realism regarding the existence of immaterial essences of things,[11] and on the idea that thinking has an unrestricted scope: namely, that it can think everything, including itself. From an Aristotelian point of view, we may describe this account as a *non-natural* account of thinking, since it hinges on a conception of thinking devoid of all core features of nature: namely, matter, material affection, change, and motion. From a modern point of view, and despite the causal language Aristotle uses in formulating it, we may describe it as a *non-causal* account of thinking. However, having said this, it is worth

[10] More on this in Chapter 3.
[11] For more on immaterial essences, see Section 3 below.

recalling that this account pertains only to thinking *qua* thinking and not to the (numerous and various) physical enabling conditions of human thinking, which are antecedent to, and concomitant with, every act of human thinking.[12]

According to Aristotle's account, as we will see, the capacity of human thinking is essentially (and asymmetrically)[13] correlated to the *essences of things* as its *per se* objects, which are immaterial. The activity of thinking consists in the immediate and *sui generis* presence (or taking in) of these essences in cognitive agents, which come to be present in them in a most immediate and direct way. The thinking capacity is the bare receptivity of such *immaterial essences*, which capacity, due to its otherwise featureless immateriality, can *become* these essences. It is unrestricted in scope. It will also turn out that all acts of human thinking rest on a principle of activation, consisting in an essentially actual act of transcendent thinking. This act of transcendent thinking, as I will argue, can account for some of the prominent features of human thinking, such as objectivity, universality, and necessity. It will also turn out that thinking, understood in the narrow sense as the thinking of essences of hylomorphic compounds, is not devoid of structure, which can likewise be fully transparent to thinking agents. I will discuss the above five sections in turn.

2. A preliminary account of the thinking capacity (Section I: *An.* III 4, 429a13–b9)

The hypothetical analogy with perception and the resulting account of the thinking capacity

Aristotle's distinction between *phantasia* and thought in *An.* III 3 to some extent deprives the phenomenon of thinking of its familiar features. Aristotle must somehow compensate for this, or so I have argued. Having established this, though, I should add that there are two basic assumptions about thinking that Aristotle never doubts, however controversial they may be. They do very important work in his account of the thinking capacity. This is the assumption that thinking is some kind of reception of its cognitive object, and the assumption that thinking is unrestricted in scope: it can think everything, including itself.

Aristotle at no point argues for this latter assumption, which from a modern perspective is, to say the least, optimistic.[14] He simply takes this feature of thinking for granted, notwithstanding his occasional honorary references to Anaxagoras. But what he has in mind is perhaps less optimistic than what one might think at first. His view is that thinking has an unrestricted scope in terms of the objects of *thinking*. In other words, Aristotle is not saying that thinking can think, for

[12] See above and Chapter 1 (Section 2).
[13] In a way to be discussed later in this chapter, Section 6.
[14] For Aristotle's perceptual optimism, see Gregoric 2019.

instance, the objects of perception in the same way in which perception perceives them but only that the human capacity for thinking can think all *thinkable aspects* of perception and its objects,[15] just as it can think the thinkable aspects of everything else as well, albeit one at a time (and not all of them at once).[16] But of course, the thinkable aspects of things are their most important aspects, as we will see below in more detail. The unrestricted scope of the capacity for thinking qualified in this way will be a (if not *the*) central structuring principle of Aristotle's discussion of human thinking in *An.* III 4. It is no overstatement to say that his account of the thinking capacity in a way *results* from this assumption combined with what we already learned about cognition generally in the previous chapters in *De anima* on perception. This becomes clear in this first section of *An.* III 4, where Aristotle develops his preliminary and hypothetical account of the human capacity of thinking. The argument there goes as follows:

(i) [All cognition consists in the reception of the relevant objects by a capacity that somehow is these objects in potentiality.]
(ii) *If thinking is like perceiving,*[17] it will consist in an affection (or in something like an affection) by the object of thinking.
(iii) It will follow that the thinking capacity, prior to the act of thinking, will be, just like the capacity for perception is in relation to its object, *unaffected by its object so as to be receptive of it.*[18] [(i), (ii)]
(iv) The thinking capacity has an unrestricted scope: *it can think all beings.*[19]
(v) Any physical (material) implementation of a cognitive capacity, as in the case of perception, must lead to "blind spots" that restrict the scope of the reception of its object.
(vi) The existence of "blind sports" for thinking as in (v) is incompatible with the unrestricted scope of thinking expressed in (iv).
(vii) It follows that the thinking capacity has no physical implementation but only the immaterial feature of being capable of receiving its objects. [(iii), (iv), (v), (vi)]
(viii) [Beings are either physical (i.e., material), or they are immaterial.]
(ix) It follows that the thinking capacity, *before it thinks, will be none of the beings at all in actuality.*[20] [(vii), (viii)]

This argument hypothetically establishes—see the "if" in (ii) which sets the modality for the entire argument—the immateriality and complete featurelessness of

[15] See Politis 2001.
[16] See Chapter 5.
[17] *An.* III 4, 429a 13–14.
[18] *An.* III 4, 429a15–16.
[19] *An.* III 4, 429a18.
[20] *An.* III 4, 429a21–22.

the thinking capacity except for the bare receptivity of the objects of thinking, by way of the combination of three factors. They are:

(1) *a general theory of cognition* as the reception of cognitive objects by something that has the capacity to receive them in (i);
(2) *the claim of the unrestricted scope of the thinking capacity* stated in (iv); and
(3) *the (transformative) modification of the account of perception*, which strips it of all the features that are in conflict with the unrestricted scope of thinking stated in (2), while at the same time retaining its receptive nature as introduced in (1).

In effect, the hypothetical argument advanced in the first section offers an account of the thinking capacity by way of a modification of the account of perception offered in *An.* II 7–12. The result is an account of the thinking capacity as the bare and otherwise featureless capacity to receive the objects of thinking in (vii) and (ix). Let us look at the three factors and their impact on the argument in turn.

The general theory of cognition—(1)—is the common ground of Aristotle's approach to all forms of cognition. It consists in a minimal account according to which cognition is the reception and resulting internal presence of a cognitive object in a cognitive agent. Most probably, the account is incomplete. The mere internal presence of an object would not suffice to distinguish cognition from other kinds of internal presence as, for instance, in the case of nutritive ingestion. But we can safely assume that Aristotle takes his account of perception in *An.* II 12, which entails a clear distinction between perceptual and nutritive reception, still to be fresh in the reader's mind. This is clear from his reference to his own account of perception early on in our chapter in *An.* III 4, 429a13–18. Aristotle does not spell out (i) explicitly as a premise of his argument, but it is clear that he assumes it (or at least something equivalent to it), since otherwise the analogy between perception and thinking would not allow him to draw the consequences stated in steps (iii), (vii), and (ix).[21] Alternatively, we can take the general theory of cognition not so much as common ground for all kinds of cognition but rather as the bare bones of Aristotle's account of perception which we are left with in our analogy once the account is stripped of all of its physical features. In that case we should perhaps not speak of an analogy between perception and thinking but of a more radical dependence of Aristotle's account of thinking on his previous account of perception. Both ways of describing what is going on in this first section seem permissible.

The unrestricted scope of thinking—(2)—is an axiom of Aristotle's discussion of the thinking capacity. Aristotle invokes Anaxagoras' *nous*, but not to derive any justification for the claim advanced in (iv). Rather, the axiom is a crucial premise

[21] Step (viii) is not explicitly stated by Aristotle. Most likely, he takes it to be trivial. Still, without it, step (ix) could not be derived.

of the argument serving as the main criterion for the (transformative) modification of the account of the perceptual capacity in *An.* II 5–12 in (3). The claim that thinking is unrestricted in scope has vast and partly (for me at least) unforeseeable philosophical consequences. It implies not only that there is nothing that could not be made an object for thinking so as to be intellectually grasped, but also that thinking is, or at least can be, entirely transparent to itself. This feature of thinking in the narrow sense seems to form the basis for the possibility of scientific knowledge and of the awareness of principles as *sui generis* states of objective truth, which are set apart from opinion or other, more subjective, cognitive states. And given that Aristotle's methodology consists in defining the most fundamental capacities of the soul so as to ground the less fundamental capacities, actions, and affections "common to body and soul" in them, we have good reason to think that our capacity to think everything including itself should also provide the ground for the objectivity of human thinking more generally. Examples of what I have in mind include our ability to make statements of fact ("it is the case that . . ."), which imply an attitude toward the world that determines how the latter is independently from us, our needs, desires, and so on. Our ability to grasp the essences of things, which is thinking in the narrow sense, then, provides the ultimate ground for our intellectual capacity to assess things as they are in themselves. And it is reasonable to suppose that it should also provide, even though Aristotle does not say so explicitly here, the ultimate ground for our other intellectual features, including for example our moral capacity to put ourselves in someone else's place. Aristotle, by his own methodology, is committed to the claim that the unrestricted scope of thinking, and its capacity to think everything including itself, is fundamental for *all* our intellectual states.

The transformative modification of the account of perception—(3)—does away with the causal affection model of perception by stripping it of all of its material features.[22] If the thinking capacity is to be capable of thinking all beings, it cannot have any material features as these features would prevent it from being receptive of all beings, which, of course, includes being receptive of itself as an object of cognition.[23] To see why this is so, recall the basic account of perception as the

[22] Not everyone agrees with this. Busche (in Busche 2001: 67 ff., and Busche and Perkams (in Busche and Perkams 2018: 132–139, 817–831, 856–863, following Kampe 1870: 14–49)), argues that there is a material substrate of human *nous* after all: namely, something like a "materialized point" of ether (cf. Kampe 1870: 45). However, the arguments of these authors, many of which have been attacked already by Zeller (Zeller 1921: 569n3), are far from cogent. More importantly, on their interpretation, it becomes very hard to make sense of Aristotle's argument in *An.* III 4–5. I especially fail to see how being a body external to the sublunary world could be of help in accounting for the cognition of the non-material features of things (their modes of composition and intelligible forms; cf. *An.* I 5, 409b23–29), for its capacity to think itself, and for the objectivity of thinking (unless all of these features are somehow identical with ether, which would however make Aristotle look like a Stoic).

[23] Provided one does not allow for an interpretation of Aristotle's claims concerning the perception "that one sees or hears," outlined in *An.* III 2, 425b12–15, as immediate and without affection, as argued in Caston 2002. See also footnote 63.

reception of perceptual qualities without their matter in *An.* II 12. To be receptive of a quality such as hotness, for instance, requires the physical implementation of the cognitive apparatus of the cognitive agent. More specifically, it requires the cognitive agent to be equipped with the relevant perceptual mean. In this case the perceptual mean is a neutral position on the relevant qualitative scale between hot and cold, whereby the neutral position is both located on that scale and neither hot nor cold. This physical implementation of the sense of touch makes it receptive of qualities such as hotness and coldness. The receptivity for these qualities is, so to speak, a qualitative potentiality, or a qualitative "blank," constituted by the range of potential perceptual qualities between the extremes on the relevant scale. But the same physical implementation that makes it receptive of perceptual objects in the first place also produces its cognitive limitations (also known as "blind spots"). In fact, there are two kinds of hot and cold things that the sense of touch cannot perceive. They are (1) all those values of hot and cold that exceed the limits of the relevant qualitative scale, and (2) those values of hot and cold that match the value of the perceptual mean. This is an immediate consequence of what above I have called the *qualified difference thesis*.[24] Perception is always of *differences* between the perceptual mean and other values within the relevant qualitative scale. Perceptual stimuli that exceed the limits of the receptivity of the perceptual capacity, therefore, will either fail to be perceived (because they fail to meet the minimal threshold of perceptibility), or destroy the corresponding organ, while those values that coincide with the value of the perceptual mean will fail to generate the required difference (contrast), and thus also fail to result in perception. Only the values that fall within the relevant scale and that do not coincide with the perceptual mean will generate such differences. So, in effect, what the transformative modification of the account of perception in (3) does is to purge Aristotle's account of the perceptual capacity of the cognitive limitations that result from the fact that perception is essentially a physically implemented kind of cognition. This leaves us with the bare general theory of cognition stated in (i) plus the explicit denial of the physical character of the corresponding capacity stated in (vii) and, indeed, of any other positive nature as stated in (ix). What is said in (ix) is the converse of the claim made in (2): if thinking has an unrestricted scope—if it can think everything—and the corresponding capacity is the mere capacity for receiving the objects of thinking, then that capacity cannot have any positive features in actuality, as that would create a "blind spot," which would bar it from receiving what it already is.

This, then, is the basic line of the hypothetical argument: Aristotle purges his account of perception of all its physical features, reducing it to the bare and otherwise featureless immaterial receptivity of the objects of thinking.

[24] See Chapter 1 (Section 6).

2.1 Making the hypothetical statement factual

The rest of the first section offers confirmation, as well as some elucidation, of the main hypothetical conclusion that the human capacity for thinking is the *bare capacity for taking in essences* as per steps (vii) and (ix). Aristotle uses this confirmation to turn his hypothetical conclusion into a statement of fact.[25]

This starts with the argument advanced in *An.* III 4, 429a24–27. Aristotle seeks to establish the truth of the claim stated in (vii) by way of an indirect argument. For the sake of the argument, Aristotle assumes the (for him, counterfactual) thesis that the intellectual capacity is physically implemented ("mixed with the body"). On these grounds he generates the thesis that the capacity for thinking has a determinate physical quality (*poios*) or an organ, which for him is manifestly false. Since, as he claims, none of this is actually the case, it makes no good sense (*ouk eulogon*) for the thinking capacity to be physically implemented in the way perception is. What this means is that thinking has no dedicated organ or substrate; it is not the *energeia* of any kind of body (*An.* II 1, 413a5–6).[26]

A second point is advanced in *An.* III 4, 429a27–29. I take it to be an elucidation of the claim that the capacity for thinking is immediately receptive of the essences of things. Aristotle says that those (presumably, Plato and his followers) who said that the soul is the "place of [essential] forms" got it right, but only with two very important qualifications. First, the soul as a whole is not the place of essential forms, but only that part of the soul that is capable of thinking; second, the capacity for thinking is not the place of actual essential forms, "but it is only potentially the [essential] forms." This formulation is interesting because it confirms an immediate realist picture of the thinking capacity according to which the essences literally come to be present in those who think them: intelligible essences and the thinking of essences are the same ("identity claim" in what follows).[27] As we will see, in what follows Aristotle will qualify this identity claim significantly.

[25] Aristotle offers a general ontological argument for the reality of potentialities for actualities that are not currently existing in *Metaph.* IX 3, 1047a17–24. According to that argument, it should follow that what is none of the beings in actuality but is the potentiality of them—as in (ix)—*is* a reality.

[26] Aristotle does think that our thinking takes place in our bodies. More precisely, he thinks that thinking takes place in our heart, which is the organ of our perceptual capacity (e.g., *An.* I 4, 408b15–29; *Sens.* 1, 436b6–437a17; *Mot. an.* 7, 701a34–703a3). But that does not make the heart an *organ* of thinking. For that to be the case, thinking would have to be *essentially* embodied, which is a thesis Aristotle rejects in *An.* III 4 and elsewhere (e.g., *An.* I 4, 408b18–30; *An.* II 2, 413b24–27; *Gener. an.* II 3, 736b28–29). Thinking, thus, is existentially dependent on the human body (only a human being can engage in human thinking and humans do necessarily have a certain kind of body), but thinking does not depend on the human body for its essence and definition; in other words, thinking is not essentially physically implemented. This is also what Thomas Johansen (in Johansen 2012: 235) and David Charles (in Charles 2021: 220–223) say about human theoretical thinking.

[27] This claim is made explicitly with relation to knowledge and its objects in *An.* III 5, 430a19–21 and *An.* III 7, 431a1–3. See also *Metaph.* XII 8, 1074b38–1075a5.

A third point is offered in *An.* III 4, 429a29–b5. Aristotle appeals to certain facts of experience about our thinking something or other. His immediate goal is to offer additional confirmation for the thesis that the thinking capacity is not physically implemented and thus transcends physical reality. He compares the unaffectedness (*apatheia*) of the perceptual capacity with the unaffectedness of the thinking capacity, arguing that in cases of exposure to intensive perceptual objects the affection of the physical implementation of the former capacity can lead to a temporary incapacitation of our receptivity to further perceptual input, to then infer from the absence of such incapacitations in the case of the thinking of intensive intelligible objects that the thinking capacity is not physically implemented. Whenever we have very intense perceptual experiences—for instance, when having been exposed to extremely loud sounds or to extremely bright colors—then this leads to the temporary incapacitation of our corresponding senses to register minor perceptual differences in these same modalities. This observation is meant to show that the unaffectedness of our perceptual capacity—that is, the qualitative "blank" along a range of qualities around our perceptual mean within a given scale, the unaffectedness of which constitutes our receptivity to those perceptual qualities in the first place—is essentially physically implemented. It is also meant to show that its physical implementation is the reason why our capacity to perceive can be disturbed or even destroyed by the very same kind of object it is supposed to be receptive of. This physical implementation is, of course, our perceptual apparatus. Perception is essentially a physically implemented kind of cognition, which entails that the capacity for perception is inseparable from the body and hence (as all things physical) susceptible to destruction. This, argues Aristotle, is not the case with our thinking capacity, given that we can observe that after having had very intense thoughts, we are even better at thinking less intense objects of thinking. This is supposed to be a datum of experience, from which Aristotle wishes to generate support for his claim that the thinking capacity is separate (*chôriston*) from the body.

The final remark advanced in *An.* III 4, 429b5–10, offers a more positive description of the capacity for thinking, albeit from a different angle. And the fact that Aristotle here uses his distinction between different kinds of potentiality and actuality seems to indicate that he is no longer hypothesizing but speaking in a factual mode. This is confirmed by the fact that he provides us with additional information about thinking going beyond what he has said in his initial hypothetical argument. Aristotle here invokes his doctrine of first and second potentiality and actuality—the so-called *Dreistufenlehre*.[28] As we have seen, the knower who possesses a body of knowledge in the way envisioned by Aristotle is an actual knower insofar as she has realized her innate, basic, and generic capacity to know

[28] See the Glossary (*s.v.* ACTUALITY) for additional information about this doctrine.

through continuous intellectual training, learning, and even successful research (whatever this requires).[29] Having knowledge in this way is having acquired the capacity to immediately exercise knowledge at will.[30] Such a skilled knower is a knower in the sense of the first actuality (i.e., second potentiality) of knowing. At the same time, this knower is not currently exercising knowledge, which is to say that this person is a potential knower. The actual exercise of the second potentiality of knowing (i.e., first actuality) is the second actuality of knowledge, which is the actual contemplation of a particular item of knowledge. But here Aristotle seems not so much interested in the second actuality of knowledge. His comparison with the knower is specifically with the knower in the state of first actuality (i.e., second potentiality), because this allows him to make clear that on his account the thinking capacity as described above is not equivalent to the general human capacity to think we are born with and which everyone possesses simply by virtue of being a member of the human species (i.e., first potentiality). Rather, this capacity is what we possess as the result of having learned and researched everything necessary so as to be *immediately capable* of contemplating essences. Aristotle adds that the thinking capacity is capable of thinking itself only once it is in that state of first actuality, and not before that. This statement, I take it, implies that the thinking capacity, when actual in the sense of second actuality, even though immaterial and none of the beings at all, has some kind of *structure* which can be known.

In sum, this series of remarks shows that Aristotle accepts his hypothetical account of the thinking capacity as the immaterial bare receptivity of the objects of thinking also as non-hypothetically true. The thinking capacity of the soul has no physical implementation—that is, no dedicated organ—and is in this sense separate from the body. Again: this is not to say that there are not all sorts of bodily conditions for thinking to take place. But these bodily conditions will be accidental to thinking *qua* such. The capacity for thinking in the relevant sense of second potentiality is an acquired state of bare receptivity to the essences of all things. When fully actual, it exhibits some kind of structure so that it can itself be made an object of thought.

[29] In this sense of potentiality—the sense in which, for instance, a boy has the potentiality to be a general—human *nous* is no doubt an innate capacity possessed by every human being. Jiménez (in Jiménez 2017: 31 and elsewhere) vehemently denies that. He also argues that in the whole of section I (*An.* III 4, 429a13–b9) Aristotle is not speaking *in propria persona* (Jiménez 2017: 20 ff.), and that the argument there is "dialectical," whereas *An.* III 5 is "demonstrative" (32). There is no basis whatsoever for this in the text. Jiménez's main argument for this is that Aristotle rejects the initial claim of the passage according to which thinking is like perceiving (Jiménez 2017: 22). This is true enough; Aristotle does not believe that thinking works in the same way as perception does (as is clear from *An.* I and III 3). But why should that prevent him from making the hypothetical claim that thinking is like perceiving, as he does in *An.* III 4, especially if that claim helps him generate an account of the thinking capacity?

[30] This is a claim about the volitional enabling conditions of thinking on the level of personal agents. Aristotle is not saying here that the *capacity* for thinking can initiate its own actualization (as claimed by Michael Wedin in Wedin 1988, 1993, and 1994).

3. The objects of thought and the capacities with which we cognize them (Section II: *An.* III 4, 429b10–22)

Thinking has an unrestricted scope for Aristotle. It can think anything, including itself. Still, Aristotle does not claim that all beings are the *per se* objects of thinking but that *essences* alone are. Essences are the being or, more precisely, the "what-it-is-to-be" (*to ti ên einai*) of things. As will become apparent later on in *De anima*, it is in virtue of our capacity to think essences that we have the capacity to think other things as well.[31] How the scope of thinking broadens out from the thinking of essences to propositional thinking is discussed in *An.* III 6.[32] For the time being, Aristotle introduces essences as the *per se* objects of thinking, distinguishing three basic types of them: essences of things without matter, and two kinds of matter-involving essences. He also discusses how we, as cognitive agents who are equipped with a plurality of cognitive capacities, can cognize them by clarifying which cognitive capacities we use to think each of the different types of essences. This discussion is necessary because, as it will turn out, thinking the essences of things that are inseparable from their matter cannot be done by thinking alone. Such things are in fact more than just their essences. More specifically, they are their essences plus their matter, which is why thinking by itself, which is the capacity of taking in essences, will not be able to fully grasp them, and why the thinking of them must be a joint cognitive effort of thinking and perception, which is the cognitive capacity responsible for the cognition of materially extended things. The section ends with the important statement that there are *corresponding degrees of separation* in the objects of thinking on the one hand and in the corresponding cognitive capacity on the other: essences not separate from matter (i.e., essences that essentially involve matter because they are the essences of things that have matter) can only be grasped by a kind of thinking that is not separate from perception, while essences separate from matter can only be grasped by a kind of thinking that is separate from perception. The separation of essences from matter strictly corresponds to the separation of the correlated capacity for thinking from the perceptual capacity.

Some basic features of Aristotelian essences should be noted at this point. This will help us appreciate just how specific and far removed from an everyday understanding Aristotle's conception of the *per se* objects of thinking is. First, Aristotelian essences are *simple* entities.[33] Linguistically, they correspond to terms ("names"), not to propositions. However, they can be defined by way of propositions.

[31] This is to say that Aristotle claims that we can think other things in virtue of our *capacity* to think the *per se* objects of thinking: namely, the essences. He does not claim that we could not think other things without having had thoughts of essences. On the contrary, he thinks that most of us are very unlikely to ever engage in the proper thinking of the essences of things, as that would require that most of us were philosophers or scientists.

[32] See Chapter 3.

[33] More on this in Chapter 3.

Definitions are the linguistic expressions of essences. As such, they are not isomorphic in structure with the essences they express.[34] Propositions are always complex for Aristotle. They consist of combinations (*suntheseis*) of a subject with a predicate term, while the essential beings they express do not exhibit such a complex structure.[35] And since the truth and falsehood of propositions for Aristotle lies in the correct or incorrect *combination* of terms, the thinking of an essence *cannot* be false: either one thinks it and then the thought will *eo ipso* be true or one doesn't think an essence at all.[36] The objects of thinking we are dealing with in *An.* III 4 are the *per se* objects of thinking: simple and non-extended beings (essences), the thinking of which is necessarily true. Of these *per se* objects, Aristotle distinguishes three different types.

3.1 Three types of essences

The types of essences Aristotle distinguishes differ in accordance with just one criterion. This is the degree to which they involve, or are separate from, matter.[37] To forestall a possible misunderstanding, it is important to be aware that for Aristotle *all* essences are immaterial. So, the types of essences cannot differ from each other in virtue of the fact that some of them are immaterial while others are not. The types of essences Aristotle distinguishes in this stretch of text are different from one another insofar as they are the (immaterial) essences either *of* material or *of* immaterial things; moreover, if they are the essences of material things, they can still differ according to the particular way in which the things they are the essences of are materially extended.[38] The types of essences Aristotle distinguishes according to that criterion are three in number.

(1) *Essences without matter*: these are the essences that are in no way distinct from the things whose essences they are. They are separate substances, in the sense of "substances separate from matter." As such, strictly speaking, they have nothing attached to them *of* which they are the essential being; rather, they are fully identical with their essential being (*An.* III 4, 429b11–12).

[34] See the discussion in *Metaph.* VII 10–12 (especially, *Metaph.* VII 12).

[35] See the Glossary (*s.v.* SUNTHESIS).

[36] For a full discussion of these claims, I refer the reader to Chapter 3.

[37] Aristotle's conclusion toward the end of the section makes it very clear that he thinks that separation from matter comes in degrees.

[38] The kind of separation, or separability from matter, Aristotle has in mind here is *unqualified separation* or separability, according to which *X* is separate, or separable, from *Y* whenever *X* can exist without *Y* (Corcilius and Gregoric 2010: 114; see also Cohoe 2022: 239). Miller, in his article on the separability of the intellect, calls it "ontological separability" (Miller 2012: 309). Separability without qualification, or ontological separability, is an asymmetrical relation. *X* can be separate in existence from *Y* without this implying that *Y* is separate in existence from *X*.

(2) *Essences of natural, material objects*: these are the essences of natural hylomorphic compounds, which are compounds of essential forms and matter. Such essences are inseparable from their matter. The being of a cat, for instance, is not separable from a certain kind of living body (i.e., the body of a cat), and wherever there occurs the essential form of a cat there will also be a corresponding body as its matter (having potentially the feline soul as its essential form). In this respect, natural hylomorphic compounds are like the snub, which is "concavity in nose-matter"[39] and thus a "this-in-that" (*tode en toide*), which is Aristotle's standard locution for an essential form that occurs always and only in a given kind of matter.[40]

(3) *Essences of abstract mathematical objects*: of these Aristotle also says that they are like the snub, and thus in some way hylomorphic compounds, even if not in the same way as natural objects are. His example is "the straight" (*to euthu*); the straight is supposed to be different from its essence in that straight lines involve continuous extension (see *Phys.* VI 1, 231a25), while its essence is without extension. Aristotle says: "let it be duality (*duas*)."[41]

By way of which capacities are we able to cognize the different types of essences?

Aristotle says, without any ambiguity, which cognitive capacities we use to grasp essences of types (2) and (3). By contrast, he does not tell us how we grasp essences of type (1). But this is presumably because he takes it for granted that they are grasped by thinking alone.[42] His example for natural material objects—that is, natural hylomorphic compounds—is flesh. Flesh and the essence of flesh are not the same thing (*An.* III 4, 429b10–11), and each of them is grasped by a different cognitive capacity. We cognize flesh with our perceptual capacity. For Aristotle, flesh is a certain proportion of warm and cold and the like, which are perceptual qualities which we discriminate with our perceptual capacity. The essence of flesh ("the being of flesh"), by contrast, we cognize not with perception but with some other capacity.

Instead of simply saying that we cognize such matter-involving essences by way of our thinking capacity, Aristotle makes an intriguing and perhaps only tentative statement about how perception and thinking may relate to each other so as to be capable of jointly cognizing essences of type (2). The way he conceptualizes the

[39] *Metaph.* VII 5, 1030b31–32; for the claim that physical objects generally are like the snub in the respect of being a "this in a that," see *Phys.* II 2, 194a12–15. Cf. *An.* I 1, 403b1–9.

[40] Form and matter are inseparable from each other, and the only way they can be regarded as separable is in the metaphysical account of the philosopher (*Phys.* II 2, 194b12; *Metaph.* VIII 1, 1042a28–29). It should be noted, however, that even this is controversial (see Charles 2021, who argues that the forms of natural objects contain a specific reference to perceptual matter as their parts, 46).

[41] *An.* III 4, 429b20. This is not his own doctrine, but it is taken over and assumed for the sake of argument from certain holders of a theory of forms (cf. *Metaph.* VII 11, 1036b12–16).

[42] He may even think that separate objects of type (1) cannot be grasped by any capacity at all. More on this below.

relation between the two cognitive capacities in their joint effort is in terms of their *separability from each other*:

> one discriminates what it is to be flesh with something other, which is either separate [from perception] or with something [which is not separate from perception and] that stands in the same relation [to perception] as a bent line stands to itself when it has been straightened out.[43]

With this statement Aristotle spells out his earlier remark at 429b13, where we are told that we "discriminate the being of flesh and flesh either by way of something else or *by way of something that is in another state* (*ê allôi ê allôs echonti*) [presumably that same perceptual capacity when it is in another state]." The expression is repeated almost *verbatim* with relation to the capacity responsible for the thinking of abstract mathematical objects further down the text in 429b20–21.[44] These are puzzling remarks. Aristotle here speaks of the cognition of the essences of natural material objects as in some way the result of a joint effort of perception and thinking. The main issue is whether with this additional clause he somehow wishes to revise his claims regarding the definitional separability of the different parts of the soul. How can perception and thinking be separate parts of the soul while relating to each other in the same way that one and the same line relates to itself when it is first bent and then straightened out? Aristotle's either/or formulation leaves open the question whether the two capacities involved in the cognition of such matter-involving essences are separable from each other or not. At the same time, the hypothesis that these capacities might relate in the way a bent line relates to itself when it has been straightened out spells out a scenario in which perception and thinking are not separable from each other. And the specificity of the scenario additionally suggests that this, or something like this, may indeed be Aristotle's favored option. This would also be in line with his general views about the corresponding unity of the object and the subject of cognition earlier in *De anima* (*An.* III 2, 426b16–427a9) and their corresponding separability from matter further down in our chapter (*An.* III 4, 429b21–22). But given how elliptical the text is, we cannot assert anything about this with great confidence.

Still, if Aristotle thinks that perception and thinking are in fact related in the aforementioned way when they are jointly engaged in the thinking of essences of type (2)—that is, as one and the same item in different states, in the way a bent line relates to itself once it has been straightened out—we should be careful not to take this as a remark about thinking *per se*. Most probably, Aristotle is speaking only about the inseparability of thinking and perception *insofar as they jointly engage in*

[43] *An.* III 4, 429b16–18.

[44] The difference is that 429b13 reads *allôi ê allôs echonti*, whereas 429b21 has *heterôi ê heterôs echonti*.

grasping the essences of natural hylomorphic compounds. He makes no claim about thinking and perception *per se* and without further qualification. This, at any rate, is what I would like to suggest: Aristotle is not identifying perception and thinking as fundamentally being one and the same capacity; he merely points out that perception and thinking, when they jointly engage in the thinking of matter-involving essences, share a common ground which makes them inseparable from each other *qua* thinking such essences. Thus, whenever we think the essence of a natural hylomorphic compound, our thinking of it relates to our perception of that same thing in the same way as a bent line that has been straightened out relates to itself before it has been straightened out (about which formulation see below), which is to say that perception and thinking, even though different cognitive capacities with their own respective objects, somehow are capable of grasping the same object *as* the same object. This would not be possible if they did not relate to each other in such a way as to be able to function as some sort of unity. Otherwise, it would be difficult to see how different capacities could yield the cognition of one and the same object.

At any rate, two things seem clear. To begin with, the essences of natural hylomorphic compounds can be grasped neither by perception nor by thinking alone. The essence of flesh is the essence of a perceptible object (flesh), and there is no way of grasping the perceptible qualities that materially constitute flesh without perception. And it also seems clear that there can only be one unitary cognitive correlate for every object of cognition. This follows from Aristotle's previous general statements about cognition, according to which each act of cognition must be unitary (*An.* III 2, 426b16–427a9). With these two claims in place, we obtain the result that the cognition of the essences of things like flesh—namely, essences of type (2), which are inseparable from their matter—requires that thinking and perception somehow come together to form a unitary cognitive entity.

But does this require that the *capacities* for thinking and perceiving be one and the same capacity, albeit in different states? I do not think so. First, this would bring Aristotle into obvious conflict with his own arguments to the effect that perception and thinking are not the same capacity (most notably, in *An.* III 3).[45] Second, and no less importantly, it would imply that thinking and perceiving are mutually inseparable—not only conceptually (in definition) but also in extension, which is to say that they would necessarily co-occur. This would be parallel to the way in which, for instance, a man and his courage (a state of his) could not be separated from each other extensionally. Wherever the man is, his courage will be there too (even if it may not be constantly displayed by the man), and wherever his courage is, the man will be there as well. But this contradicts Aristotle's repeated statements that thinking *can* be separated from the body (and therewith also from perception, which is inseparable from the body).[46] Third, it is difficult to see how Aristotle

[45] See Chapter 1 (Section 7).

[46] See, e.g., *An.* II 2, 413b24–27; *An.* III 4, 429b5. See also the frequent statements to the effect that thinking is accidentally related to perception (e.g., *Sens.* 1, 437a12–14; *Mem.* 1, 450a22–25).

could possibly account for a double actuality of one and the same capacity in simultaneously perceiving and thinking the same object, as would be required for instance in the cognition of the essence of flesh. I conclude that Aristotle's claim about thinking and perception relating in the way a bent line relates to itself after it has been straightened out in *An.* III 4, 429b16–17, is not a claim about the capacities for thinking and perception being one and the same, but about them being one and the same *qua* being different cognitive capacities *of one and the same cognitive subject*—namely, a human thinker—and that collaborate in the cognition of one object. If this is right, then perception and thinking are not the same capacity in different states; rather, they remain different capacities, which, however, are possessed by one and the same cognitive subject who employs both capacities in a *common cognitive effort*, in the course of which they relate to each other in the way a bent line relates to itself after having been straightened out (in a way to be discussed presently). What I have in mind is what in this book we refer to as the *operational fusion* of perception and thinking in the *cognitive soul*.[47]

What, then, is the relation of the bent line to itself when it has been straightened? For Aristotle, if *X* can be either straight or bent, then the absence of the bending will make *X* simpler: that is, more of a unity (*Metaph.* V 6, 1016a12–13). This simpler unity, moreover, stands in an *explanatory relation* to the bent line. It explains what the bent line essentially is—namely, a line—and it also helps to explain what the bent line is: namely, a line in a certain condition.[48] This already suffices for regarding the line when it has been straightened out as the equivalent to the thinking of essences and the perception of bodily features as the equivalent to the bent line.[49] Essences are simple, while the hylomorphic compounds they are the essences of are not. Essences are the simple principles of the multifarious features of the hylomorphic compounds they are the essences of. They explain why the hylomorphic compounds possess their many features.[50]

What does it mean, in this context, to be a cognitive capacity "in a different state" (*allôs echonti*; *An.* III 4, 429b21)? This statement is probably best taken as a claim about the state *perception* is in when it is involved in the thinking of essences of hylomorphic compounds (see *An.* III 4, 429b15: *tôi aisthêtikôi*).[51] Perception, when it is part of a joint cognitive effort with the thinking capacity in grasping the essences of natural hylomorphic compounds, acts in the service of theoretical thinking. And insofar as this is the case, perception is *not* doing what it usually does outside of such collaborative contexts. In other words, in such contexts, perception is not,

[47] I refer the reader to the Glossary (*s.v.* COGNITIVE SOUL).

[48] This has already been observed by Trendelenburg: "*Si inflexam [scil. lineam] in rectam rursus extenderis, princeps illud et causa restituitur*" (Trendelenburg 1877: 393).

[49] See below for additional reasons why this is probably what Aristotle has in mind. For the history of the interpretation of this difficult comparison, see Hicks 1907: 486–488.

[50] Aristotle's essentialist conception of scientific explanation is based on that relation. See Chapter 1 (Section 1).

[51] What follows could also be applied *mutatis mutandis* to thinking.

or is not entirely, acting according to its own nature. Perception is in this case in a state different from the normal state it is in when it acts in accordance with its own nature outside of acts of theoretical thinking. But while embedded in such theoretical contexts, it makes sense to say that perception acts *according to something else*: namely, thinking. It makes sense to say that because to say that perception is part of a joint theoretical effort with thinking really is to say that the directing principle of perception's cognitive engagement is not determined by perception itself. Perception in such contexts is *used* in the service, and in the interest, of theoretical thinking, which is the grasp of the essence. It is in this sense *teleologically subordinated* to thinking. We could thus say that perception in such contexts is "possessed" by thinking in a way that is comparable to the way we are possessed by a fever, which directs us according to *its* nature rather than according to our own nature. (This is the first meaning of "having" (*echein*) Aristotle lists in the corresponding entry in *Metaph.* V 23, 1023a8–11.)

If this suggestion is on the right track, then saying that perception is in a state different from itself when engaged in the thinking of essences of type (2) is compatible with, and perhaps even equivalent to, saying that it ceases to act just as perception, because it has become attached to thinking in a way that *transforms* it into something else: namely, into a subservient part of thinking. Thus, the locution of perception being "in a state different ('other')" from itself when it (merely) perceives may well imply some sort of change of identity—but, again, not because thinking and perception are one and the same *capacity* but because, in such contexts, perception will be "possessed" and teleologically subordinated to thinking. There will, then, ultimately be only one cognitive capacity responsible for the cognition of essences of type (2)—namely, thinking—but thinking will use perception as a cognitive means, or as a kind of extension, to access them. It will use, or co-opt, perception to grasp the perceptual features of, for instance, flesh but the corresponding act of perception will take place in the service of thinking the essence of flesh. And when that happens, the act of perceiving the perceptual features of flesh will stand in a relation to the thinking of the essence of flesh similar to the relation in which a bent line will stand to itself when it has been straightened out. Such teleological subordination may well be *natural* for the relevant living things (humans in our case) possessing these two cognitive capacities. The point is only that *for perception as such* this is not natural but accidental:[52] perception and thinking are not the same capacity—they are and remain definitionally separate, but perception, when used in the context of the thinking of essences of type (2), is in a state in which it acts as a kind of cognitive extension of

[52] *EE* I 2, 1219b36: *kata sumbebêkos*. Compare the discussions in *EN* I 13, 1102a28–32, and *EE* II 1, 1219b28–36, about the way in which perception/desire and thinking form a natural unity of what remain definitionally separate parts of the soul (*tôi logôi duo esti achôrista pephukota* in *EN* I 13, 1102a30–31, and *adiachôriston . . . ouk ousia tou autou* in *EE* II 1, 1219b34–36).

thinking. And insofar as, and to the extent to which, it is engaged in such contexts, it is inseparable from it.

Aristotle seems to think that a similar joint cognitive effort of thinking and perception under the guidance of thinking is required for our cognition of essences of type (3) as well. Grasping the essences of mathematical objects (Aristotle's example is "the straight") involves continuous extension (*meta sunechous*; *An.* III 4, 429b19). That continuous extension makes the straight (and all abstract mathematical objects) like the snub and thus like natural material objects. Even if their continuous extension is a mere residue of the abstraction from the physical extension of natural hylomorphic compounds, such abstract objects are still hylomorphic compounds. They do have matter after all. Hence, if the straight and the being (i.e., the essence) of the straight are not the same thing (the essence of the straight has no extension; Aristotle says "let it be duality"[53]), and the one is cognized *per se* by perception and the other *per se* by thinking, then the thinking of abstract mathematical objects will involve a similar joint effort of perception and thinking as in the case of the thinking of essences of type (2). The upshot is the same. Either we cognize the essences of abstract mathematical objects with another capacity, separate from perception, or we cognize them with a capacity which is not separate from perception and in a state similar to the line that has been straightened out relates to its own former state of being bent—which is to say that in the act of grasping such mathematical essences, and insofar as they grasp them, perception and thinking are inseparable from each other.

I have described the joint effort of thinking and perceiving as a teleological subordination of perception under the interest of grasping the essences of hylomorphic compounds. Thinking guides perception and "uses" it to access essences of things with matter that it otherwise could not access. This is why Aristotle says that, during such acts, thinking and perception stand in the same relation as a bent line relates to itself when it has been straightened out. However, it should be added that this talk of one capacity "using" the other to some extent is only figurative speech. It should not be taken to imply that in humans thinking is somehow a separate cognitive subject that uses perception in a way comparable to the way in which a person uses a tool. It is important not to apply a homuncular conception of the teleological subordination of perception. Aristotle may well have something different in mind and below I will suggest a conception of teleological subordination that is not homuncular.[54]

In the concluding sentence of this section, Aristotle says that generally (*holôs*) there is a *corresponding degree of separateness* among the *per se* objects of thought from matter (i.e., the different type of essences) and the corresponding kinds of

[53] *An.* III 4, 429b20.

[54] This will be an asymmetrical conception according to which the agent of the subordination is not thinking but the thinking *person*.

thinking from perception (which involves matter) (*An.* III 4, 429b21–22). This, as we have seen, entails that the thinking of essences of type (1) is done by separate thinking, while essences of types (2) and (3) (i.e., the essences of different kinds of matter-involving objects, either physical or abstract) can only be grasped by way of a joint effort of perception and thinking.

If the above suggestion about the nature of that joint effort as teleological subordination is correct, then, in the course of grasping matter-involving essences, and insofar as it is thinking them, thinking will indeed be inseparable from perception and vice versa perception from thinking, and generally thinking will be separate or inseparable from perception to the same degree to which the essences it thinks will be separate from matter; but this is not so because the *capacity* for thinking is the same as the capacity for perception. Aristotle's statement about the corresponding degrees of separateness of thinking and its objects from matter and perception in *An.* III 4, 429b21–22, does not say or imply that the thinking of separate essences of type (1) is carried out by a fundamentally different kind of capacity for thinking than the capacity for thinking essences of types (2) and (3)—one inseparable from perception, the other separate from perception; rather, the statement regards only the respective *acts* of thinking.

What all of this amounts to is that (i) we cannot think the essences of matter-involving objects without simultaneously engaging our perceptual capacity because the (physical, qualitative) extension these essences involve can only be cognized by perception and other perception-based representational states, all of which involve *phantasia*;[55] and, therefore, (ii) during the cognition of such essences, thinking and perceiving cannot be separate from each other (just as hylomorphic compounds cannot be separated from their essences). Moreover, if the above suggestion about the character of the inseparability of thinking and perceiving during such acts is correct, we can also infer that (iii) it will be one and the same capacity of thinking that is engaged in the thinking of all three types of essences.

The most important difference between the three kinds of thinking of essences is that in the case of the thinking of essences of types (2) and (3), the thinking capacity *co-opts* the perceptual capacity to access the corresponding objects. Hence, on this interpretation, there is only one capacity for thinking in a human cognitive agent, and this capacity can, but need not, be separate from the capacity for perception. While in thinking essences of type (1), thinking is separate from perception, in thinking essences of types (2) and (3), it is not. In sum, perception and thinking remain fundamentally different capacities. Another upshot of the proposed analysis is that essences of type (1) are fully transparent to thinking, while essences of types (2) and (3) are less so. They involve some sort of extension

[55] *An.* III 7, 431a16–17: "soul never thinks without a *phantasma*." For a discussion of this claim, see Chapter 1 (Section 7), Chapter 4, and the Glossary (*s.v.* PHANTASIA).

(to different degrees), the cognition of which is not transparent to thinking and is to be grasped by perception. In terms of separateness from matter, therefore, the cognitive capacities are exactly parallel to their objects, as Aristotle says they are in 429b21–22. The thinking involved in grasping the essences of material objects is inseparable from perception to the same degree to which the corresponding essences of these objects are inseparable from their matter.[56]

3.2 The structure of Aristotle's account of thinking, the role of matter, and the problem of the subject of thinking

Aristotle's thesis of the corresponding separateness of essences from matter and the thinking of these essences from perception in *An.* III 4, 429b21–22, structures his entire account of thinking. It is the structure of a *continuum* of degrees of corresponding separation from matter and perception.[57] On the one end of the continuum, there is pure thinking, completely separate from perception and concerned with an essence as its object that is entirely separate from matter (type (1) essences). This pure and separate thinking is maximally transparent from a cognitive point of view. The object and the thought of the object fully coincide in this kind of thinking, and there is nothing left either in the object or in the thinking of it that is not fully cognized. Further down the continuum, there are essences of types (2) and (3). Such essences are inseparable from matter, and the degree to which they are so corresponds to the degree of their cognitive opacity/transparency. With this, Aristotle posits a strong structural parallel between the ontological structure of things in terms of the separateness of their essential forms from their matter and their transparency/opacity to cognition. While the pure thinking of separate substances is maximally transparent to cognition, essences that are not separate from matter are not fully transparent to cognition. In the latter case, object and subject of thought do not coincide (to different degrees). Such matter-involving essences, due to the matter or extension they involve, cannot be made objects of

[56] The inseparability of form and matter and the corresponding inseparability of thinking and perception are important anti-Platonic tenets for Aristotle. They ensure that form and matter of hylomorphic compounds are form and matter *of one and the same thing*, and that the thinking of the essences of such compounds is really the thinking of the compound's essence. Both results are problematic on the Platonic account of essential Forms as ontologically separate from the things they are supposed to be the forms of. How will they form a unity? How can we cognitively access essences of hylomorphic compounds and be sure that they are really the essences of these compounds? While Plato seems to deny the former point (Forms are separate), the latter remains problematic for him.

[57] It is of no importance for present purposes whether Aristotle thinks that separability from matter/perception is literally continuous or thinks that there simply happen to be different kinds of essences whose separateness from matter can be arranged along a continuum (his language in *De anima* seems to suggest the latter, while he does seem to entertain the idea of a continuum of separability from matter in *Meteor.* IV 12). What is important is that there are different kinds of thinking which either involve no matter at all or involve matter to different degrees, and that the degree to which they and their objects involve matter strictly corresponds to their cognitive transparency/opacity.

thought without perception, which is the kind of cognition responsible for the cognition of material objects. The cognition of material objects and their essences thus always contains elements that remain cognitively opaque. The reason for this is that perception involves matter. So, in the case of matter-involving essences, on both sides of the cognition relation, it is matter that obstructs the identity of a thing with its essence and therewith its cognitive transparency.[58]

But for all the structural unity across cognitive kinds that Aristotle's thesis of corresponding degrees of separateness from matter brings with it, this thesis also creates a serious interpretative difficulty. The problem is that there seems to be a shift in the subject of cognition along the different degrees of separateness from matter. While in pure matterless thinking the cognitive subject is identical to its object, in the thinking of enmattered essences subject and object of cognition come apart. Is it still the same cognitive subject of thinking in both cases? This is an important interpretative difficulty of the chapters devoted to thinking in *De anima*, which, even if perhaps not always identified by them, has beset interpreters since antiquity. While it seems relatively clear and uncontroversial that we human thinkers, who are hylomorphic compounds, are the cognitive subjects of all kinds of thinking of essences of types (2) and (3), the identity of the cognitive subject of the thinking of essences of type (1), which are separate from matter, is less obvious. If we as hylomorphic compounds can think separate essences—a question that Aristotle does not clearly settle in *De anima*—then is it still *us* as hylomorphic substances who think them?[59] Or is it rather the case that only separate essences can think separate essences? What about us hylomorphic thinkers, then? Can we think separate essences, or can't we?[60]

The structure of corresponding degrees of separateness on both sides of the cognitive relation along a continuum with a pure and separate self-thinking subject of cognition at the top would suggest that we as hylomorphic compounds could not cognitively access separate essences. The very fact that we are hylomorphic compounds should imply that our cognition will involve bodily perception. And Aristotle's often repeated statements that we cannot think without a *phantasma* would seem to say just that, or something very close to that. So, according to

[58] "Matter in itself is not a possible object of cognition" (*hê de hulê agnôstos kath' hautên*; *Metaph.* VII 10, 1036a8–9. That perception and *phantasia* involve matter and are not separable from body and matter is a standing theme in Aristotle's *De anima* (see, e.g., *An.* I 1, 403b5–10).

[59] Even toward the end of his treatment of the thinking capacity, in *An.* III 7, 431b17–18, Aristotle tells us that "the question whether or not it is possible [for the capacity for thinking] to think any of the separated entities, when it is not itself separate from magnitude, must be investigated later." Cf. also *An.* I 1, 403a3–b16, 413a6–7, 413b24–27 (explicitly speaking of the *possibility* of the thinking part or capacity of the soul being separated from the body "like the eternal from the perishable," which seems to imply that at least temporarily our thinking capacity is not separate from the body; is this meant to be during our entire lifetime?).

[60] On that very question, see Chapters 4 and 5. Gerson 2004 also speaks of a "difficulty of identifying the subject of cognitive activities." However, he wishes to resolve that difficulty by introducing the concept of a *person* as the "essentially self-reflexive" underlying subject of both embodied and disembodied acts of thinking (2004: 366, 371). Below I argue that purely matterless thinking of essences of type (1) is not personal.

Aristotle's thesis of corresponding degrees of separateness on the object and the subject side of cognition, we should be barred from thinking separate substances as a matter of principle. On the other hand, the thesis also seems to establish that there is only one capacity for thinking in each of us along a continuum of separability from matter. Aristotle clearly does not believe that we think the different types of essences with different kinds of capacities for thinking. On the contrary, he speaks of only one thinking capacity and that seems to be the capacity for thinking essences of all three types. And of these three types, essences of type (1)—that is, essences separate from matter—are more fundamental than essences of types (2) and (3). And this seems to suggest that we as hylomorphic compounds are capable of thinking essences of hylomorphic compounds of types (2) and (3) only by virtue of somehow being attached to, or by somehow being continuous with, separate thinking.[61] Would this not suggest that we do have access to separate thinking, after all? We will return to these issues below.[62]

4. Two difficulties (Section III: *An.* 4, 429b22–29)

Aristotle has presented us with an account of the capacity of human thinking as a pure, immaterial, and otherwise featureless capacity for taking on the objects of thinking. This account avoids the cognitive limitations that his account of the perceptual capacity brought with it: that is, the "blind spots" that come with the fact that that kind of cognition is physically implemented. Indeed, as we have seen, this account basically consists in purging the account of the perceptual capacity from its physical features. With this, Aristotle seems to be in a good position to account for the unrestricted scope of thinking, while at the same time preserving the structure of his general account of cognition that underlies his account of perception. So, this seems like a simple and viable way of accounting for the human capacity of thinking and its alleged unrestricted cognitive scope. However, in what follows Aristotle raises two difficulties (*aporiai*) which cast fundamental doubt on his basic strategy of purging his account of perception of its physical features. Both difficulties result more or less immediately from Aristotle's application of the physical (i.e., causal) model of perception to the case of thinking, a model which works on the assumption of an affection of the cognitive agent by the cognitive object.[63]

[61] The fact that perception is attached to separate thinking is accidental to the latter. Hence, our attachment should be conceived of as asymmetrical. We as hylomorphic compounds are attached to separate thinking but separate thinking is not thereby attached to us. See this chapter, Section 5.2.

[62] The distinction between cognizing separate thinking *per se* as it is in itself and cognizing it *per accidens*—namely, as a cause and principle of other things—will play an important role in that context. See below (Section 6).

[63] There is the view in the literature that "perceiving that we see or hear" is a kind of self-perception of perception that does not involve self-affection (most notably, Caston 2002). I do not share this view, however. Given that it does not occur even in thinking, I find it more likely that for Aristotle perceiving

The first difficulty questions the possibility of there being an affection of something immaterial; the second questions the possibility of self-affection, which would seem to be necessary on the causal model of affection if thinking really should be able to think itself. How can anything affect itself, unless it has different parts affecting each other? But thinking is supposed to be partless and simple. So, in this case self-affection seems a real problem for Aristotle's account of thinking. Both difficulties are entirely reasonable and therefore serious, and their discussion will keep Aristotle busy for the rest of *An.* III 4 and eventually, as we will see, up until the end of *An.* III 5.

4.1 First difficulty (*An.* III 4, 429b22–26)

If the thinking capacity is immaterial and unaffected and shares nothing with any of the beings, as Aristotle says it is, how will it think, if thinking is being affected by a cognitive object? Affection (*paschein*), as we learn in Aristotle's general physics, is the transmission of a form from an agent who is the bearer of that form to the patient who is receiving it. For that to occur, agent and patient need to meet two basic criteria. First, they need to be sufficiently different from each other, as there can be no affection of the same by the same (what is already *F* cannot be acted upon by *F*). Second, there must be a common element (*koinon ti*) in both the agent and the patient, since without a common element there would be, as it were, nothing common for them so that they are able to encounter each other and interact. Thus, affection can only occur among ordered pairs of agents and patients that, while pertaining to the same genus, are specifically different from each other.[64] This is why there can be no affection of, for example, white by hot nor of sweet by loud, as there is nothing in the white that the hot could act upon, nor is there anything in the sweet that could possibly be affected by the loud. Nor can there be an affection from white to white or from hot to hot, but only from white to some other color on the color spectrum (the genus) and so on. It is this ontological order of things that makes affection possible in the first place. Aristotle's account of the thinking capacity, however, seems to violate that order. His postulate, that there is an affection of something devoid of any feature apart from potentially being the object of thinking, violates the criterion of sameness in genus between agent and patient. In this respect Aristotle's account seems similar to the impossible case of an affection of white by hot. How can *X* be affected by *Y*,

that we see or hear is a kind of affection of one part of the perceptual system by another. I cannot argue for this claim here.

[64] *Gener. Corr.* I 7, 323b30–324a9.

if *X* falls under genus *G*, but *Y* falls under no genus of being at all? If *Y* falls under no genus of being at all, then surely it will not fall under genus *G* either. Hence, Aristotle's idea of an affection of something that is none of the beings at all before it thinks seems obviously incompatible with the account of affection advanced in *Gener. Corr.* I 7. There simply is no substrate, nothing to be acted on by the agent of the affection.

4.2 Second difficulty (*An.* III 4, 429b26–29)

This difficulty takes the form of a reductive dilemma. Supposing Aristotle's model of thinking as an affection, according to which the capacity for thinking is made actual by way of being affected by its cognitive object, and supposing further—with Aristotle—that thinking can think itself, it should follow that the thinking capacity affects itself. But how is this possible? How can anything affect itself? As we have just seen, the very idea of affection is based on the distinctness of agent and patient, since what is already *F* cannot be acted upon by *F*, and Aristotle would certainly be the first to point out that self-affection in the strict sense is not possible.[65] Hence, given that this is so, we are left with two options, neither of which seems acceptable: either thinking is contained in the objects of thinking (429b27)[66] or thinking is somehow mixed with matter, which makes it an object of thinking just like any other ordinary object of thinking: that is, a hylomorphic compound. Both options seem unacceptable. It is absurd to hold that all objects of thinking contain thinking and hence somehow are thinkers; and it is utterly unacceptable, at least from an Aristotelian point of view, that thinking should be mixed with matter and thus somehow itself be a hylomorphic compound, since this would entail that thinking could not fully grasp itself, which would destroy the core tenet of his account of thinking as an unrestricted cognitive capacity. It seems, then, that thinking could not possibly think itself in the way Aristotle envisages.[67]

[65] See *An.* II 5, 416b35–417a20 (with cross-reference to *Gener. Corr.* I 7); see also his many arguments against a similar possibility advocated by Plato of there being self-movers in the strict sense in *Phys.* VIII 5.

[66] Aristotle makes this claim dependent on two conditions, both of which he thinks are clearly fulfilled: namely, (i) that thinking is not an object of thinking "according to something else (*kat' allo*)" and (ii) that all thinkable objects share the same form insofar as they are objects of thinking (*An.* III 4, 429b27–28). The first condition demands that thinking be an immediate object of thinking: i.e., that it is not made an object of thinking *indirectly* by way of thinking other things but that it be directly thinkable. The second condition demands that "object of thought" is not an ambiguous expression but has the same meaning both in the case of thinking's self-thinking and in the case of the thinking of other objects.

[67] The difficulty is a difficulty about the self-thinking of thinking; it is *not* a question about self-awareness. On this point, see Gregoric and Pfeiffer 2015.

5. Solutions (Section IV: *An.* III 4, 429b29–430a10)

5.1 Solution to the first difficulty

Aristotle meets the first challenge by introducing his famous analogy of the wax-tablet. The analogy does no more than providing a concrete example to help us in conceiving of the unaffectedness of the thinking capacity introduced in the first section of *An.* III 4. The example illustrates and thus elucidates the account of the thinking capacity as a mere, and otherwise featureless, capacity for taking in the objects of thinking.

> Or is it rather that we have previously made a distinction about "being acted upon in virtue of something common"—namely, that the capacity for thinking is potentially in some way the objects of thinking, but it is none of them in actuality before it thinks? It must be just as in a writing tablet, on which nothing is written in actuality, which is exactly what happens in the case of the capacity for thinking.[68]

Aristotle can preserve his account of thinking as a case of affection (*paschein*) because he does not conceive of the affection of the capacity for thinking by its object as a case of *physical* affection to begin with. On his conception, there is indeed no common element or genus that underlies as the substrate of affection. Unlike a physical affection, where an underlying and persisting substrate takes on the form of the agent, there is nothing underlying. Rather, there is only the bare, and otherwise featureless, potentiality of an essence. It is a mere "blank" with no further intrinsic feature of its own (which is why Aristotle has likened it to the "place of forms" in *An.* III 4, 429a24–29). The "affection" of that "blank," therefore, consists not in a physical affection in which a property of an underlying substrate gets replaced by another property (change), but in the replacement of that intellectual "blank" by an actual essence.[69] This involves no physical affection whatsoever because there is nothing actual there for the essence to act upon. Essences, we may say, simply come to be present in human thinkers without this involving any kind of change or affection other than the actualization of an immaterial capacity for that essence.

[68] *An.* III 4, 429b29–430a2. We are following the generally accepted reading at 430a1 γραμματείῳ ᾧ μηθὲν ὑπάρχει (with Förster and all the recent editors of *De anima*). For a discussion of the textual issues and a different interpretation of the example, I refer the reader to Crubellier (forthcoming).

[69] The above quotation refers to Aristotle's distinction between two kinds of affection in *An.* II 5, 417b2, in which he (prospectively) used his account of thinking from *An.* III to explain the kind of affection (*paschein*) that occurs in perception according to his theory. In perceptual affection, there is a perceptual "blank," which gets replaced by a perceptual object as well (see Chapter 1, Section 6). But, unlike thinking, that perceptual "blank" *is* physically implemented.

On Aristotle's account, then, thinking episodes in the narrow sense consist in the presence of an essence in a subject capable of receiving it, without this presence involving any change or affection of a substrate. The capacity for thinking is not physically implemented, yet it is capable of receiving the essence. The reception consists in the presence of the essence where there previously was nothing but the potentiality for that essence. This, I take it, is what the wax-tablet is supposed to illustrate. So, Aristotle in a way concedes to his imaginary objector that the physical model of affection collapses in the case of thinking. And this appears to be part of the *point* Aristotle wishes to make in introducing the example of the wax-tablet. Adapting the physical model of affection in perception to the account of thinking at the beginning of the chapter resulted in stripping that account of its physical features. Aristotle's answer to the first problem does little more than remind us of the fact that this applies also to the concept of "affection" relevant in this case. It should not be understood as a physical affection along the lines of *Gener. Corr.* I 7, but rather as a "popping up" of an essence where there previously was a mere intellectual blank: that is, an immaterial capacity for receiving the essence. Nothing gets changed in the cognitive subject *qua* affection by the object of thinking. "Affection," therefore, has the very specific meaning here of switching from an intellectual and otherwise featureless blank into the actuality of an essence.[70] Note, however, that this mere cognitive blank will be the result of a long and arduous process of scientific education. And since there is no underlying subject that would "become" that essence, but just a previous bare potentiality for it, that switching is not a continuous process; it is an instantaneous "popping up."[71] Aristotle, we may say, has used the analogy with perception in *An.* I, 429a13–b9, as a ladder to establish his positive account of the thinking capacity as the immaterial and featureless bare receptivity of the objects of thinking. Now he, as it were, throws that ladder away.[72]

5.2 Solution to the second difficulty

The difficulty was this: how can the capacity for thinking ever think itself, if thinking is some kind of affection and nothing can possibly affect itself (in the strict sense)? If thinking's self-thinking is to be possible at all, either all other things

[70] This of course only holds *qua* thinking itself: i.e., *qua* the presence of the essence in the soul, and not *qua* the representational, linguistic, volitional, and otherwise necessary conditions of thinking. Also, as we have already seen in *An.* III 4, 429b5–10, thinking is a second actuality and as such an acquired, and indeed highly "educated," capacity. The acquisition of that capacity involves all sorts of changes (see *An.* II 5, 417a31–b2).

[71] See, *Phys.* VII 3, 247b1–248a6 and, e.g., *Metaph.* VII 15, 1139b20–27; IX 6, 1048b23–36.

[72] Alexander of Aphrodisias captures this idea rather well when he says that the writing-tablet is not so much about a tablet with nothing written on it as it is about its "unwrittenness" (*mâllon de tês pinakidos agraphôi* [*sc. eoike*]; *An.* 84.25 f.). See also Trendelenburg 1877: 399 and Rodier 1900: 455–456.

will be thinking as well, or the capacity for thinking will be mixed with the body so that it can be an object of thinking just like the other hylomorphic compounds. Aristotle responds to this difficulty in a nuanced way. He distributes his solution over the three kinds of *per se* objects of thinking he has distinguished previously: namely, essences of types (1), (2), and (3). The answers turn out to be different for the thinking of essences of type (1) on the one hand, and the thinking of essences of types (2) and (3) on the other. However, while there will be a satisfying answer to the problem of self-thinking in the case of essences of type (1), *An.* III 4 will not offer a satisfying answer with regard to the self-thinking of essences of types (2) and (3).

> And it [i.e., thinking] is also itself an object of thinking just like the [other] objects of thinking.[73] That is to say: in the case of objects without matter, that which thinks and that which is thought are identical, because theoretical knowledge is identical with what is known in this way. (We will have to inquire into the reason why it does not always think). In [the domain of] things that have matter, however, each thing is [only] potentially an object of thinking; so that the capacity for thinking will not belong to them (for the capacity for thinking is a capacity for such objects without matter), but it will belong to it [i.e., to the capacity for thinking] to be an object of thinking.[74]

In the case of essences separate from matter—essences of type (1)—Aristotle is happy to accept the first horn of the dilemma, which must have seemed an absurd consequence to the imagined objector when the difficulty was posed with relation to all kinds of thinking in *An.* III 4, 429b27. In other words, Aristotle accepts that the objects of thinking of type (1) are themselves actually thinking. In the case of objects of type (1), subject and object of thinking are the same and hence the object of thinking will be a thinking act and the subject of thinking will be a thinkable object. Essences separate from matter are thinking acts and the thinking of them is what they are; it is identical with them. In this case, we have a full-blown identity of the subject and the object of cognition and consequently no need for an affection by an object that is not currently in possession of thinking. Here Aristotle employs his thesis of the identity of the subject and object of theoretical science as an example for his identity thesis with regard to the subject and object of cognition of essences of type (1).[75] But it is not the case that all Aristotelian theoretical sciences can provide such full-blown identity. For instance, physics, understood as the science of things insofar as they change and

[73] This formulation takes up the claim about the non-ambiguous meaning of "object of thinking" in *An.* III 4, 429b28.

[74] *An.* III 4, 430a2–9.

[75] See also *An.* III 5, 430a19–20; *An.* III 7, 431a1–2; *Metaph.* XII 9, 1074b38–1075a1.

have matter, cannot because it is concerned with the essences of hylomorphic compounds.[76] What Aristotle seems to have in mind here, then, is not all theoretical sciences but first philosophy, and theology in particular.[77] So much for the self-thinking of essences of type (1).

Aristotle's answer regarding the self-thinking of essences of type (1), however, raises the question of why, when "it"—presumably the thinking capacity of a thinker—engages in such theoretical thinking, it does not remain engaged in thinking forever. Given the nature of essences of type (1) as essentially thinking themselves, this is a natural question to ask. For if there is an immaterial essence that not only happens to think itself, but *is* the thinking of itself, as Aristotle says immaterial essences are, then it is very hard to see how the corresponding act of thinking could partake in potentiality. The object of thinking will be fully present to it and there will be no potentiality on the side of the thinker that is not fully realized in that act. In such a scenario it becomes a real question why thinking of this kind should ever stop. For how could it do so and stop thinking if it doesn't have the potentiality not to think? Aristotle says here that this is a question to be investigated (*episkepteon*; *An.* III 4, 430a5–6). The answer will not be apparent before the end of *An.* III 5.

In the case of the other objects of thinking (type (2) and type (3) essences: i.e., the essences of either physical or mathematical hylomorphic compounds, which are grouped together here under one common heading as "things that have matter"), Aristotle does not give a clear indication as to how or even whether the thinking of such essences can think itself. Hylomorphic compounds clearly are not a kind of thinking. Thinking does not belong to them because hylomorphic compounds essentially have matter, while both the act and the capacity for thinking are supposed to be immaterial (as Aristotle says about the thinking capacity in *An.* III 4, 430a7 and 8). Essences of types (2) and (3), by virtue of their ontological makeup as essences of hylomorphic compounds, therefore, cannot possibly be active thinkers. But they are potential objects of thinking: that is, they are potential objects of thinking for a thinker who is external to them. Aristotle applies this same status also to the corresponding capacity for thinking essences of types (2) and (3); it too is a potential object of thinking. So, while objects of type (1) are straightforwardly cases of thinking, which is why in their case we can see how thinking can be its own object and think itself, objects of types (2) and (3) clearly are not. All hylomorphic compounds are potential objects of thinking, and the same goes for the

[76] *Phys.* II 2, 194a12–b14; *An.* I 1, 403b7–12; *Metaph.* VI 1, 1026a10–18. Menn (Menn 2020: 116–118) offers interesting arguments for why one could think of Aristotelian physics as different from purely theoretical sciences (despite Aristotle's classification of physics as theoretical science in *Metaph.* VI 1, 1025b26–1026a7).

[77] See *Phys.* II 2, 194b14–15; *An.* I 1, 403b15–16; *Metaph.* VI 1, 1026a10–18; and especially *Metaph.* XII 9, 1074b38–1075a5.

corresponding capacity for thinking. From the information given so far, then, it is unclear how the thinking of essences of hylomorphic compounds can think itself. What we have heard so far is only that the thinking of such essences is a potential object of thinking, which suggests that its self-thinking is possible. But how? This is where *An.* III 4 stops.

Beyond the unanswered puzzle about the self-thinking of the thinking of the essences of hylomorphic compounds, however, the end of *An.* III 4 leaves us with a question that is even more critical. Aristotle does not raise the question explicitly. But this should not mislead us into thinking that the question is not an important one in that context, especially since Aristotle has already raised it at the very beginning of the chapter (*An.* III 4, 429a13). The problem is this. Based on all the information given so far in the chapter about the thinking of essences of hylomorphic compounds, there are passive potentialities on both sides of the cognitive relation, one being an essence of a hylomorphic compound (which is not actually but only potentially an object of thinking for a thinker), the other being the capacity for thinking (which is only the potentiality of being affected by an actual object of thinking). Therefore, the following question poses itself: how does the thinking of essences of hylomorphic compounds come about?[78]

For Aristotle this must be a most serious and pressing question, given that in this case—and unlike the case of physical affection—physical contact (*haphê*) between the bearers of the relata of affection will not suffice to make the relevant potentialities actual: neither the potential object of thinking nor the capacity for thinking is materially extended, as Aristotle insists time and again, so there is no underlying substrate of affection (hylomorphic compounds are, of course, materially extended, but their essences are not). More importantly still, there is no active potentiality involved on either side of the cognitive relation. Neither the potential object of thinking nor the capacity for thinking can play the active role that the actualization of the two passive potentialities requires: the capacity for thinking is "none of the beings" at all before it is passively "affected" by the object of thinking (the essence), while the essence is only potentially being thought by a thinker; it has no actual features that would endow it with the power to act, and impose itself, on a thinker. How, then, if neither the potential object nor the potential subject of thinking is an active potentiality, will the thinking of hylomorphic essences come

[78] *Contra* Caston 1999: 203–205, who says that there is no question left unanswered by the end of *An.* III 4. Likewise, Willy Theiler claims that without *An.* III 5 one would not miss anything from Aristotle's "naturalistic Psychology" and that the chapter is probably a later insertion by Aristotle (Theiler 1959: 142). But, as argued above, there is an open question: namely, the question of how actual thinking comes about in the sense of *second actuality*. I agree with Wedin who observes that: "... one could say that the chapter [*sc. An.* III 5] is almost exclusively interested in the topic of $actual_2$ thinking" (Wedin 1988: 222). Gerson 2004 also argues that *An.* III 5 continues the argument from *An.* III 4 (Gerson 2004: 361) and that *An.* III 5 is concerned with the second actuality of thinking (364).

about?[79] This, as the reader will remember, was the second of the two questions Aristotle asked at the beginning of *An.* III 4.[80]

6. Two modes of thinking, and the intrinsic nature of the active cause of thinking (Section V: *An.* III 5, 430a10–25)

6.1 Two modes of thinking

The first part of *An.* III 5,[81] with its distinction between two modes of thinking and its doctrine of active thinking, seems to offer an answer to this further, and indeed more critical, question—namely, the question of how thinking comes about:

> Since, just as in all nature, there is something which is matter for each kind of object (this is what is potentially all these things) and something else which

[79] The solution of the latter problem may offer a perspective on the first problem of the self-thinking of the thinking of essences of type (2) and (3) as well. Once we can explain how thinking comes about, we may also explain how it can think itself. More on this in the next section.

[80] Stephen Menn (2020: 109–111, 127, and especially 120) argues that the object of thinking is to thought like the art is to its matter (namely, a way of being an *efficient cause* of affections such as Aristotle discusses them in *Gener. Corr.* I 7, 324a30–b14), which is to say that the object of thinking in cases of essences of types (2) and (3) is always an actual object of thinking and is in potentiality only so far as it can, but does not as of yet, act as the *efficient cause* of the act of its being thought (where the idea is that the object acts as the *unmoved mover* of the act of its being thought by a cognitive agent). Presumably, that is why Menn—agreeing with Caston 1999—thinks that there is no question left unanswered at the end of *An.* III 4 with respect to how thinking comes about. I do not see how this can be the case for human thinking of essences of hylomorphic compounds. First, I am not aware of any direct textual evidence for the claim that hylomorphic compounds are actual (immediate) objects of thinking before they are made objects of actual thinking by a thinker (on this, see the above discussion of *An.* III 4, 429b5–10, the discussion below, Schmitz 1985: 229, and Kelsey 2022: ch. 7). Menn neutralizes the positive textual evidence for the claim that essences of types (2) and (3) are only potential objects of thinking before they are being thought by cognitive agents in *An.* III 4, 430a6–7, by way of a new translation. In our translation the passage says that "in [the domain of] things that have matter, however, each thing is [only] potentially an object of thinking;" Menn, by contrast, translates "in things that have matter, [the *nous*] is potentially each of the νοητά," making *nous* the subject of the sentence. However, without further passages that positively affirm or otherwise support the thesis that the essences of hylomorphic compounds are actual objects of thinking even before they are made objects of thinking by a thinker, Menn's translation of the sentence in 430a6–7 is no good support for his interpretation, especially since the question Aristotle appears to address in this passage is not whether *nous* is potentially the essences of hylomorphic compounds—this has been stated several times at this point—but the second difficulty concerning the possibility of the self-thinking of *nous* raised in 429b26–29, whether its self-thinking requires that the objects of thinking will have *nous* as well or that *nous* will have something "mixed" like ordinary things. It also seems that the underlying idea of Menn's interpretation—that there are actual objects of thinking "out there" that constantly act on us each time we perceive the corresponding hylomorphic compounds—is intrinsically difficult to maintain. Actual objects of human thinking are universals and universals do not exist in materially extended things, at least not *as such*, but only in human souls (*An.* II 5, 417b22–24; cf. *An.* III 4, 429a27–29); note that the claim that materially extended things are not actual objects of thinking before they are made actual by suitable thinkers does not in any way imply that they do not have actual essences. That materially extended things have actual essences is fully compatible with the fact that these essences are only potential objects of thinking.

[81] Our division of Aristotle's treatises into chapters dates to the sixteenth century. Although it was carefully made, this division has no special authority, so it is in no way binding for us.

> is the cause and producer because it makes them all, as art stands in relation to its material, it is necessary that there be these different [factors] in the soul as well: and there is one such kind of thinking on account of becoming all things and another [such kind of thinking] on account of making all things, like a state, as light does: for in a way light also makes potential colors colors in actuality.[82]

Very roughly, Aristotle makes three claims about thinking (*nous*) in this first part of *An.* III 5:

(i) There are two modes of thinking: potential thinking and active thinking.
(ii) Potential thinking becomes all things, while active thinking is the cause which produces all things.
(iii) Active thinking acts like a state (*hexis*) does, in a way that is similar to the way in which light (which is a state of the transparent medium) turns a potential color into an actual color.

Aristotle says that active thinking makes potential thinking become all things in intellectual actuality by acting on it. Given the general context of the passage, it is highly reasonable to assume that potential thinking is the capacity for thinking that Aristotle has just defined in *An.* III 4. "All things," then, refers to all *per se* objects of thinking—namely, essences of types (1), (2), and (3)—whereas active thinking seems to be the item responsible for making the capacity for thinking actual. This is the item we have been looking for at the end of *An.* III 4. Now since Aristotle, as we have seen, is as direct a realist as one can possibly be with respect to the thinking of essences—for him the essences of things are literally present in the thinker's soul—making the capacity for thinking actual is tantamount to making the essential forms of things actual objects of thinking.[83] Before we engage further in the interpretation of these claims, we should glance at the reasoning Aristotle adopts to establish the first two of the above three claims. In the text, he seems to argue as follows: because all of nature exhibits a matter/maker distinction, these same differences must also occur in the soul; therefore, necessarily (i) and (ii).[84] So far this seems straightforward.

[82] *An.* III 5, 430a10–17. See also the discussion of that same passage in Chapter 6.

[83] Essences of types (2) and (3), therefore, are only potentially existent objects of thinking before they are made actual objects of thinking by being thought by an epistemic agent. Their potential existence, as we have seen above, was also the solution to the second difficulty with regard to essences of types (2) and (3). Hermann Schmitz takes this line of thought to the extreme by claiming that active thinking does "the making or the creation of the essences themselves (*das Machen oder Schaffen der Ideen selbst*)" (Schmitz 1985: 229), identifying it with "being as such (*mit dem Seiendem schlechthin*)" (1985: 237). See also his commentary on *An.* III 5, 430a22–25 (1985: 236–239). But there is no reason to suppose that the essences of things do not exist before they are thought by epistemic agents. They exist in actuality, but they are potential as objects of thinking.

[84] The Greek expression "in all of nature" (*en hapasêi têi phusei*) can also be given a distributive reading ("in each nature"). This is how Stephen Menn takes it, especially on the ground that the

Before we can move on, however, there are two initial questions we need to get out of the way. The first has to do with the meaning of the formulation "in the soul." Does Aristotle speak of the human soul to the exclusion of any super-personal aspect of human thinking? That would immediately decide the above-mentioned interpretative problem of the cognitive subject of thinking. However, such a subjective understanding is certainly not necessitated by that formulation, and it is also not suggested by it. The expression "in the soul" may very well refer to the acts that take place in the human soul, without implying that all the factors that play a role in these acts are entirely internal to the human soul. Such an implication would not even be true of the most trivial physical changes as they occur in nature, in which the agent of change under normal circumstances is external to the patient. Take, for instance, the heat of a stove, which affects the cold body of a dog sleeping next to it. A natural change occurs in a natural substance (the dog), but the active factor in the change (the heat, which serves as the agent in our example) is not internal to the dog. Thus, it neither follows from, nor is suggested by, the formulation "in the soul" that all the factors that contribute to the actuality of the thinking capacity in the human soul are internal to the soul. But the formulation does not rule that out either. Therefore, we should not let our interpretation be restricted by our preconception of what "in the soul" may mean, apart from the fact that it is referring to something that takes place in the human soul. The interpretative problem of the cognitive subject remains.

The second question we need to get out of our way is whether Aristotle wishes to establish (i) and (ii) by way of deduction or not (it seems clear that he does not offer arguments for (iii) here). In the former case, thinking would have to fall within the boundaries of nature. The advantage of the deductive reading is that we can easily understand why the conclusion to (i) and (ii) is supposed to follow with necessity, as it would logically follow from the premises "all natural domains exhibit a matter/maker structure" and "the soul is a natural domain." But the shortcoming of this interpretation is that we know from other passages, including the previous chapter and what will follow in the immediate sequel to this very passage, that Aristotle does not believe that thinking is part of nature, at least if thinking is taken in the narrow sense in which it is discussed in *An.* III 4–5, by ignoring not only its bodily and representational aspects but also its volitional and scientific enabling conditions. But if the argument is not a deduction, it is no longer clear what necessitates the conclusion. Is Aristotle arguing by mere analogy? And if so, why is the conclusion necessary?

Perhaps there is less of a problem here than one might initially think. Since *An.* III 4–5 speaks about a transition from potential thinking into actual

formulation *hekastôi genei* in the very next line, 430a11, seems to suggest exactly this (Menn 2020: 125), and I agree with his motives. Aristotle is clearly not saying something that holds of nature only globally and as a whole; rather, he is saying something about each nature within nature as a whole. However, I think this is one possible way of taking the "all."

thinking, there is sufficient grounds for Aristotle to appeal to nature in the broad sense of the locus of transition, or—more plausibly perhaps—to appeal to nature only as the most perspicuous subclass of the larger class of all the things involving transition. Here "transition" is to be taken in the general sense of *metabolê*, which covers all kinds of transitions, including full-blown changes and mere relational ("Cambridge") changes. This is how Aristotle speaks of *metabolê*, for example, in *Metaph.* XII 9, 1074b26–27: that is, as "some kind" of change (*kinêsis tis*).[85]

This interpretation has the advantage of including art (*technê*) as a subclass in the relevant class of things mentioned in *An.* III 5, 430a12–14. And it has the further advantage of covering the immediately relevant case of immaterial and extensionless transition mentioned previously in *An.* III 4. Recall that, in this sort of transition, (a) there is no affection of an underlying subject or substrate, since the thinking capacity is just a (highly educated) intellectual blank and none of the beings before it thinks, and (b) the object of thinking, which is supposed to come to be present where there was previously this blank, is not a natural thing but an immaterial essence. On this interpretation, Aristotle would be speaking of nature only as the most prominent subclass of things that involve transition quite generally. His point then would be that wherever there is transition there must also be potentiality and actuality,[86] including the entirely immaterial transition from potential to actual thinking. This interpretation would also allow us to preserve the deductive reading of the passage. Aristotle would apply a general principle about all transitions—not only physical ones in the narrow sense, but also immaterial ones, such as the change of relational properties. According to that principle, all transitions require an underlying potentiality (matter, passivity) as well as a productive cause. At any rate, since it is clear from *An.* III 4 that thinking is a non-standard case of affection, which I have interpreted as a non-natural, instantaneous presence of an essence (or the replacement of an immaterial, intellectual, blank by an immaterial object of thinking), we can rule out an inclusion of

[85] For more on this interpretation, I refer the reader to Chapter 6 (Section 3).

[86] Aristotle does discuss transitions that are not transitions in the strict, physical, sense in *Phys.* VII 3, especially 247b1–248a9 (Ross). There he argues that thinking states (*noêtikai hexeis*) are not physical changes but like relational states in that they come about instantaneously *when certain qualitative changes occur*: "what is potentially knowing becomes an actual knower not by itself undergoing change in any way but by virtue of the presence of something else. For when the particular happens, [the knower] knows in a way the universal by way of the particular" (*Phys.* VII 3, 247b4–7). To be sure, *An.* III 4–5 does *not* speak of this relation between underlying natural processes and the acts of thinking they underlie (which bears some resemblance to the relation of supervenience: see, e.g., Everson 1999, Wedin 1993, and Caston 1993) but solely about the transition from potential thinking to actual thinking: i.e., about what happens once all the underlying processes that enable thinking occur in the appropriate way. *Physics* VII 3 does *not* talk about this. The chapter is devoted to the physical changes that *underlie* thinking acts, one of its main points being that these acts are not themselves physical changes.

thinking in the domain of nature in the narrow sense of the realm of matter and change.[87]

When understood in this way, claims (i) and (ii) are quite straightforward.[88] The capacity for thinking is potentially its object, and for every potentiality there is a corresponding actuality. Hence, necessarily, since there is potential thinking, there is active thinking, which produces all thoughts by acting on the corresponding capacity. This, if straightforward, is of course a very abstract statement. It tells us nothing about the specific way in which active thinking is supposed to act on its passive counterpart. This is where claim (iii) becomes relevant. For it seems that claim (iii), which Aristotle does not argue for, gives us some information about the particular way in which active thinking makes the capacity for thinking actual.[89] According to that claim, active thinking does not act on the capacity by way of an episodic affection, either by changing it or by imposing a form or specific content on it, but rather like a state (*hexis*) that is exclusively responsible for making it actual. This is at least what the comparison with light suggests.

In Aristotle's theory of vision, light (*phôs*) is defined as the actuality of the transparent body insofar as it is transparent. Light is not a body but a state (*hexis*; *An.* III 5, 418b19) of the transparent body that either is, or perhaps results from, the presence of some fiery body in it. This presence makes the transparent body actually transparent: that is, it makes it possible for the transparent body to be seen through so that the outer boundaries of the transparent body (the colors) become visible (*An.* II 7, 418b9–20). Light so understood is a state of the transparent medium that makes potential colors become colors in actuality. But how exactly does the state of light act as a productive cause of the actuality of colors? It does so by its presence (*parousia*; *An.* II 7, 418b16 and 20) in the transparent body which serves as the

[87] Another way to take the argument is to understand it as Hermann Bonitz suggested: namely, as deriving the claim about the existence of a maker/matter distinction in the soul as *emerging from* the fact that all nature exhibits this distinction (on the basis of a parallel formulation in *Pol.* I 3, 1254a31–32: *ek pasês tês phuseôs*. See *Index Aristotelicus*, *s.v.* φύσις, 835b56–58). But that interpretation makes the necessity claim look rather weak.

[88] Here I am cutting a long story short. But to me it seems obvious that Aristotle is not introducing two different things but rather two modalities of one and the same thing: namely, thinking. The unfortunate tendency in the literature since antiquity to reify different parts of *nous* or even *nooi* (cf. Cassirer's complaints about this 1932: 168) may go back to Alexander of Aphrodisias who—no doubt only in order to be as clear as possible—enumerates different kinds of thinking and gives them different names, three altogether, both in his own *De anima* (*An.* 80.24 ff.) and in the *De intellectu* (*De Int.* 107.11 ff.).

[89] I would like to remind the reader of what I stressed in Chapter 1 as well as at the beginning of this chapter: namely, that Aristotle is not concerned with the explanation of the volitional preconditions of thinking in *De anima*. These preconditions (i.e., our wishing to think) pertain to us as acting persons (i.e., as psycho-physical unities); they are "common to body and soul" and are an *explanandum* of his theory of the soul (see *An.* I 5, 409b13–17, which lists *logismous* "reasonings"—i.e., some sort of rational thinking—among its *explananda*). On why the light example is not an illustration of the cause of the transition from first potentiality to second potentiality, or not primarily, I refer the reader to Kosman (1992: 346–348).

medium of sight.[90] This means that light makes potential colors actual not like episodic change does. In an episode of change, as we have seen, a form gets transmitted from the agent to the patient of change. It is an episode of change because it is finite and limited. In other words, it has a *terminus a quo* and a *terminus ad quem*, which mark the beginning and endpoint of the episode respectively. Once the patient of change possesses the form transmitted by the agent, the process ends. Light, by contrast, makes potential colors actually visible not by conveying any visible content or a given form to them but simply by being present in their environment as a standing condition of their visibility. If we apply this to active thinking in a manner that abstracts away from the physical implementation of the state of light, then the idea of the comparison must be that active thinking makes potential thinking actual by its sheer presence and not by conveying any content to it. For, if active thinking did convey the content of thinking (the actual essential forms of things) to potential thinking, then active thinking would not behave in the way light does but rather in the way colors do. But Aristotle did not compare the causality of active thinking with colors but with light.[91]

The comparison with light makes it clear, then, that active thinking does not act on potential thinking in an episodic way by conveying the essential forms of things or other intellectual content to it; active thinking acts on potential thinking simply by being present as a standing condition for thinking. Since there are, furthermore, no causal conditions for the existence of active thinking that are comparable to the fiery body in the analogous case of light, we can safely assume that the presence of active thinking does not depend on any conditions. Its presence is a standing condition for thinking that does itself not depend on any other condition.[92] What the comparison with light is supposed to show is the way in which active thinking is responsible for turning potential thinking into actual thinking, and not more. If I am right, even to say that active thinking "illuminates" potential thinking, as many commentators do,[93] would go beyond what the comparison is supposed to show. Is active thinking a state (*hexis*)? This is not what Aristotle says. Rather, he says

[90] A discussion of the meaning of the term in Aristotle and its subsequent reception can be found in Teichmüller 1873.

[91] Still, W. K. C. Guthrie understands the comparison in precisely this way: "As the senses are called into activity by the external object perceived, so our *nous* whose objects are within it, is directly activated by the supreme, supracosmic *nous*, or God" (Guthrie 1981: 327). Light is not an external object of perception. See also next footnote below.

[92] This is confirmed by the later statement that "it is not at one time thinking and at another time not thinking" in *An.* III 5, 430a22. Michael Wedin infers from the fact that light can fail to be present during darkness that active thinking can fail to be actual as well (Wedin 1988: 178). This gets the comparison wrong. Aristotle does not compare light and active mind but rather the way in which light makes colors visible and the way in which active mind makes potential essences in the minds of thinkers actual essences. The fact that light can fail to be present when the source of light is not present is irrelevant to the comparison.

[93] See, e.g., Burnyeat 2008: 41, and Christopher Shields, who speaks of active mind "illuminat[ing] the conceptual space between an object of reason (*noêton*) and the reason (*noûs*) which grasps it" (Shields 2016: 321 ff.)

that it acts: "on account of making all things like a state (*hôs hexis tis*)." And it makes good sense not to identify active thinking with a state because, among the different meanings of *hexis* listed in the corresponding entry in *Metaph.* IV 20, there is not a single one that does not construe the term in such a way as to imply the existence of a subject of the state, which then either is a "having" of something by that subject, an accidental property, or a "having" in the sense of the actual exercise of a dispositional state of the subject, such as a virtuous or vicious state. But there is no indication in the text nor any reason to suppose that active thinking has a subject that is distinct from itself. For, if that were the case, it would be an accident of its subject and this in turn would impose a condition on its existence and its actuality.[94] Hence, what the statement in *An.* III 5, 430a15, about active thinking acting "like a state" says is that active thinking acts on the capacity for thinking in a non-episodic kind of way, without conveying any determinate content to it, and only by way of its sheer and unconditioned presence. The expression "like a state," on this reading, qualifies only the way in which active thinking acts on potential thinking.

This, however, is not how the comparison with light is usually understood in the literature. The comparison is often taken to be a rich analogy between colors, sight, and light on the one hand, and potential thinking, essential forms, and active thinking on the other. Such readings clearly go well beyond what the text says.[95] But

[94] Active thinking is not a virtue either. Virtues are states possessed by entities that can also fail to act virtuously (for passages, see *Index Aristotelicus, s.v.* ἀρετή, 92a55 ff.). So, while theoretical thinking by human beings is surely an intellectual virtue for Aristotle, the active thinking we are talking about here as the cause of the actuality of our capacity for thinking is not a virtue. Franz Brentano took Aristotle's usage of the expression "*hôs hexis tis*" in *An.* III 5, 430a15, as decisive evidence for his thesis that active thinking is part of the human soul arguing that active thinking is an accidental property of the human soul (Brentano 1867: 170). But he also thought that it is a human capacity (1867: 171). Apart from simply sounding wrong (why would active thinking, which according to 430a18 is essentially actual, be a capacity?), this interpretation relies on a contextually questionable reading of "like a state" in *An.* III 5, 430a15. *Hôs hexis tis* can, of course, be taken to mean "as a certain kind of state." But if Aristotle were in this context talking about the possession of an accidental attribute, the example of light would be ill-chosen.

[95] Here are notable examples (with no pretension to exhaustiveness). Michael Frede compares the light in 430a15 to the intelligibility of things, which he takes to be equivalent to their conceptual order and, ultimately, to their first principle. This principle, according to Frede, is God taken as the source of the intelligibility of everything. Thus, he argues, the fact that we have an adequate thought (a "concept" in his parlance) of something (a human being in his example) is made possible by the conceptual order of things and by the first principle of that order in particular. He writes: "Ce qui fait que le concept est adéquat c'est son appartenance à tout un système de concepts, parmi lesquels apparaissent des concepts antérieurs et plus fondamentaux, qui nous rendent capables non seulement d'expliquer le concept d'un être humain, mais aussi d'expliquer les êtres humains eux-mêmes et leur comportement. Ainsi toute pensée présuppose tout un système de concepts, d'hypothèses, d'explications" (Frede 1996b: 389–390). This sounds right: we do not come to understand essences in isolation from other essences and all knowledge presupposes an intelligible order of things. And both for Plato and for Aristotle the first principle of that order is plausibly something divine. What I do not see, however, is how Frede's epistemic story can be justified with reference to the light example in *An.* III 5, 430a15. The example illustrates the way in which the active intellect acts so as to turn the potential essences in the minds of potential thinkers into actual essences. I do not see how the *content* of an actual thought—i.e., the supposition that God exists as the first principle of the intelligibility of things ("la présupposition de son existence, et les explications par rapport à lui," 390)—can help to answer that question. Having an actual thought

however that may be, the particular way in which active thinking turns potential thinking into actual thinking—namely, as a standing, non-episodic condition ("like a state")—makes the thesis that active thinking is a part of the human soul, which is not always active, extremely unlikely. And Aristotle's statement, a little later in the text, that active thinking is actual "by its essence" (*An.* III 5, 430a18) rules it out altogether, given that being essentially actual for Aristotle is incompatible with being a capacity. Now, typically, interpretations of *An.* III 5 are classified according to whether they conceive of active thinking either as a part of the human soul or as an impersonal and divine kind of thinking.[96] I agree that this is an important difference

about the existence of God presupposes that there is an actual thought in one's mind. But the question was how we come to have actual thoughts in the first place. Aristotle's account of thinking in *An.* III 4–5 *presupposes* the possession of the relevant knowledge to be activated (*An.* III 4, 429b5–10). Aristotle's light example does not regard the *content* of thinking. The same objection applies to Myles Burnyeat, who says: "How does the immortal intellect help us? How does it make things intelligible to our mortal minds? Simply by existing, I would suggest, by being what it is: an eternal intellect constituted, like any other intellect, as a system of concepts. The difference is that the divine intellect is a system (better, perhaps, *the* system) of absolutely correct concepts. As such, the deity does not need to act on us from up high, but merely to illuminate the intelligible forms, somewhat in the way light, simply in virtue of being what it is, illuminates colours and makes them actually visible to us" (Burnyeat 2008: 40–41). David Charles identifies active thinking with the *order* of universals: "If the analogy is sustained, what it is for a universal to be active will be for it to occupy a given niche in an organized structure in which each of the relevant universals is active. The active intellect, so understood, will be the organized structure in which each of the relevant universals is active. As an intellect, it is the appropriate locus, the 'place for such forms' (*An.* III 4, 429b2 ff.). However, unlike Plato's sun, the active intellect is not itself a distinct object. By analogy with light, its role is as the abiding and structured space in which distinct universals themselves are active" (Charles 2000: 134). This interpretation is vulnerable to the same set of objections. The fact that there is an order of universals does not address the question how potential thoughts come to be actual. Charles also speaks of universals as being like thoughts "in God's mind" (Charles 2000: 134n34; Charles 2021: 222n41). As a thesis about Aristotle's conception of God's thinking, this seems intrinsically doubtful (unless one, with *Metaph.* XII 9, *identifies* God with these universals, which however is difficult to maintain with matter-involving essences of types (2) and (3)). It is more likely that the intelligible order of things, for Aristotle, is a consequence, or a side-effect, of the order of actual things. All the above interpretations (with the possible exception of Frede, who is not entirely clear about this) assume that God's thinking is rich in content beyond the thinking of its own self, and even comprises all essences/universals. But there is no positive evidence in the text for this reading either in *An.* III 5 or in *Metaph.* XII 9 (on which see Menn 2012: 443 ff.; Wedin 1988: 241 ff.). I submit that, on Aristotle's account of active thinking, this reading is also impossible. Active thinking, as we will see, is an essence of type (1). As such, it is completely devoid of matter, while the thinking of essences of types (2) and (3) necessarily requires matter. God, if understood as an essence of type (1), would be prevented from thinking such essences. Lindsay Judson, in his commentary on *Metaph.* XII, suggests that God can think all essences of things because they form an essential unity which can be thought indivisibly on the alleged grounds that the essences of natural hylomorphic compounds are likewise taken to be unitary objects by Aristotle in passages such as *Metaph.* VII 12 and VIII 6, in spite of consisting of parts (Judson 2020: 238). But Aristotle does not argue in those chapters that the *essences* of hylomorphic substances consist of parts but only that their *accounts* (*logos*) do. Essences and their accounts are not isomorphic in their structures (see this chapter, Section 3).

[96] Alexander of Aphrodisias famously argued that active thinking is divine thinking itself (*An.* 89.17–91.06; *De Int.* 110–113). Other more recent interpreters in this camp are Guthrie 1981: 322–330 (with a short overview of positions in the literature), Schmitz 1985: 236, Lear 1988: 135, Johansen 2012: 239 ff., and Buchheim 2016: 277. Most interpreters since Themistius (at least) are inclined to think otherwise, however. They either conceive of active thinking as a part, or in some way an aspect, of the human soul (102.30–103.19)—to name only a few: Thomas Aquinas (*In An.* § 734), Brentano (1867: 171), Ross (1961: 45), followed by Horn (1994: 104), and Wedin (1988: 179–195)—or they conceive of it not as an

by which to classify interpretations of *An.* III 5.[97] But I would like to add a further, perhaps more important, criterion by which to classify the relevant interpretations. This is whether or not they conceive of active thinking as conveying any specific content (objects or forms), and actual essences of types (2) and (3) in particular, to potential thinking. On the interpretation advanced here, as we have just seen, this is not possible. On this point the proposed interpretation departs both from most recent and from most of the older interpretations. On the proposed interpretation, active thinking, in making potential thinking actual, does not convey any content or object to it.[98] At the same time, as the light example shows, active thinking is supposed to be responsible for the actual presence of the essential forms in epistemic agents. It remains to be seen how this can be the case.

Let us return to the text. On the above account of the way in which active thinking acts on potential thinking—as a standing condition, not in an episodic way, and without conveying the object of thinking—it should become a pressing question how Aristotle can say that the object of thinking, which in the case of essences of types (2) and (3) is only potentially present, acts on the capacity of

active thinker at all, but as the body of knowledge items that "constitutes the patrimony of knowledge belonging eternally, as Aristotle believes, to the whole of humanity" (Berti 2016: 144, 148, who traces his view back to an anonymous view reported by Themistius, *In An.* 102.30–33) or, like Ronald Polansky (2007: 646–665), as first actuality knowledge possessed by a human thinker acting as an unmoved mover of their knowledge. For a discussion of this family of views (labelled the "social interpretation" by him), see Zucca 2019, 146–149. Zucca's own view that the active intellect is not the knowledge, but merely the *content*, of the knowledge of the "system of first principles" (150–153) is open to objections similar to those made against Menn's interpretation discussed above (Menn 2020). A further problem is that an eternal presence of the actual essences of all things (or their principles) does not go together well with Aristotle's claim that active thinking is separate from matter, as that would seem to entail that active thinking cannot think hylomorphic essences.

97 For a concise and judicious overview of the main historical interpretations in terms of that difference, see Shields' commentary (Shields 2016: 312–317) and Caston 1999: 199–201. For a scheme of classification plus an informative overview of the relevant interpretations, see Miller 2012: 321 combined with endnote 47. The views according to which active thinking is either the body of eternal scientific truths or the first actuality knowledge of an individual cognitive agent are, in my judgment, incompatible with the text of *An.* III 5, which says that active thinking is both thinking and actual by its essence. For a concise, chronologically ordered report of the major interpretations since antiquity (up to his time), see Kurfess 1911.

98 Here is an alternative argument for the same thesis. My contention that active thinking does not act in an episodic way on potential thinking leaves us with two interpretative options. *Either* active thinking thinks all the essences of types (2) and (3) actually and eternally (all essences are "thoughts in the mind of God") *or* it does not think essences of types (2) and (3) at all. On the former option, active thinking would, as it were, constantly "broadcast" all the essences of things and the job of human thinking would be equivalent to "tuning in" to receive the right information appropriate to one's mental representations. This cannot be right, however. In his solution to the second difficulty Aristotle has affirmed that the essences of types (2) and (3) before they are actually thought by human thinkers exist only potentially (*An.* III 4, 430a6–9). In addition, there is no textual evidence that active thinking thinks essences of types (2) and (3). By contrast, there is evidence for the thesis that it is thinking only itself, to the exclusion of things with matter. This leaves us with the second option as the only viable one. On the earlier history of the conception of ideas as thoughts in the mind of God and especially the relation of that conception to Aristotle's conception of *nous*, see the still very interesting discussion offered in Krämer 1967: 127–191.

thinking (*An.* III 4, 429a14–15, 429b24–25; *An.* III 5, 430a24–25), and how he can maintain that the thinking capacity is affected by the object of thinking (*An.* III 4, 429a14–15, 429b3–5). As we have already seen in the discussion of the first difficulty in *An.* III 4, one part of the answer is that in the case of thinking "acting" and "affection" acquire a special, non-physical meaning. What remains to be seen is how this affection is supposed to work, what the role of active thinking amounts to: that is, how thinking comes about.

But before I come to discuss this, let us take stock of what has been established so far from *An.* III 4–5:

(i) Potential thinking (i.e., the human capacity for thinking) is the capacity to take on all objects of thinking. It is a mere blank (even if highly educated, it is "none of the beings" before it thinks), but potentially all the objects of thinking (*An.* III 4).[99]
(ii) Active thinking brings it about that this potential thinking becomes actual thinking; the former acts on the latter so that the latter becomes the objects of thinking (*An.* III 5).
(iii) Active thinking acts on potential thinking (makes it actual) in a non-episodic way by its sheer presence and without conveying any particular content of thinking (*An.* III 5).

This set of claims is quite abstract, and it does not help us very much in seeing how active thinking can make our capacity for thinking think in actuality. But if we add, as a further claim, a thesis that Aristotle will make explicitly later in *An.* III 8, 431b22–23[100]—namely, that all things are either materially extended objects of perception or immaterial objects of thinking—and if we further add the thesis that active thinking is an essence of type (1)—that is, a self-thinking essence (*An.* III 4, 430a3–5; *An.* III 5, 430a17–23)—we obtain a more interesting set of claims. Together with the above, these claims will allow us to construe an informative account of how active thinking turns potential thinking into actual thinking:

(iv) Active thinking is an essence of type (1). It is exclusively thinking itself as its object.
(v) All beings are either material objects of perception or immaterial objects of thinking.

The most important difference with respect to the previous set of three claims is that now, with the addition of (v), there are only two kinds of beings, so that we can say that for each being, if it does not fall into one class, it will have to fall into

[99] Of course, this is the second actuality.
[100] See the discussion of *An.* III 8 offered in Chapter 5.

the other. And, with the addition of (iv), something important about the character of active thinking is introduced: namely, that it is an eminent thinking being (i.e., an essence of type (1)), which is to say that it is an entirely immaterial and cognitively completely self-transparent thinking act. Claim (iv) makes it clear that active thinking has no object or content whatsoever other than itself. From (i) we know that potential thinking is "none of the beings at all" in actuality but potentially all the objects of thinking, which potentiality we here described as an "intellectual blank." Applying the bifurcated ontology of (v), we can furthermore say that potential thinking is neither a materially extended being (this has been explicitly denied by Aristotle in *An.* III 4) nor, as of yet, any object of thinking in actuality. However, it is also not equivalent to a nothing at all, given that it is the pure and immediate potentiality of an object of thinking. This, as I will argue now, opens up the possibility for an interpretation according to which potential thinking is receptive of the object of thinking in virtue of the fact that it is neither materially extended nor any object of thinking in actuality.

In what follows I will try to sketch an account of how human thinking of essences of types (2) and (3) comes about. I will ask two questions: what does "potentially the object of thinking" mean? and: what is the role of active thinking in human thinking?

6.2 What does "potentially the object of thinking" mean?

To address this question, I will have to briefly recall what Aristotle says elsewhere about the necessary enabling conditions of human thinking. This is not because I think that potential thinking is identical with the enabling conditions of thinking (as tend to do those who identify potential thinking with *phantasia*)[101] but because I want to contrast the potentiality of thinking with its enabling conditions as sharply as possible. Strictly speaking, accounting for these conditions—like accounting for psychophysical episodes generally—falls outside of the purview of *De anima*, as I have argued above. This presumably is also why Aristotle does not mention the enabling conditions of thinking in our passage. However, as we will see, a minimum of information about them is necessary to see in which direction Aristotle's argument is heading.

For all we know about Aristotle's conception of the second potentiality of human thinking, we can be fairly certain that he thinks of it as involving highly specific acquired states. They are acquired through painstaking and time-consuming processes of education, intellectual training, learning, and scientific research. The second potentiality of thinking, apart from its bodily preconditions (which are

[101] See, e.g., Philoponus, *In An.* 11.9–10; Brentano 1967: 167, 173 ff.

on the level of first actuality), as we have seen, also requires highly specific volitional, representational, and linguistic conditions. At least in standard cases of the thinking of essences, the cognitive agent must have the right mental and linguistic representations and must have the actual wish to know.[102] Potential thinking, as in (i), is the state that *results when all enabling conditions of thinking are in place*. Now, in his account of thinking in the *De anima*, and especially in *An.* III 7–8, Aristotle focuses almost exclusively on the representational conditions of thinking: namely, on what he calls *phantasmata*. But he chooses to do so not because he thinks that the other conditions of thinking are unimportant. Rather, I suggest that he focuses on them because this is where the bodily enabling conditions of thinking and actual thinking come "closest" to each other. Apparently, Aristotle thinks that the right mental representations result as achievements of the other enabling conditions of thinking and that they are in this way "proximate" to actual thinking. He seems to think that the right language, learning, and scientific research all contribute toward forming the right mental representations in the minds of potential thinkers, so as to make them immediately receptive of the essences of things. On this hypothesis, the mental representations of essences are, as it were, only the tip of the iceberg of all the other necessary conditions for actual thinking, which importantly include previous successful scientific research.[103] In addition, potential thinking in (i) is not to be conceived as potentially being all objects of thinking at once but rather as potentially being one object of thinking at each given point of time.[104] Hence, the intellectual blank that results from the matterlessness of the cognitive agent is not likely to be simply matterlessness without further qualification. Put differently, it is not a nothing at all but a highly qualified and very specific matterlessness of a cognitive agent's educated representational state, which will moreover have to have some determinate object. The cognitive agent's educated representational state prior to actual thinking will have to be about some specific thing.[105] And if this state regards essences of types (2) and (3), it will have to be about a certain kind of material object.

[102] "Wish" here translates *boulêsis*: namely, rational desire. See *An.* III 4, 429b5–10; *An.* II 5, 417b24–25.

[103] Cf. *An.* III 4, 429b9 (*prin mathein ê heurein*). This same thought is nicely put by Trendelenburg: "*omnes illas, quae praecedunt, facultates in unum quasi nodum collectas, quatenus ad res cogitandas postulantur, νοῦν παθητικόν dictas esse iudicamus*" (1877: 405). On that—reasonable—hypothesis, Aristotle is certainly not an "abstractionist" in the sense of someone who thinks that universals are contained in perceptual content and only need to be isolated by way of abstraction (for a classical criticism of that view, see Geach 1957: 11 ff.). Rather, he thinks of abstraction as one among many necessary conditions for thinking to come about. Much less does Aristotle think that abstraction is something that is done by active thinking itself, as was famously maintained by Thomas Aquinas (*In An.* § 730). On research as an enabling condition of actual thinking, see below.

[104] For more on this, see Chapter 5 (Section 2).

[105] The capacity for thinking is the underlying capacity for the thinking of each of the different types of essences. They are different kinds of what fundamentally is one and the same capacity of receiving immaterial essences.

Such highly qualified "matterless" representational states about material objects are abstract mental representations. By Aristotle's lights, "abstracting" means "taking away" features from our mental representations which originate in the perception of external physical objects, so as to isolate certain other features of these objects that one wishes to focus upon. This is achieved by taking away the features that are accidental to what one wishes to focus upon. Thus, when we "take away" features in abstraction, there is a criterion at work by which we distinguish relevant from irrelevant features. This criterion is the aspect of the objects we wish to focus upon, the "insofar as" (*qua*) we contemplate the object. In the case of our mental representation of the essence of a given perceptual object, *x*, the criterion under which we select, or deselect, its perceptual features is what *x* is *qua* itself: that is, *qua x*. The moving cause of that process of abstracting away from all the features of *x* that *x* does not possess insofar as it is *x* is our wish (*boulêsis*) to know the essence of *x*. Below I will have to say more about that wish and how it allows us to relate to essences even before we actually contemplate them.[106] If successful, the result of such a process of abstraction is the mental presence of only those perceptual features of *x* that it minimally possesses insofar as it is *x*.[107] In this way, mental abstractions are matterless (in the highly qualified way of not exhibiting features over and above the features they possess *qua* being what they are) and they are about something determinate: namely, *x*. In the *Physics*, Aristotle describes mathematical abstractions as "separating in thought" (*chôrizein têi noêsei*). And his examples for features we "take away" in mathematical abstraction are "movement" (*kinêsis*) and "matter" (*hulê*), which presumably leaves us with quantitative features of things.[108] The science of physics, by contrast, abstracts from physical objects to isolate the features they possess insofar as they are physical: which is to say, insofar as they are subject to motion and composed of matter and form (*Phys.* II 2, 194a12–17; see *An.* I 1, 403b9–19, which is also what we get in *An.* III 4, 429b14: *tode en tôide*). What is important is that both mathematics and physics work on the basis

[106] On the so-called "*qua*-operator," see *Metaph.* XIII 3, 1077b17–1078a17; *An.* III 7, 431b12–17; *Phys.* II 2, 193b22–194b15. For Aristotle, all intellectual thinking requires abstraction. An important difference between kinds of scientific abstraction lies in the way and degree to which material features are separated from their matter. For an overview of the issues around mathematical abstraction and the *qua*-operator in Aristotle, see Mendell 2004. Bäck 2014 offers a monographic treatment of abstraction in Aristotle.

[107] One can immediately see that to perform such an operation successfully requires much more than simply leaving irrelevant perceptual features out of our mental representations. It will also involve comparisons, induction, and many other complex mental operations that I cannot go into here. As mentioned above, certainly, abstraction from perceptual features by itself is not *sufficient* for the immediate receptivity to essences. It will also require volitional, linguistic, and many further conditions such as experience, induction, and trial-and-error research methods of defining the items one desires to know as they are partly described in sections of the *Posterior Analytics*. But, as I have argued above, Aristotle seems to think that these other conditions are all preparatory for, and productive of, the right mental representations. Abstraction and scientific research are certainly not incompatible ways of reaching essences (as Jiménez seems to think; Jiménez 2017: 4).

[108] *Phys.* II 2, 193b30–35. The passage in *Metaph.* XIII 3, 1077b17–1078a17 contains many examples of aspects *qua* which we can engage in abstraction.

of such abstractions. (The discussion in *Phys.* II 2 also suggests that we can isolate in thought whatever aspect we wish to.) This allows us to conceive of our educated cognitive "blank" or matterlessness, which we said was the immediate potentiality for an object of thinking, as the outcome of such a process of abstraction (or separation in thought): that is, as a mental representation that is devoid of matter; not, however, unqualifiedly so, but devoid of matter only within a certain domain—namely, within the domain the cognitive agent wishes to isolate in their process of abstraction. For instance, a cognitive agent's potentiality for thinking the essence of cats would consist in the specific and highly qualified matterlessness of the relevant mental representations (*phantasmata*) of cats as they result from her having abstracted away from all the perceptual features that are not characteristic of cats *qua* cats. These will be only those perceptual features of cats that are jointly necessary and sufficient for capturing the being of cats. To be sure, this would have to involve some modicum of matter (via quasi-perceptual *phantasmata*), since these abstract representations will have to be of cats, a materially extended species, after all, with an essence of type (2).

On this hypothesis, the human capacity for thinking (i.e., the potentiality of the object of thinking) of essences of type (2) would be "none of the beings at all" only in the highly qualified sense of being none of the beings at all with reference to the particular domain the cognitive agent is focusing upon. With regard to the potentiality for thinking the essence of cats, for instance, this entails reference not to any particular cat, or to any particular feature of any particular cat, but only to those perceptual features of cats that are jointly necessary and sufficient for capturing cats *qua* cats. Such would be the mental representations human thinkers typically employ when they actually think the corresponding essence of cats. They are the immediate potentiality for the thinking of the essence of cats. Or so I have argued.

Two qualifications are in place here. First, the focusing on these isolated ("abstract") features would not be a part of the immediate potentiality of thinking, which is only the qualified "blank" resulting from it, but it would be part of the enabling conditions of thinking, the explanation of which falls outside of the scope of *De anima* and is part of the explanation of the "actions and affections common to body and soul" (about which more below). This qualification is important because it preserves Aristotle's claim that the human capacity of thinking is "none of the beings at all before it thinks." It would, moreover, still be the case that the potentiality for thinking essences of type (1), should there be such a potentiality, would require an unqualified matterlessness or intellectual blank—unlike the thinking of essences of types (2) and (3). This preserves the principle of the corresponding degrees of separateness from matter in the thinker and the objects of thinking presented in *An.* III 4, 429a21–22, extending it (as is plausible) to the capacity of thinking. Second, as we have seen as well, the matterlessness or intellectual blank in cases of essences of types (2) and (3) is relative to a certain matter-involving essence. This means that focusing on a particular type (2) essence by abstraction necessarily involves some modicum of matter (in the case of mathematical objects, mathematical extension) in the corresponding *phantasmata*. But this should not present a problem since Aristotle has qualified his initial claim of the matterlessness of the capacity of thinking in *An.* III 4, 429a21–b5, by introducing matter-involving essences of types (2) and (3) in *An.* III 4, 429b10–21, and corresponding degrees of involvement of matter on both sides of the thinking relation in 429a21–22, thus making the matterlessness of thinking a matter of degree. The fact that Aristotle does not bother to explain how the thinking of matter-involving essences of types (2) and (3) takes place, I submit, is most likely due to the fact that in *De anima* his interest is, first and foremost, to offer an account of the *capacity* of thinking *per se* rather than a full account of how human beings come to think. In sum, I argued that, for Aristotle, the immediate potentiality of the object of thinking of essences of types (2) and (3) is the qualified matterlessness as it issues from adequate abstract mental representations of objects of the kinds corresponding to (2) and (3), while the potentiality of thinking essences of type (1), if there is such a thing, is an unqualified matterlessness.

6.3 What is the role of active thinking in human thinking?

As we have seen, active thinking acts "like a state" by its sheer presence. I have also argued that active thinking is active thinking of type (1), a self-thinking separate essence. If we now suppose (a), the thesis that the intellectual blank of the immediate capacity for thinking, by virtue of its specific matterlessness in relation to a certain domain (cats in our example), is immediately receptive of the corresponding essence, what account of the actualization of potential thinking results? How does the thinking of the essence come about?

Let us recall two previously introduced assumptions. First assumption: what is not materially extended, but is not a nothing at all, must be an object of thinking (this is claim (v) above). Second assumption: there are corresponding degrees of separateness from matter in the *per se* objects of thinking and the corresponding kinds of thinking (*An.* III 4, 429b21–22). Hence, if an object of thinking has no matter at all, then it must be an essence of type (1) and be thinking itself.[109] How, then, does the thinking of essences of types (2) and (3)— the essences of given hylomorphic compounds—come about? I have argued that the qualified matterlessness of our mental representation of a given hylomorphic compound *x qua x* is equivalent to the immediate potentiality for the presence of *x*'s essence.

[109] See also the previous discussion of the different types of essences in *An.* III 4, 429b10–21. The different kinds of essences differ along a continuum with respect to their separability from matter. Objects without matter are identical with their being (*An.* III 4, 429b11–12); in their case thinking and the object of thinking are the same (*An.* III 4, 430a3–6).

I have also argued that—somehow—active thinking is responsible for the essence of *x* coming about in the cognitive agent's soul, provided the cognitive agent is in a state of immediate potentiality for the essence of *x*. But how does the presence of a self-thinking essence of type (1), "like a state," bring about the essence of *x* in the mind of a potential thinker? How can its presence explain the presence of the essence in a cognitive agent as an object of thought, which is to say as possessing the typical qualitative characteristics of the content of human thinking, such as universality, necessity, and objectivity?[110] To be sure, Aristotle does not tell us *expressis verbis* how he thinks the presence of active thinking can have that effect on human thinking agents. But he offers us the conceptual resources to understand how this can be the case, which is what I will try to explain in the next paragraph.

From the above assumptions it is possible to infer the following role for active thinking in the actualization of potential thinking. Suppose that there is an immediate potentiality (i.e., a capacity) for thinking the essence of cats in a human cognitive agent. This immediate potentiality, as we have seen in (a), will be a highly qualified and abstract sort of educated matterlessness with relation to the agent's representational states about cats *qua* cats. Such abstract representations involve matter, but only as much matter as an adequate abstract mental representation of cats *qua* cats requires.[111] In all other respects, that abstract mental representation of cats *qua* cats is an intellectual "blank," and so is matterless in the aforementioned qualified way. Now, our first assumption derived from claim (v) has it that whatever is matterless, if it is anything at all and not a nothing, must be an object of thinking. This means that our abstract matterlessness in relation to cats is an immediate potential object of thinking.[112] If we now add the "state-like" presence of active thinking, then there is both active thinking, which is thinking itself, and the immediate potentiality of an object of thinking, which results from the (qualifiedly) matterless abstract mental representation of cats *qua* cats. With this, both the agent and the patient of the (immaterial) actualization relation Aristotle has introduced in *An.* III 5, 430a13–15, are present. Therefore, necessarily, the agent will act on the patient[113] and active thinking will bring it about that the immediate potentiality of the object of thinking in the cognitive agent will be made actual. It will be made actual by active thinking's presence, which presence will obtain in the cognitive

[110] This list of features is meant to be representative, not exhaustive. For the feature of unity, see Chapter 3 in this volume.

[111] Of course, such mental representations are not to be confused either with the essences they represent or with universals. Aristotle is a realist about essences (see below, Chapter 5), which are the causes of the observable features of the things whose essences they are. Aristotelian essences of hylomorphic compounds are also not constitutive parts of these compounds. Essences are not elements, as Aristotle famously argues in *Metaph.* VII 17; rather, they are immaterial causes and principles for their organization. Universality is a feature of thinking (in the narrow sense), not of mental representations.

[112] I say "immediate" or "proximate" because no further preparation of the mental representation is required for the act of thinking the essence to come about (cp. *Metaph.* IX 7). In a mediated sense—i.e., allowing for further intermediate preparatory steps—it is, of course, also true of the objects of perception that they are potential objects of thinking (*noêta*).

[113] See *Metaph.* IX 5, 1048a11–15.

agent's soul to the degree in which the object of her thinking is without matter (given that only its matterlessness is the immediate potentiality for thinking; see *An.* III 4, 429a21–22). The result of this, I suggest, should be the presence of an actual object of thinking of type (2) or (3) in the soul of the cognitive agent, which was what thinking was supposed to be from the very beginning of the discussion (i.e., from 429a13 onward). Note that active thinking's role here is strictly confined to making the potential object of thinking an actual object of thinking in the cognitive agent's soul; there is no suggestion that active thinking thinks that object (the essence of cats in our case) as a content of its own thinking. Rather, the content of the object of thinking is determined by the mental representation of the object whose essence the cognitive agent wishes to think (cats). The mental representation, provided it is well formed, then, is responsible for both the content of the object the cognitive agent wishes to think and its (qualified) matterlessness.

The cognitive agent's capacity for thinking is not affected by the essence of cats in the way in which a cognitive agent who perceives a cat is affected by that external cat. This is so, first, because there is no actual intelligible essence of cats before that agent engages in thinking it and, second, because even if there were such an actually existing essence to act on the cognitive agent, there would be nothing in the agent to be positively affected by it, as the immediate potentiality of the object of thinking was said to be a matterless blank (which, as we have seen, cannot be affected). Instead, the essence of the cat comes to be in her instantaneously and without literal physical affection. This non-literal (non-physical) character of the affection of potential thinking, as I've argued above, was the very point Aristotle wanted to drive home with the wax-tablet example in the solution to the first difficulty at the end of *An.* III 4: the affection of the capacity for thinking consists in the "popping up" of an essence where there was previously a qualified intellectual blank. The presence of the essence in the thinker should therefore result from the combination of the qualified matterlessness of the mental representation of cats *qua* cats and the presence of active thinking in some other way, not by physical affection. Active thinking, as we have seen, is a self-thinking essence of type (1), which is entirely transcendent: that is to say, none of the things in the physical world. That, however, should already suffice to explain why thinking takes place in the cognitive agent: given Aristotle's bifurcated ontology, to create the appropriate kind of qualified matterlessness in the mind of a cognitive agent just is the removal of (material) obstacles that prevented her from accessing active thinking, given that the qualified matterlessness resulting from the mental representation of the cat *qua* cat is not nothing at all but the immediate potentiality for the thinking of the essence of the cat. At the same time, the resulting episode of thinking will fall short of being an episode of active thinking of essences of type (1) for as long as her intellectual blank will not be completely devoid of matter. The result, I suggest, is the presence of an essence of types (2) and (3). Note, however, that in cases of qualified matterlessness, such as in our example of the thinking of the essence of cats, the presence of active thinking does not contribute anything to the specific content of the object of thinking, to what it is concerned with; it only acts as the cause of the actual presence of the essence of cats in the cognitive agent; it does not cause her to think of *cats*. But how can active thinking explain the actual presence of the essence of cats in a thinker if it does not think, or otherwise contain, the essence of cats, so as to affect the thinking agent with that essence? On the interpretation advanced in this chapter, Aristotle holds that adequate abstract mental representations of *x qua x*, provided they result in the right "intellectual blank," lead, to the extent in which they are matterless, to the presence of active thinking in the thinker, while at the same time exerting a filtering (or screening) effect on active's thinking's full presence (by being specifically about *x*). The suggestion is that the result of that filtered and qualified presence of active thinking in her should be the presence of the essence of *x* in her. This is so because it is *x*'s matter *qua x* that is supposed to filter the presence of active thinking in her. Active thinking thus contributes not with the object of thinking—what hylomorphic essence it is concerned with—but with the objectivity, universality, and necessity that characterize her thinking of *x* as the thinking of *x*'s essence. And that same presence of a (highly qualified) matterlessness in the cognitive agent that explains what essence her thinking is concerned with can also explain why the mental presence of essences of types (2) and (3), in spite of its actualization by an essence of type (1), fails to be self-transparent: namely, because it involves matter.[114]

This is the most viable account of how the thinking of essences of types (2) and (3) comes about that I can construe on the basis of Aristotle's doctrine of corresponding degrees of separateness from matter in the objects and kinds of thinking expressed in *An.* III 4, 429b21–22. All in all, Aristotle's statements in *An.* III 4–5 strongly suggest that active thinking will be present in cognitive agents *to the extent* to which their corresponding potential objects of thinking are free from matter (in the aforementioned, highly qualified and domain-restricted way).

6.4 Objectivity, universality, and necessity

How can a qualified matterlessness as it results from the mental representation of *x qua x*, as just described, plus the presence of active thinking account for human thinking in the sense of the presence of the universal, objective, and explanatory essence of *x* in the soul of a cognitive agent? Regarding explanatoriness, Aristotle says

[114] See *An.* III 4, 429a20–27. We can, of course, further speculate as to how active thinking can have that effect on a human thinker. But Aristotle does not give us much to speculate about in this regard. What we can be fairly confident about, however, given the doctrine of corresponding degrees of separateness from matter in the objects and the kinds of thinking introduced in *An.* III 4, 429b21–22, is that active thinking will be present *to the extent* to which the corresponding potential object of thinking is free from matter.

many times that essences are causes and principles of the things whose essences they are. He is an ontological realist about essences of hylomorphic compounds, and he thinks that they exist independently from our thinking (before they are actually thought, however, they exist only in potentiality as objects of thinking, as is said in *An.* III 4, 430a6–9).[115] Given this, the question of how active thinking can account for the explanatory features of essences seems ill-posed to Aristotle. The world simply is such that there are essences of things. Active thinking does not make the essences of things have their causal and explanatory power (at least not *qua* its role in human thinking), but rather only reveals it. But the other features of human thinking—universality, objectivity, and necessity, which no doubt are no less prominent features of human thinking—do seem to bear important relations to active thinking. They add, as it were, a new quality to human thinking over and above the mental representations (*phantasmata*) that bring about the immediate potentiality of thinking. In what follows I will try to tentatively sketch a possible way in which active thinking may contribute toward the explanation of these features.

Let us recall the basic ingredients of Aristotle's account: active thinking is entirely transparent self-thinking, essentially actual, and separate (i.e., transcendent). The separateness of active thinking is important here because it may explain why our thinking can take a standpoint that is not the standpoint of any of the things in our physical world or of any combination thereof. The separateness of active thinking has the potential to account for the objectivity of our thinking. It can provide our mental life with a position or a dimension that is, as it were, located outside of all materially extended things. It makes the content of our thinking factual in the sense of holding *per se* and independently of the point of view of any particular person. And since we as thinkers, according to Aristotle's theory, can access this dimension at least to some extent, we can to some extent take a perspective on things that will be different from the perspective of any materially extended thing, while at the same time being numerically one and the same for all of us. We can achieve this intellectual feat because we all have the capacity to bring ourselves into the state of qualified matterlessness which is the immediate potentiality for thinking one thing or another, while the active thinking we thus can have access to is the only other thing there is. The objectivity of any act of human thinking of essences, therefore, may be explained with reference to the transcendent

[115] This is understood differently, e.g., by Jung who maintains that the essences of hylomorphic objects are "always actual because they are the formal principles of things" (Jung 2011: 101), while the hylomorphic objects of thinking are potential only in the sense that they are not themselves engaged in actual thinking (80). But the fact that the essences of hylomorphic objects are always actual as the formal principles of things does not mean or entail that they are actual objects of *thinking*. And the fact that actual objects of thinking are universals, and universals are in the soul, additionally confirms that the essences of hylomorphic objects are not actual objects of thinking before they are thought by a thinking agent.

standpoint of active thinking.[116] This, or something like this, is how Aristotle's account of active thinking could contribute toward accounting for the objectivity of human thinking. It could do so by way of its transcendent uniqueness in connection with the fact that it is accessible to all thinkers.

These same features of active thinking may also contribute to the explanation of the universality of human thinking. Universality is a characteristic feature of the objects, and therewith also of the acts, of human thinking. In the case of essences of types (2) and (3), the universal is not just that which is predicated of many or of all;[117] rather, it is the "one besides the many" in the sense of the one essential being of *x* that is common to all *x*-things insofar as they are *x*.[118] Aristotle's account of thinking as interpreted here has the resources to account for this feature too because, in his theory, human thinkers have the capacity to bring themselves into the state of potentially thinking the essence of *x* by way of abstract mental representations. These representations, as we have seen, capture only those perceptual features of *x* that are characteristic of it *qua x*, and not *qua* being any particular instance of *x*. In this sense, the mental representations capture features that apply to all and any given exemplar of *x*. That by itself does not make these representations universal, to be sure. Still, it seems to me that contact between immediate potential thinking of *x* and active thinking, which is numerically one, could account for the presence of the one essential being of *x* in the sense of the one besides the many *x*. In this way, the combination of active thinking's singularity with the general applicability of our mental representations could account for the universality of human thinking.

As for necessity, we have seen that Aristotle conceives of essences as causes of the being of the things whose essences they are. Thus, in scientific explanations, we can explain why *x*-things are thus and such with reference to the definition of the essence of *x* as their cause.[119] Such scientific explanations are necessary and universal. Aristotle says many times, explicitly and unequivocally, that the universal is explanatory, and he even says that the more universal an account is, the more explanatory it will be.[120] Where does he think that the necessity of the universal thoughts of essences comes from? We will hear below that active thinking is essentially actual (*An.* III 5, 430a22). It always thinks in the sense that it is not the case that it thinks at one time and not at another, which is to say that it thinks eternally.[121] With this, active thinking is necessary in the strongest sense of "necessary"

[116] I leave out the question whether, and if so why, and in which way Aristotle does conceive of a plurality of acts of active thinking.

[117] *Int.* 7, 17a39 ff.

[118] *Posterior Analytics* II 4, 73b26–74a4, and II 19, 100a7; cf. *An.* III 4, 429b10–21.

[119] *Posterior Analytics* I 3, 23–25.

[120] E.g., *Posterior Analytics* I 2 and I 24, 85b23–86a21; cf. *Metaph.* I 1, 981a5–b6.

[121] It is *not*, *pace* Berti, a way of saying that it does not think at all (Berti 2016: 144). All ancient and modern interpreters took this sentence as an attribution of thinking to active thinking. Some of those, however, who advocated the idea that active thinking is a part of the human soul excised the negation *ouch* in 430a22 and read: "But it sometimes thinks and sometimes does not think." (Sophonias reads it

that Aristotle allows for: namely, in the sense of not allowing for the possibility of being otherwise.[122] Given that the objects of human thinking are actual only for as long as human cognitive agents have contact with active thinking, the latter's absolute necessity can account for the necessity in human thinking.

Hopefully, in this (or some other similar) way Aristotle's theory of human thinking can be seen as offering the resources to account for the aforementioned prominent features of thinking: contact between the qualified matterlessness that results from our representations of *x*-things insofar as they are *x*, which produce the immediate potentiality for our thinking *x*'s essence, and active thinking can account for the mental presence of *x*'s objective, universal, and necessary essence in the soul of a cognitive agent.

On the above account, active thinking is a non-physical and entirely self-transparent thinking act of type (1). It is neither personal nor episodic but an eternal and transcendent act of thinking. Its eternal presence "like a state" makes it that the potential objects of thinking that we produce via our abstract mental representations become actual objects of thinking. Also, all human intellectual thinking depends on the transcendent presence of active thinking.[123] Without it there would be no human thinking of essences, including the thinking of essences of types (2) and (3), and there would be no objectivity in human cognition either. If what I have suggested is along the right lines, Aristotle explains the fact that we human thinkers can think essences by way of our access to active thinking. On his account, we can access active thinking to the extent to which we are able to free our mental representations of hylomorphic compounds from their matter. This, as I have argued, happens when we focus and prepare our abstract mental representations in such a way as to produce what I have called a qualified intellectual blank with relation to a given kind of hylomorphic compound (provided, of course, all other enablers and necessary conditions of thinking are in place). That matterless intellectual blank, due to its specific and highly qualified domain-specific matterlessness, is the immediate receptivity and potentiality for the actual presence of the essence of that kind of compound (where the essence is the simple cause of the manifold features such hylomorphic compounds exhibit insofar as they are what they are: i.e., insofar as they are of such an essence). In short: in Aristotle's bifurcated ontology, either things are materially extended hylomorphic compounds or they are entirely immaterial active thinking (= essences of type (1)).

without negation and so does Ps-Simplicius; Torstrik excises it; for a full report, see Siwek 1965: 333, who also excises it and claims that seventeen manuscripts do not read the negation.) Rodier has a judicious discussion of the issue (Rodier 1900: 446–465). See Szlezák 1979: 185 ff. for the possible influence of the passage on Plotinus; see Blumenthal 1996 and Perkams on interpretations of the passage in late antiquity (Perkams 2008: 134 ff.).

[122] *Metaph.* XII 7, 1072b11–14.

[123] This is also what Alexander of Aphrodisias seems to claim (in *An.* 89.6–8), even if (apparently) for different reasons.

While the latter are entirely transparent for thinking, the former are potential objects of thinking only, which, due to their material extension, are moreover not fully transparent for thinking. And the essences of hylomorphic compounds are possible objects of thinking only because there is active thinking of type (1), which is unqualified matterlessness.[124] This is so because its presence actualizes the immediate potentiality for thinking which is produced by our abstract mental representations of hylomorphic compounds, turning it into actual thinking of an essence of type (2) or of type (3). When all other necessary requirements are fulfilled, and we prepare our mental representations of a given hylomorphic compound *x* in such a way as to bring about the right qualified matterlessness with regard to *x*, then that qualified matterlessness will not be a nothing at all but the immediate potentiality for the essence of *x*; due to the presence of active thinking, which is always actual "like a state," our potentiality for the essence of *x* will be made actual and the essence of *x* will be present in us. In this way, on Aristotle's account, active thinking makes all things intelligible to us. But it does not act on us by imposing *x*'s essential form on us (it does not have, or otherwise contemplate, that essence), but merely by providing the actuality of our thinking, bringing objectivity, universality, and necessity to our qualified matterlessness with regard to *x*; what our thinking will be concerned with—the essence of *x*—is determined not by active thinking but by us.

Education and learning, the shaping of our abstract mental representations, volitional attitudes, linguistic abilities, experience, research activities, and everything else that jointly lead us to the second potentiality of our capacity for thinking, are, in a way, processes that rid us (or, rather, our mental representations) of matter. But they do so in a highly refined, controlled, and educated way. On Aristotle's bifurcated ontology, the goal of these processes is to remove the material and perceptual obstacles in our cognitive apparatuses that prevent us from accessing matterless, active thinking. Given the material implementation of our cognitive apparatuses, and their dependence on perception and perception-dependent mental representations (involving *phantasia*), that removal will be gradual and probably never fully completed during our lifetime. Indeed, to grasp active thinking *per se* will most probably be impossible for us.[125] And the cause of this would lie in our very condition as materially implemented intellects, as Aristotle seems to imply in the following passage:

[124] Or, as *An.* III 6, 430b2–26, puts it in a similarly contrastive way, separate self-thinking is a "cause without opposite." See Chapter 6.

[125] Even if Aristotle never says so in so many words, see *An.* III 7, 431b17–19, where he says that the question whether it is possible for us to think a separate object of thinking with a capacity which is not separate from the body should be investigated later. This is likely to refer to a corresponding investigation in first philosophy. More on this front in Chapter 4. Johansen interprets *An.* III 5, 430a22–23, in such a way that we can think separate substances of type (1) *per se* (Johansen 2012: 240–241). More about this below.

> For as the eyes of bats are to the blaze of day, so is the thinking capacity (*nous*) in our soul to the things which are by nature most evident of all. (*Metaph.* II 1, 993b7–11, trans. Ross, slightly modified)

Nevertheless, and however indirect our access to active thinking may turn out to be, it is by virtue of our capacity for accessing active thinking that we are capable of having objective thoughts, so as to grasp things as they are in themselves (as opposed to how they appear to us). So much for my hypothesis about how Aristotle explains how human thinking of essences of types (2) and (3) comes about.

Is it Aristotle's theory? There are good chances that it is. All the claims that are relevant to the formulation of this hypothesis can be extracted from *An.* III 4–5 and *An.* III 8, and the hypothesis does not conflict with any other primary text. Most importantly, the proposed reconstruction allows us to attribute to Aristotle an explanatory account of how thinking comes about with its characteristic features of objectivity, universality, and necessity.[126]

Meanwhile, there is still the open problem of the self-thinking of the thinking of essences of types (2) and (3), which is left unanswered at the end of *An.* III 4. I have argued that the account of how human thinking comes about is a prerequisite for addressing this problem. Now, with the above hypothesis in place, I can venture to give an answer. Above I argued that the mental presence of essences of types (2) and (3) in an actual thinker, because it involves matter, is not self-transparent. The thinking of such essences is not an act of thinking that thinks itself.[127] Still, Aristotle believes that there is a way in which the thinking of essences of types (2) and (3) can be an object of human thinking. The answer I would like to propose is that the structure intrinsic to our capacity for thinking the essences of hylomorphic objects becomes apparent to our thinking *ex post facto*: that is, as a result of us having had many thoughts of essences of types (2) and (3). That structure will consist in the features that our actual thoughts of such things exhibit as they emerge from thinking other objects: namely, essences of types (2) and (3), and all other objects of thinking as they emerge from the exercise of our capacity for thinking such objects. They will be features that emerge in the actual thinking of such objects, without being, however, properly speaking features of the objects that we

[126] What is intellectual error on the suggested account? It is to engage in *false* abstractions. which fail to access active thinking in the right way. A false abstraction is an abstraction in which we abstract away from certain material or perceptual features of a given hylomorphic domain in such a way that the resulting mental representation does not adequately capture, or correspond to, the essential being of that domain. How do we know whether we have gotten it right? I suppose that the answer to this question lies in Aristotle's account of scientific explanation. Real essences have explanatory powers that false abstractions do not have, even if they at first may appear to have them.

[127] Of course, while we are thinking we are usually aware that we think. That awareness should, however, not be confused with the transparency of thinking thinking itself; rather, it seems to be our *perception* that we think.

think but of our thoughts of them.[128] Examples: contrariety, unity, serial order, the rules of inference, and so on. They will, to be sure, be true of things, whose ordering structures they are, but they are neither hylomorphic objects nor their essences.[129]

6.5 The intrinsic nature of the active cause of thinking

What follows in *An.* III 5 is a direct continuation of the previous text. Aristotle lists the intrinsic features of pure and matterless active thinking:

> And this kind of thinking is separate, unaffected, and unmixed, it being an actuality by its essence. For what acts is always more valuable than what is acted upon, and the principle is more valuable than the matter. Actual knowledge is identical with its object, and potential knowledge is prior in time in the individual; however, on the whole [it is] not even [prior] in time, but it is not at one time thinking and at another time not thinking. When it is separated, it is only what it really is,

[128] This is how I understand *Metaph.* XII 9, 1074b35–36, where Aristotle says that the thinking (i.e., of ordinary objects, not active thinking) seems to be of itself "*en parergôi*," as a side-effect of its thinking of other objects. The facts of logic, for instance, do not seem to be objects in the way things are, and neither do ordering principles such as oppositions, ordered series, and so on; they seem to be the structures that emerge from the actual thinking of things. Arguably, then, these are examples of structures that are intrinsic to the thinking of hylomorphic objects.

[129] Lewis 1996 has mounted an impressive battery of philosophical objections (and some solutions) to different conceptions of the alleged identity of the subject and the object of thinking in Aristotle. But most of them lose their bite once it becomes clear that Aristotle maintains only that an essence of type (1) can (and also necessarily will) think itself directly. Human thinking of essences of types (2) and (3) does not think itself in any other way than indirectly, as has been pointed out above (it is not "straightforwardly reflexive" in Lewis' idiom). And Aristotle also nowhere claims that it does. It seems to me that many of the problems Lewis discusses arise because there is a tendency in the literature not to distinguish with sufficient clarity between the matterlessness of essences, on the one hand, and the matterlessness of the things they are the essences of, on the other. All essences for Aristotle are matterless; but that does not mean that they are all essences of type (1). That, however, is what, e.g., Miller seems to take it to mean when he invokes consciousness to account for the self-knowledge of thinking (Miller 2012: 320). Consciousness and self-knowledge are different things (see also the discussion in Gregoric and Pfeiffer 2015). In *An.* III 4, 430a3–6, and its parallel passages (*An.* III 5, 430a20; *An.* III 7, 431a1; *Metaph.* XII 9, 1075a2–5), Aristotle claims direct self-knowledge exclusively for essences of type (1). Now, unlike the latter, essences of types (2) and (3) do involve matter because they are the essences *of* material objects, which means that the thinking of them involves mental representations. This makes them, to some extent at least, cognitively opaque. The thinking of them therefore fails to be a candidate for direct self-thinking. As regards the alleged identity between the object and subject of thinking, on the account here proposed, an episode of human thinking, say, of the essence of flies, will, for the duration of that thought, not be identical with any fly but with the actual intelligible essence of flies. Thinking the essence of flies (*pace* Miller 2012: 320) is not an instance of thinking's self-thinking, even if the cognitive agent may be conscious of her thinking. What if two human individuals simultaneously think the essence of flies? In that case, the thinking of both will be identical with the actual intelligible essence of flies. Is this a problem? Their mental representations will still be different, perhaps not only numerically but also qualitatively, even if perhaps only slightly, and to that extent their subjective thinking will be different as well (even if their linguistic representations of that essence in their definitions should be the same). But even if they were perfectly identical, I can still see no problem in saying that both have the exact same thought. On the contrary. On this point, see also Gregoric and Pfeiffer 2015.

> and this alone is immortal and eternal. But we do not remember, because this is unaffected, whereas passive thinking is corruptible; and without the former, it does not think anything.[130]

"This kind of thinking" clearly takes up the "and another [i.e., kind of thinking]" (*ho de*) in line 430a15, which is the grammatical subject of the previous clause, so there can be no doubt that Aristotle is speaking about active thinking in the sense of type (1) thinking here. To say that active thinking is separate, unaffected, unmixed, and an actuality by its essence is to say what active thinking intrinsically is, even if the bulk of the predicates consist of negations.[131] This is apparently meant to contrast with the short description in the previous section where Aristotle pointed out what active thinking does extrinsically: namely, insofar as it acts on potential thinking. The last sentence ("But we do not remember . . .") then returns to a very brief discussion of the relation of human thinking to active thinking.

The features that apply to active thinking *per se* are separateness, unaffectedness, unmixedness, and being actuality by its essence. While unaffectedness and unmixedness are very close to each other, they are not exactly the same thing. Unaffectedness amounts to the feature of not being affected by any agent (see *An.* III 4, 429a15, 429a29–b5), whereas unmixedness entails purity in the sense of not having anything in common with anything else (see *An.* III 4, 429a18, 24; 429b23–24, 28). I have already spoken about active thinking's specific kind of separateness (i.e., non-physicality).[132] While its intrinsic essential actuality has not been mentioned previously, we can see that this feature connects with the causal role active thinking plays in relation to potential thinking and also how it does so: namely, in the way a state does. The disanalogy with the state of light (and indeed, as far as I can tell from the list in *Metaph.* V 20, with any state) lies in the fact that all such states occur in nature and as such are contingent, whereas active thinking is not a natural state but a transcendent, necessary, and immutable *act.* This is captured by the formulation "an actuality by its essence." Again, there is a sharp contrast with potential thinking.

Presumably, for Aristotle, all these predicates of active thinking are eminently positive from an axiological point of view, which is probably why he adds that the active part and principle is always more valuable than the passive part.[133] All these features so far are well motivated by what has been said in the first part of *An.* III 5, so it is not absurd to say that they can almost be inferred to be intrinsic properties of active thinking from the effect that active thinking has on potential thinking as described in the previous section. Active thinking is an entirely non-physical and

[130] *An.* III 5, 430a17–25.
[131] As has been observed by Cassirer (in Cassirer 1932: 176).
[132] I refer the reader to the discussion of the first part of *An.* III 4 offered in this chapter, Section 2.
[133] I take the *gar* to introduce a piece of background information. I do not think that it introduces an explanation of the previous clause.

essentially actual thinking act. I add that it is thinking itself in the sense of being an essence of type (1), even though Aristotle does not say so explicitly here (though in the next sentence he will). He also does not have to say so, given that being an act of thinking implies having an object of thinking, which, considering both the unaffectedness and unmixedness of this active thinking, can only be identical with itself.[134]

The next sentence is repeated *verbatim* at the outset of *An.* III 7 (431a1–3).[135] It underlines the identity of the act of thinking with its object in scientific thinking (which is to be understood here in the ontological sense discussed above, as the thinking of objects of thinking that are separate from matter). It says that in scientific knowledge, when actual, thinking and the object of thinking are one and the same (see the similar formulation in *Metaph.* XII 9, 1074b38–1075a5), which is to say that it is a *per se* feature of active thinking that it is an essence of type (1).

Another *per se* feature of active thinking is that it is eternally and uninterruptedly (or continuously) thinking. But before Aristotle turns to this feature, he apparently wants to get a familiar objection out of the way. This is the objection that active thinking's eternity seems to clash with the familiar observation that, from an ontogenetic perspective, potential thinking comes before actual thinking. It is a trivial observation that individual thinkers are potential thinkers before they think in actuality. Aristotle's response consists in a change of perspective away from individual thinkers to a global perspective. From this global perspective ("on the whole"), the seeming temporal priority of potential thinking vanishes because it is true to say that (the ontogenetic histories of individual thinkers notwithstanding) there was never a moment in time at which active thinking was not actual. Active thinking is not sometimes thinking and sometimes not: that is, it is always actively thinking and has no potentiality (see the parallel of this argument in *Metaph.* XII 9, 1075a7–10).

This underlines eternal continuity as a *per se* feature of active thinking. Aristotle's brief discussion most likely picks up at least part of the implicit question posed above in *An.* III 4, 430a5–6, where it was said that the reason (*aition*) for the fact that "it does not always think" has to be investigated. This remark followed immediately on a statement very similar to the one made in *An.* III 5, 430a19–21: namely, that in things without matter object and the thinking of the object coincide. The reason would seem to be twofold. There is a kind of thinking that does always think: namely, active thinking. But our human thinking of essences of types (2) and (3) involves potentiality and this makes it discontinuous and episodic. The reason for this is that the subject of human thinking is different from its object, and that prior to the act of thinking both subject and object of thinking are in a

[134] See the similar argument in *Metaph.* XII 9, 1074b22–1075a5.

[135] Which is not to say that Aristotle cannot repeat himself, and especially in the case of a slogan-like statement about the structure of the thinking of separate essences. For more on this doublet, see Chapter 4 (Section 2).

state of potentiality. This is why human thinkers require both the presence of active thinking to bring them into actuality, and mental representations (*phantasmata*) to present the object of thinking to them in a quasi-perceptual way. Presumably, it is the frailness of the latter—not of thinking itself—and generally the weaknesses of our physical enabling conditions of thinking that are responsible for our inability to think continuously.[136]

The ensuing clause "when it is separated, it is only what it really is, and this alone is immortal and eternal" has presented interpreters with difficulties. What is the subject of "when *it* is separated" (*chôristheis*)? On our interpretation, the subject is the same active thinking which Aristotle has been speaking about in the previous section: the separate eternal thinking act of an essence of type (1). The expression "when it is separated" must not be taken to imply that active thinking of type (1) was ever in a state in which it was not separate and mixed with the human soul *per se*. Rather, Aristotle, in continuation with his list of *per se* features of active thinking, *contrasts* these *per se* features of active thinking with human thinking and with the effect (extrinsic for it) active thinking has on human thinking in particular. He has taken this comparative perspective already in the previous sentence, where he has said that active thinking is not sometimes thinking and sometimes not thinking, which comes with the implicature that our human thinking is episodic in this way of sometimes thinking and sometimes not thinking.[137] Hence, the meaning of "separated" here is not to be taken as entailing that non-separation can be a *per se* feature of active thinking. Rather, it is an accidental feature of active thinking that there are human thinkers who access it via their qualified matterlessness in the way canvassed above. Active thinking remains unaffected throughout, acting "as light" does. This means that "separation" and "non-separation" in the case of the separation and non-separation of human thinking from active thinking are to be conceived *asymmetrically*. Active thinking is in no way affected by the fact that there are human thinkers whose potentiality for thinking is made actual by it. "When it is separated," therefore, need not imply that active thinking has at some point been united with human thinking or even that human thinking *is* active thinking; it only serves to signal what active thinking of type (1) is *per se* and not in relation human thinking. In this respect, the affection of human thinkers by active thinking of type (1) works just like other cases of causation by unmoved movers:[138]

136 See, e.g., *EN* VIII 15, 1154b24–31, where this is pointed out quite clearly; cf. *EN* X 8, 1178b33–35.

137 Caston 1999 observes that all the *per se* attributes of active thinking listed in *An.* III 5 are also attributes of God in *Metaph.* XII 7–9 and elsewhere. In his *De anima* Aristotle does not discuss the question whether active thinking and the God of *Metaphysics* XII are identical. But the list of attributes offered in *De anima* strongly suggests an affirmative answer, as Caston has pointed out.

138 As explained, e.g., in *Gener. Corr.* I 6, 323a12–33, where Aristotle explains that not all kinds of contact need to be reciprocal. If *X* has contact with *Y*, then this does not necessarily imply that *Y* also has contact with *X*. On the causation by way of unmoved movers, see Primavesi and Corcilius 2018: cxlvv–clx. Johansen (2012: 242n48) has an interesting, somewhat tentative discussion of the way the first unmoved mover causes thinking in Aristotle.

ASYMMETRICAL AFFECTION BY ACTIVE THINKING:
X is affected (actualized) by *Y*, but *Y* is not thereby affected (actualized) by *X*.

This asymmetry is possible in this case because active thinking of type (1) acts on the human potentiality of thinking as a state does "like light": that is, without acting on it specifically and/or by bestowing any content or form on it. It acts just by being there. Nothing changes in it in virtue of the fact that the human potentiality for thinking is actualized by its presence. There is no reciprocal interaction, only an asymmetrical "affection" of human thinking. The only affection in the literal sense that occurs in cases of human thinking should be the affection of the perceptual system by the mental representations involved in the thinking of essences. But this is a necessary condition of actual human thinking and part of its causal ancestry. The essences themselves exert no physical effect on human thinkers; they just come to be present in them.[139]

But, if this is correct, how do human thinkers establish *contact* with active thinking, if active thinking always remains in the same state? Put differently: how does our thinking "use" our perceptual capacities for the purpose of grasping essences, if active thinking does not, and could not, act on human thinkers (or on their perceptual apparatus) in the way human agents typically act on the tools they use: namely, by touching them with their hands? The short answer I would like to suggest is "by way of being a *goal* of human action." Humans can *desire* to cognize essences and they can desire to know them even when they are not currently cognizing them intellectually.[140] The motivational structure of such desires is asymmetric. It is that of a rational wish (*boulêsis*) for the *solution or an answer to a problem*, a kind of wish Aristotle calls *zêtêsis* (intellectual search, investigation). According to that motivational structure, an agent desires to know the answer to a theoretical problem of the following form: "what is the explanatory ground of phenomenon *X*?" This will relate the agent's desire to an object of thinking that is still unknown to the agent at the time: for example, the essence of *X*. Indeed, the agent will rationally desire to know this object of thinking *because she is ignorant of it*. Such asymmetrical rational desire is the motivational condition, and also the moving cause, of the mental representations and the other conditions that are up to us and that enable us to engage in actual episodes of thinking (in our example, to think the essence of *X*).

This yields the following conception of how thinking functions asymmetrically as a goal of human action and how our thinking thus "uses" the perceptual capacity (the idea being that this is how perception, in our endeavor of grasping the essences of things, is *teleologically subordinated* to thinking):

[139] See *An.* II 5, 417a27–29, 417a32–b2, 417b22–28; *An.* III 4, 429b5–10. Aristotle nowhere says that the enabling conditions of thinking necessitate actual thinking to come about. But he may have thought so. See *Phys.* VII 3.

[140] For more on how this works from a motivational point of view, see Corcilius 2009.

ASYMMETRICAL TELEOLOGICAL SUBORDINATION TO THINKING

X, the human thinking of an essence *E*, is "using" *Y*, a human agent's perceptual capacities (and everything that follows from it, including *phantasia*), by virtue of the fact that (i) *X* is the goal of the human agent's desire to grasp *E* as the solution to a problem, and (ii) that desire is the moving cause of the internal events and mental representations in the human agent that are the necessary conditions for the potentiality for the reception of *E* to come about in the agent.

On this asymmetrical conception of teleological subordination, human thinking can co-opt the capacity for perception without physically intervening in the natural world. It "uses" perception in virtue of being the *goal* of a human desire to grasp the essence of *E*. The important feature of this conception is that *X* can use *Y* by virtue of a desire for *X* in the agent who possesses *Y*, so that *X* uses *Y* as a means *via* the human agent's usage of *Y* for the sake of *X*, which is the object of *Y*'s desire. Thinking "uses" perception in virtue of the fact that human agents act for thinking's sake: they desire to think *E* and therefore do everything in their power that will make them think *E*.[141] Human thinkers establish contact with an active thinking by wanting to think.

The last bit of *An.* III 5, makes the famous statement: "but we do not remember." How can Aristotle say this, if he has just spoken of the *per se* features of active thinking? Why does he speak of us human thinkers here? What could be Aristotle's motives to speak about remembering here, given that we've just heard that active thinking of type (1) is not concerned with anything other than the thinking of itself? The answer is probably that he is trying to ward off the Platonic idea of recollection.[142] This becomes a natural suggestion as soon as we realize that Aristotle agrees with Plato that there is an immortal aspect of thinking *per se*, and that active thinking, moreover, is in some highly qualified way accessible to us (in the way mentioned above). The crucial difference is that Plato, unlike Aristotle, appears to have a conception of the immortal aspect of our thinking that is rich in content over and above the self-transparency of active thinking. On Plato's doctrine of recollection, the rational soul has acquired its non-empirical (in the sense of

[141] On teleological subordination of the perceptual part of the human soul under its rational part, see Corcilius 2023. Note that asymmetrical teleological subordination can by no means render superfluous the asymmetrical affection of the human thinking capacity by active thinking. *Both* are required for human thinking to take place. One is the motivational mechanism on a personal level to engage in a mental process which culminates in the actual thinking of an essence of types (2) and (3); the other is the actualization of the immediate potentiality for thinking in the cognitive agent. *EE* VIII 2, 1218a18–29, clearly talks about the former, even if about a special case thereof. Wedin—erroneously, I think—takes that passage to be about the latter (Wedin 1988: 218–220).

[142] See Cassirer 1932: 177–178, Fronterotta 2007, and Menn 2020: 140, who even writes: "the translation of *ou mnêmoneuomen* is 'the theory of recollection is false.'" Schmitz suggests an additional connection to the *Eudemus* fr. 5 (in Schmitz 1985: 240–243).

"non-perceptual") content prior to its descent into the body. This content is somehow stored in us as latent knowledge, and the process of learning consists in the retrieval of that content so as to bring it to consciousness again. Therefore, on Plato's view, the rational soul is a kind of storage place for non-empirical mental content; indeed, the soul possesses *all* such content, and it seems that it somehow possesses it as knowledge (this, at least, is how Aristotle construes Plato's doctrine in *Posterior Analytics* II 19, 99b26–27). Aristotle, unlike Plato, does not believe that active thinking thinks anything apart from itself. And neither does he think that the contents of our thinking of essences of types (2) and (3) are anywhere stored. He has already made this clear in *An.* I 4, 408b24–30: the contents of our thinking are our possessions as psychophysical compounds, and they are so only *insofar as we possess* the capacity for thinking. The intellect itself remains unaffected by our thinking. This is why there is neither memory nor any other surviving psychophysical affection after death. Aristotle is an actualist with respect to the content of thinking.[143] The final statement of *An.* III 5 ("because this is unaffected, whereas passive thinking is corruptible") states the reason why there is no content for human thinking to retrieve in active thinking. It is because active thinking has no content beyond itself, since to have any content beyond itself would imply being affected by, or mixed with, something else, which Aristotle has denied. Active thinking is not subject to affection, and hence not even to corruption: it is eternal and immortal. Our passive thinking, however, which Aristotle here again contrasts with active thinking, is affectable, at least to the extent that it can perish and cease to exist.[144] This happens when *we* cease to exist.[145]

[143] Of course, *we* do remember our thoughts, and memory has an important part to play in the psychophysical causal ancestry of human thinking. But the memory items corresponding to them are part of our perceptual system, which is bodily; they are not actual thoughts, and they stand in contingent relations to our thinking (*kata sumbebêkos*; *Mem.* 1, 450a22–25).

[144] The expression "*pathêtikos nous*," I submit, here refers to what above I have called the immediate potentiality for thinking, including its operations (and which I take to be the object of the definition in *An.* III 4; see also this chapter, footnote 107). Against this, Paul Siwek (following Brentano 1867: 175), claims that *pathêtikos nous* cannot be the potential intellect because he thinks that the latter is separable from the body. He then conjectures that it is the perceptual faculty (Siwek 1965: 335). See Cohoe 2022: 242, for a more recent version of this view. But it is not even clear whether all kinds of separability exclude perishability. Indeed, one could perhaps argue that something like this seems to be the point of Aristotle's account of the human immediate potentiality for thinking: a non-bodily receptivity for active thinking (even if highly qualified). As such, potential thinking, even if created by a body, would be non-bodily and in this sense separate from it. But be that as it may, the claim that *nous* is *chôristos* in *An.* III 4, 429b5, which is invoked by the above interpreters, does not quite say that potential thinking is separate; the statement picks up "*nous hotan ti noêsêi sphodra noêton*" in 429a3–4, which is an *act* of thinking. And it is true for Aristotle that actual human thinking contains a separate element, and especially so when it thinks separate substances.

[145] See *An.* I 4, 408b18–25; and, most importantly, *An.* II 2, 413b24–27: "which is why if that [i.e., what has the thinking capacity] is destroyed, it [i.e., thinking] neither remembers nor loves; for these did not pertain to thinking but to the common thing [i.e., consisting of body and soul] which died." Here, the subject of the sentence is not "we" but impersonal thinking. Still, I do not think that the point Aristotle is making here is very different from the point he makes in the above quote: there is an eternal act of thinking that somehow plays an important role in our thinking but that is not part of our personal existences as human beings. See also the discussion in Chapter 6.

The very last clause "and without it, it does not think anything" is best taken as saying that our passive capacity for thinking (our immediate potentiality of receiving essences) could not think anything without active thinking of type (1). "Without it" (*aneu toutou*) could also be taken to refer to our passive capacity for thinking. That statement too would be true for Aristotle. It would be expanding on the previous point and say that we do not remember also because our *passive* capacity of thinking is corruptible. However, in Aristotle *toutou* quite often does not refer to the last-mentioned congruent noun but just stands for "the former" (which normally would be *ekeinos*).[146] And I think this reading is preferable because it is trivial to say that human beings could not engage in episodes of thinking (in the narrow sense) without having the corresponding capacity, whereas the statement that our capacity of thinking could not think anything without active thinking seems entirely appropriate in this context. Aristotle is highlighting the key tenet of his theory of thinking that our capacity for thinking depends on active thinking of type (1).

[146] See Kühner and Gehrt 1898: II § 467, 11. That is presumably also why Horn's philological study of *An.* III does not even discuss the issue and simply takes *toutou* to refer to active thinking (Horn 1994: 107). Cassirer, by contrast, argues that *toutou* must be taken to refer to *pathêtikos nous* and then finds himself forced to conclude that active thinking is not a kind of thinking at all: "*denn die tätige Vernunft ist eben nichts anders als das Moment der Vernunft, das dadurch, dass es reine Energeia ist, das Denken in Tätigkeit setzt; sie enthält aber nicht selbst ein Denken*" (Cassirer 1932: 177). This seems desperate.

3

The principles of propositional thought

The unity and the function of *An.* III 6

1. Introduction

With the human capacity for thinking having been defined in *An.* III 4–5 (after the preparatory phase of *An.* III 3), what more is there to be said? Not much in the view of most scholars, who often treat *An.* III 6–8—and especially *An.* III 6 and 7—as scrappy and disconnected appendices of secondary importance.[1] The ambition of this book is, in contrast, to bring out the unitary argument of *An.* III 4–8, in which chapters 6–8 play indispensable roles.[2]

If there is such a unitary argument, then *An.* III 6 is the obvious place for raising the question about the kind of unity involved. There is little doubt that *An.* III 4–5 contains the core of Aristotle's account of human thought. If the argument of Chapters 1 and 2 is on the right track, then Aristotle has captured here the ultimate *explanans* and the very essence of human thought—without offering any full account of the respective *explananda*—that is, the phenomena of human intellectual life—let alone providing their proper explanations. What does he intend to add now in *An.* III 6?

In comparison with the following chapter, *An.* III 6 has a fairly clear structure, dividing naturally into three parts. First, Aristotle contrasts thinking of what he calls *adiaireta*—that is, the "undivided" or "indivisible" objects of thought—with "synthetic" propositional thinking which can be both true and false (430a26–b6). Second, he draws distinctions between different kinds of *adiaireta* (430b6–26). And then, finally, he claims that in the case of certain objects, apparently falling under the class of *adiaireta*, thinking can only be true (430b26–31).

Different versions of this chapter were presented at The Warburg Institute in London in 2018, at the Gothenburg University and the Eberhard Karls Universität Tübingen in 2019, and at LMU München in 2020. Many thanks to the audiences for helpful comments, especially to Mike Arsenault, Pavel Gregoric, and Pieter Sjoerd Hasper. I am particularly grateful to those who read and commented on earlier versions of this chapter: Andreas Anagnostopoulos, David Bronstein, Klaus Corcilius, Michel Crubellier, and Andrea Falcon.

[1] See, for instance, Christopher Shields' recent judgement about *An.* III 6: "This chapter, like the two following, is a bit scrappy. It does not follow upon the preceding chapter in any obvious way; nor does it bridge in an orderly fashion to the next" (Shields 2016: 330).

[2] Besides Chapters 4 and 5 in this volume, see also Corcilius 2020a on *An.* III 7 and Crubellier 2020 on *An.* III 8.

Aristotle on the Essence of Human Thought. Klaus Corcilius, Andrea Falcon, and Robert Roreitner, Oxford University Press.
 DOI: 10.1093/9780198921820.003.0003

The content of the chapter, moreover, overlaps to some extent with Aristotle's treatment of being *qua* truth in *Metaph.* VI 4 and *Metaph.* IX 10, and with his account of simple terms in *Int.* 1. That makes *An.* III 6 sound vaguely familiar. But, in fact, this only underlines the main question: *what is the chapter doing here?* Unsurprisingly, interpreters have puzzled since antiquity over both (1) the overall point—if any—this chapter is trying to make, and (2) its place within the larger plan of Aristotle's *De anima*.

(1) It might easily seem that *An.* III 6 does not really contain much of an argument. One might think of it as a rather disordered list of different objects of thought called *adiaireta* (or, even worse, different meanings of the word "*adiaireton*"). Aristotle seems to list simple concepts, undivided lengths, objects with a unitary form,[3] geometrical divisions such as points, movers of the spheres, and, as the icing on the cake, essences. This can easily look like an entry on *adiaireton* from Borges' Chinese encyclopedia. And the chapter was, indeed, approached in such a manner by, for example, Philoponus who openly professes in his *De intellectu* that any search for an overarching notion of *adiaireton* uniting this chapter would be in vain.[4]

(2) Moreover, one might have doubts about the role of the chapter in the larger plan of *De anima*. Such a list of different *adiaireta* would perhaps better fit *Metaph.* V.[5] And if it plays any important role in *De anima* at all, then it would have been better placed *before An.* III 4–5—at least if Aristotle were to adhere to the idea that activities are prior in account to capacities, and objects to object-related activities, as professed at *An.* II 4, 415a15–22.[6] *An.* III 6 looks like Aristotle's only extensive treatment of the objects of thought, and so, if it were in any respect important for his inquiry into *nous*, it would have to precede *An.* III 4–5. Such a consideration is behind Ps.-Simplicius' and Philoponus' conviction that while investigating *nous* Aristotle in fact *reverses* the order of inquiry as described in *An.* II 4, allegedly because in this case, unlike elsewhere, the capacity is better known to us than the objects.[7] The problem is that Aristotle is not only silent about any such methodological reversal in *An.* III 4–8: in *An.* II 4, the triad of the capacity for thinking (*to*

[3] Or *infimae species* under a different understanding of *adiaireta tôi eidei* (more on that below).

[4] See Philoponus, *De Int.* 65.57–67.16 and 86.14–22; cf. Philoponus, *In An.* 543.5–17 or Hahmann 2016: 210–215. Ps.-Simplicius (*In An.* 251.14–252.24) thinks that the list of *adiaireta* in the central passage (430b6–26) is almost entirely digressive and that it at best shows what the true *adiaireta*—allegedly, Aristotle's genuine concern in *An.* III 6—are *not*. For a criticism of such "catalogue" readings, see also Trentini 2016: 182–183.

[5] As a matter of fact, there is a certain overlap between *An.* III 6 and *Metaph.* V 6.

[6] See Chapter 1 (Section 5).

[7] See Philoponus, *In An.* 542.22–27 (cf. *De Int.* 64.41–45) and Ps.-Simplicius, *In An.* 248.21–249.4, the latter being still quoted approvingly by Rodier 1900: 467–468. Ps.-Simplicius' view is, in fact, a bit more complicated than suggested above, for he thinks that in *An.* III 4 Aristotle dealt with both the passive *nous and* its objects, and III 6 treats objects of the *agent nous*, exclusively, which was as such introduced and explored in *An.* III 5.

noêtikon), the activity of thinking (*to noein*), and the object of thought (*to noêton*) was already one of the three examples to which the prescription should definitely apply. So, Aristotle clearly does *not* think that we have any immediate access to *nous* which would save us from the difficulties of inferring to it from the respective objects and activities. This is an important difference between Aristotle's inquiry into *nous* and many later inquiries into "mind" that build on the assumption, shared by Ps.-Simplicius and Philoponus, that the "mind" is most directly accessible to itself. If *An.* III 6 is in its proper place in the manuscripts, then this calls for a different explanation.

The present chapter aims primarily at addressing the two issues just canvassed. Explaining why they proved, and continue to prove, so difficult, I argue that *An.* III 6 in fact contains a coherent argument, centered around a unitary notion of *adiaireton*, and that this argument plays an indispensable role in the larger plan of *De anima*. I start with the second issue in Section 2 and argue that, far from representing any methodological reversal, *An.* III 6 has a fairly determinate role in Aristotle's inquiry into *nous*, a role that is prefigured in his treatment of perception and in *An.* II 4 itself. It expands the account of grasping of essences as developed in *An.* III 4–5 by introducing other, secondary kinds of thinking, and thus it provides an indispensable bridge to Aristotle's discussions in *An.* III 7–8 and 9–11. Indeed, without showing how this expansion can be achieved, Aristotle's account of *nous* as the principle of human intellectual life in *An.* III 4–5 could easily be suspected of lacking any genuine explanatory power. And *An.* III 6 also has an important dialectical role: the discussion of propositional thought here brings to completion Aristotle's polemic against the traditional view that like is known by like (LKL) and so clears the way for the concluding summary of *An.* III 8. Moreover, *An.* III 6 is much more intimately bound to *An.* III 5 than previously acknowledged, and this connection helps to shed light on the central notion of *adiaireton*.

This last point leads directly to the other general issue, addressed in Section 3 of this chapter. I argue that although, for good reasons, it is difficult to find an entirely satisfying unitary translation of *adiaireton* as employed in *An.* III 6, this notion does have a unitary meaning which has yet to be properly understood, because existing interpretations are all too narrow. Roughly, *adiaireton* is any object endowed with such a kind of unity that it can be thought non-compositionally. This notion accommodates, in two different ways, both objects which can be thought as subjects and predicates of propositions (whether they are thought individually or universally) and objects which, in a way, transcend propositional thought, while constituting the ultimate ground for explaining propositions: that is, essences. *An.* III 6 builds a unitary argument around this broad notion of *adiaireton*. Aristotle develops here, on the most abstract level, an account of propositional thinking as a composition of thoughts of *adiaireta* into which propositions can be structurally divided, but whose unity is derivative from the unity of propositions because only propositional thoughts are complete thoughts, whereas thoughts of structural *adiaireta* are only potential or actual constituents of such complete thoughts. But propositions can be "divided" in a yet different sense: namely, by means of the question *why?* which in Aristotle's understanding is a way of asking for a middle term mediating between the subject and the predicate. This way of dividing leads, ultimately, to the *adiaireta* of the second kind—that is, essences—and Aristotle is eager to insist that the thought of these is endowed with a kind of unity that is not derivative from the unity of propositional thoughts; rather, it is in an important sense prior to it. This idea can help us appreciate the architecture of *An.* III 4–8 and the place of *An.* III 6 in it: Aristotle confirms here that *nous*, analyzed narrowly in *An.* III 4–5 as the power for grasping essences, can, indeed, play the role of the principle of *all* human thinking. But the unifying meaning of *adiaireton* as an object that can be thought non-compositionally is also helpful on a more local level insofar as it allows us to better understand how Aristotle's treatment of undivided lengths (430b6–14) fits into the argument of *An.* III 6, and more generally what logic governs the list of *adiaireta* in the central passage (430b6–26) as a whole.

What results from the proposed analysis is a picture of *An.* III 6 as Aristotle's move from the definitory account of the ultimate *explanans* of human intellectual life (provided in *An.* III 4–5) to a display of its explanatory power, aimed at confirming that the account captures what it is supposed to capture. *An.* III 6 introduces kinds of "thinking" which are considerably closer to our factual intellectual life than the grasping of essences, while exhibiting their explanatorily derivative nature. In this way the chapter lays the groundwork for Aristotle's discussion of thought from the perspective of the cognitive soul as a whole (rather than *nous* alone) in *An.* III 7 and for the concluding summary of *An.* III 8. *An.* III 4–8 turns out to contain a single, tightly unified, argument.

2. The place of *An.* III 6 in the larger plan of *De anima*

2.1 Expansion as in *An.* II 6 and *An.* III 1 (and *An.* II 4, 416b11–20)

The above-mentioned claim that in *An.* III 6 Aristotle reverses the methodology of *An.* II 4, applied before to nutrition and perception, is not only based on a mistaken idea about the starting point and the end point of his inquiry into thinking; it also seems to betray an inadequate understanding of Aristotle's treatments of perception and nutrition.

In fact, there are good reasons for thinking that the role of *An.* III 6 with respect to *An.* III 4–5 is prefigured in Aristotle's treatment of perception: not only in the relation of *An.* II 6 to *An.* II 5,[8] but also—and in fact more clearly—in how *An.* III 1 relates to *An.* II 12. Aristotle is happy first to offer a general account of perception (*aisthêsis*) and the perceptive capacity (*to aisthêtikon*) in *An.* II 5, and only then to provide an exhaustive list of perceptible objects (*ta aisthêta*) in *An.* II 6. Moreover, in what follows he is ready to put aside, once again, the "incidental" and "common" objects, focusing on the "exclusive" objects (*idia*) characteristic of each individual sense throughout *An.* II 7–11, and offering another general account "of all perception" in *An.* II 12, still innocent of any consideration of the common or incidental objects. Only then, in *An.* III 1 (425a13–b11), does he reintroduce the division from *An.* II 6 and finally offer—on a very abstract level and in a brief outline—an explanation of how perceptible objects other than the exclusive objects are perceived. Nobody thinks that this represents a reversal of the methodology announced in *An.* II 4. The truth is that in *An.* II 5, and again in *An.* II 12, Aristotle's reflections about perception and the perceptive capacity do draw on a consideration of its primary objects: these are, roughly, objects capable of acting on the perceivers and assimilating them, qualitatively, to themselves. The underlying idea seems to be that we only need a general consideration of the primary objects, because we are first providing the core account of the activity with respect to which the capacity (or part) of the soul in question is to be defined; only after doing so should we turn to other objects, classify them, and make sure that the capacity as defined before allows for explaining how these other kinds of objects are perceived. This makes perfect sense because Aristotle's account of how the common and the incidental objects are perceived depends on the core account of perceiving and not the other way round. Aristotle's procedure is thus perfectly compatible with the methodology of *An.* II 4 and his explanatory essentialism.

In fact, one can see this procedure anticipated in the comparatively brief treatment of nutrition in *An.* II 4 itself, although the individual steps are, admittedly, less clearly articulated than in his more extensive treatment of perception. Still, we can observe that after a preliminary criticism of predecessors who thought that nutrition can be explained without referring to the soul (*An.* II 4, 415b25–416a18), Aristotle turns at *An.* II 4, 416a18–b11, to a general *aporia*, very similar to the one addressed later in *An.* II 5 and concerned with the nature of the primary objects: is it by the like or by the unlike that living beings are nourished? In answering this *aporia* he introduces his general account of the nutriment, nourishing, and the nutritive capacity: the nutriment which is first unlike is assimilated by the nourished animal *qua* ensouled (the soul, as we learn a bit later, being "what nourishes" the body "by" the nutriment). Now, after presenting this core account of nourishing

[8] Polansky 2007: 473 rightly emphasizes this parallel (see also Delcomminette 2020: 158), but without making it clear in what sense exactly the treatment of objects in *An.* II 6 and *An.* III 6 is "fuller" than the "provisional" treatment in the preceding chapters. Ross 1961, Hamlyn 1993^2, and Shields 2016, in contrast, completely avoid the question of how *An.* III 6 fits into *De anima* and what it implies about Aristotle's methodology.

with respect to which the nutritive capacity is to be defined, Aristotle turns at *An.* II 4, 416b11–20, to distinctions between different "objects" of nutrition. Besides "nutriment" (*trophê*) conceived specifically as that which contributes to the preservation of the substance of each animal, one can also speak of that which makes the animal grow (*to auxêtikon*), and—depending on how the text is construed syntactically—possibly also of that which makes the animal generate (*to gennêseôs poiêtikon*).[9] Aristotle explains why it makes good sense to subsume all these under the same "nutritive" (or "generative")[10] capacity.

The situation at the beginning of *An.* III 6 is similar to that at the beginning of *An.* II 6 or rather *An.* III 1 (and *An.* II 4, 416b11). Aristotle has already provided his core account of thinking (i.e., grasping of essences), which allowed him to define *nous* as a part of the soul distinct from the perceptive part. His definitory account of *nous* here has already been based on a consideration of its primary objects: that is, essences (most explicitly at *An.* III 4, 429b10–22).[11] In *An.* III 6, then, Aristotle is providing—perfectly in line with the methodology of *An.* II 4 and his explanatory essentialism—a more generous (and possibly exhaustive) classification of thinkable objects, focusing on propositions and their components: he is expanding the core account of thinking and displaying thereby the explanatory power of his definitory account of *nous* from *An.* III 4–5.

Aristotle seems in fact to be hinting at this structural parallelism between his inquiries into thinking and perception at the very end of *An.* III 6 (430b29–31). Here he compares the objects about which thinking cannot but be true (which, I will argue, must be the essences of *An.* III 4–5) with the exclusive objects of perception, while the objects about which our thinking can be both true and false (i.e., the objects thought by way of predicating one thing of another, introduced at the beginning of *An.* III 6) are compared with the incidental objects of perception. Just as Aristotle offered an account of incidental perception only after the perceptive capacity had been defined with reference to the exclusive objects, so he is offering an account of propositional thought in *An.* III 6 only after *nous* has been defined with respect to essences in *An.* III 4–5.[12]

[9] While most modern translators and commentators (see, e.g., Hicks 1907, Hamlyn 1993², Polansky 2007, Shields 2016, Corcilius 2017, and Reeve 2017) understand this expression as referring to the ensouled animal, I am more inclined to follow Themistius (*In An.* 52.34–53.15; cf. Philoponus, *In An.* 286.12–15) and understand it as referring to the object which thus turns out to have three different functions: the general function of that which nourishes the animal and the special function of that which causes it to grow and which, after the animal has matured, is replaced by another special function of that which causes the animal to reproduce. Such was also Moerbeke's and Aquinas' understanding, see *In An.*, lb. II, l. 9, §344; recently, Johansen 2012: 101–102 and Miller 2018 have also understood the text in this way. As an indirect support one could quote *An.* III 12, 434b20–21, and *Sens.* 4, 441b28–442a1, where Aristotle is asking whether certain objects are *auxêsin poiounta* or not. See also *Gener. An.* II 6, 744b33–36, where *to threptikon* and *to auxêtikon* are distinguished as two kinds of nutriment.

[10] As he prefers to call it at *An.* II 4, 416b25.

[11] But also elsewhere, see especially *An.* III 4, 429b3–5 and 430a3–9 (and perhaps also 429a18).

[12] If, moreover, one understands the quantitative *adiaireta* (e.g., lengths) discussed at 430b6–14 as effectively corresponding to the common objects of perception (the *megethos* being, of course, included

Accordingly, there seems to be no good reason for seeing in *An.* III 6 any reversal of Aristotle's methodology; on the contrary, having gone through *An.* II 4–III 2, one would have to be surprised if something like *An.* III 6 did not follow *An.* III 4–5 (limited to the discussion of grasping of essences).[13] That said, this picture raises several questions. First of all, why see in *An.* III 6 an expansion and a display of explanatory power rather than a transformation of the definitory account of *nous* from *An.* III 4–5?[14] Shouldn't we say that *An.* III 4–5 could not provide as such any complete definition of *nous* because it did not take propositional contents into account, and that when these are introduced in *An.* III 6 the definitory account is thereby transformed? I will argue that this is not the case. Indeed, if the parallel with Aristotle's inquiry into perception outlined above holds, it speaks against this idea: not all perceptual content counts as objects (*antikeimena*) in the technical sense of *An.* II 4, and so not every content of thought is to be expected to do so, either. Moreover, the parallel makes us expect that propositional thinking is explanatorily dependent on grasping of essences, just as perception of common and incidental objects is explanatorily dependent on perception of exclusive objects, so that the former is secondary and indeed grounded in the latter; that seems enough for an explanatory essentialist to be justified in taking the activity of grasping essences alone as the definitory activity of the thinking capacity.

But in what sense is propositional thinking derived from, or grounded in, the activity of grasping essences? Surely not in the same sense as perception of common and incidental objects is grounded in perception of exclusive objects: in order to entertain a propositional thought, I clearly need not be actually grasping any essence whatsoever. If there is to be any dependence, it would seem to be primarily teleological.[15] The idea would then apparently be that any old thought is somehow directed at grasping an essence as the full and proper realization of the capacity responsible for it—and this would have to hold irrespective of whether the subject is aware of this or not; and, indeed, irrespective of whether she believes in essences or not. Grasping essences is for our *nous* what perceiving colors is for our sight. But while sight has been granted to us by nature as a full-fledged power that can immediately exercise its essential activity, *nous* will never attain the corresponding level of perfection in most of us.[16] This lamentable fact notwithstanding, the grasping of essences constitutes the very essence of our *nous*, just as the elephant form defines what an elephant embryo is, although it has not yet attained that form. The main

among the common objects of perception at *An.* III 1, 425a15–16), the parallel becomes even more conspicuous.

[13] For more on why this would, indeed, be surprising, see the following section.

[14] Thanks to Michael Arsenault for pressing this question.

[15] But not merely teleological, to be sure; for the demonstrative thought of an achieved scientist will be based on an actual grasping of essences.

[16] Cf. *An.* II 5, 417b16–19.

difference, again, is that the development of our *nous* is not a natural process, and so it is not such a surprise that it only rarely achieves its goal. The crucial point for our present purposes is that all activities for which *nous* is responsible, even at its usual "embryonic" stage, are derivative from the activity of grasping essences in the sense that this is what they are, ultimately, aiming at, and thus, in a sense, what makes them what they are. This is a strong essentialist claim that is not easy to swallow, and if it lies at the heart of how *An.* III 6–8 relates to *An.* III 4–5 (as the parallel with perception seems to imply), we should try to better understand it. The hope is that, when properly interpreted, the argument of *An.* III 6 can help us with that; I will, accordingly, return to this issue in the final section. In the meantime, I turn to a more straightforward question.

2.2 Why is the expansion needed?

On the most general level, Aristotle's motivation for the expansion of *An.* III 6 is obvious. His definition of *nous* could hardly be successful if he failed to indicate its relevance for the phenomena of our intellectual life. And this is all but clear from *An.* III 4–5 where *nous* was only analyzed as the capacity for grasping of essences—something that most of us will never achieve. If *An.* III 4–5 is to be successful in providing the elements for a full definition of *nous*, then Aristotle's discussion of it in *De anima* cannot be limited to *An.* III 4–5. While Aristotle's immediate aim is *not* to account for mental phenomena,[17] his definition of the principles can only be successful if he shows *that* they are indeed the principles on which such an account *can* be based. That seems to be why Aristotle must explain in *An.* III 1 how our perception of number, motion or of Cleon's son is grounded in perception of exclusive objects. And that also seems to be why after *An.* III 4–5 he must turn to propositional thinking in *An.* III 6: it seems vital to show how an account of predicative thoughts, such as "the diagonal of the square is incommensurable with its side," can be based on his definitory account of *nous*. It is likely that if Aristotle wrote an inquiry aiming at explaining the phenomena of human thinking, he would repeat there some of the points from *An.* III 6 (and III 7–8), while spelling them out in more detail and supplying them with other elements indispensable to a full explanatory account.[18] But *An.* III 6 does not aim at providing anything like that; rather it is an integral part of Aristotle's inquiry into the principles on which such an account could be based.

[17] See Chapter 1 (Section 2).

[18] For a rough idea about what such an account would need to include, see Chapter 6 (Section 4). It is instructive in this respect to compare the contents of *An.* III 9–11 with Aristotle's inquiry into animal locomotion in *De motu animalium*. (I owe this parallel to Klaus Corcilius.)

There is an interesting contrast between *An.* III 4 and *An.* III 6 which suggests, in a first approximation, that Aristotle sees a difference in kind between the activity of grasping essences and propositional thinking. In *An.* III 4, "thinking" was characterized—by analogy with perception of exclusive objects—as a kind of *paschein.*[19] At *An.* III 6, 430b5–6, Aristotle describes the role of *nous* in propositional thinking in terms of *poiein*: "what produces the unity (*to hen poioun*) is in each case [i.e., in all the kinds of propositional thoughts distinguished before] *nous*."[20] This contrast seems to be linked to Aristotle's direct realism and its limits. To say that grasping an essence is a kind of *paschein* is to underline the fact that in this kind of thinking, the object, so to speak, *presents* itself to the thinker directly as it truly is: thinking defined as a kind of *paschein* is a success term, just like the perception of exclusive objects, defined as a kind of *paschein* before.[21] However, most of our thinking acts are clearly not like this: more commonly we produce, often arbitrarily, various kinds of unities, atemporal or temporal, universal or particular, theoretical or practical, in which we *represent* things, and often *not* as they are in reality.

Now this comparative imperfection of propositional thought has its other side: propositional thought is a significant enrichment because it can do things that would be unthinkable for the thinking of *An.* III 4–5.[22] It is a medium in which the *search* for essences can take place, and it can *direct* human action.[23] From this perspective, *An.* III 6 can be seen as laying the groundwork for what Aristotle will say about practical thought in the following chapters. In *An.* III 6 he introduces three crucial elements that are absent in *An.* III 4–5, but indispensable in *An.* III 7–11: (a) propositional thought as such (how we think that *S* is *P*); (b) temporal relations (how we think, e.g., that *S will be* P);[24] (c) privations (how we think, e.g., that *S* is bad and thus to be avoided).[25]

But it is not only the benefits of propositional thought that matter. From the perspective of Aristotle's overall agenda in *De anima*, its deficiencies are equally important. *An.* III 6 contains Aristotle's official account of how thinking (namely, propositional thinking) can be both true and false. As such, it provides the basis for explaining errors of reason. The question of error, I want to suggest, shows

[19] See *An.* III 4, 429a13–15, 429b24–25, 429b29–30; cf. *An.* III 6, 430a24–25.

[20] In *An.* III 5 Aristotle also characterizes one kind of *nous* as "productive." But in my understanding, this is quite a different kind of *poiein* from the one he discusses in *An.* III 6. Roughly put, in *An.* III 5 what is "acted upon" is *nous*, while in *An.* III 6 what is "acted upon" are simple thoughts *qua* elements of a propositional thought being combined into a unity.

[21] For the passivity of perception and thought, see Roreitner 2025 and Roreitner (forthcoming b), respectively.

[22] Similarly, human *nous*, which is less perfect than divine *nous*, can think essences unthinkable for the latter.

[23] This is not to say that *nous* as such does produce locomotion. Cf. Chapter 6 (Section 3).

[24] See *An.* III 6, 430a31–b6.

[25] See *An.* III 6, 430b20–24.

how intimately *An.* III 6 is embedded in *De anima* and how indispensable it is for Aristotle's overall argument.

2.3 The question of error and compositional thinking

An. III 6 opens with the question of where truth and falsity are to be found. This question was completely absent in *An.* III 4–5, but it is not new in *De anima.* It played an important role in the opening passage of *An.* III 3 (427a17–b29). There, Aristotle was criticizing the traditional view that like is known by like (LKL), which, in his eyes, improperly assimilates thinking (*noein*) to perceiving (427a26–29). As in *An.* I, Empedocles was taken to be the mouthpiece of this view. Aristotle's main objection was that thinkers who accept this view are unable to explain how thinking could ever go wrong (427a29–b6 and again b8–14).

In fact, Aristotle's objection in *An.* III 3 seems to be further developing his criticism from *An.* I 5. In *An.* I Aristotle introduced the traditional LKL view as relying heavily on a straightforward isomorphism between the soul on the one side and the elements (*stoicheia*) of reality on the other. Such a view can provide a robust account of how the elements themselves are cognized (although that account fails, too).[26] But it is utterly helpless when it comes to cognizing composite things (*ta suntheta*). Its proponents have, according to Aristotle, nothing reasonable to say about how a composition (*sunthesis*) of elements is cognized. This applies primarily to composite substances, such as man or flesh or stone. But the same can be said about the whole range of perceptible qualities between the two extremes (e.g., all the "mixed" colors between black and white).[27] And something like this will also apply to predicative relations (such as "all men can perceive") as another kind of *suntheseis*, which arguably can only be thought by a synthetic or compositional activity of *nous.*

Aristotle's argument in *An.* III 3 insists that the traditional assimilation picture can be proved wrong by a reference to the fact that thinking can be both true and false. If we leave aside his repeated insistence (which begs the question) that thinking belongs to a very limited number of animals, the main objection runs as follows:

> And thinking (*noein*) in which there is a right and a wrong—right being understanding, scientific knowledge, and true belief, and wrong being the opposites

[26] See *An.* I 5, 410a13–b16.

[27] In Empedocles' account, as reported by Theophrastus, there are two kinds of pores in the eye into which the effluences of black and white color, respectively, fit perfectly (see Theophrastus, *Sens.* 7–8). The question then is how Empedocles can explain perception of, say, red color, conceived as a certain *combination* or mixture of black and white. This is raised as an objection by Theophrastus in *Sens.* 17. Presumably, there will be a certain number of black and a certain number of white effluences. But how can the perceptive act be distinguished from another perceptive act provoked by a black-and-white object with exactly the same ratio?

> of these—this [thinking] is not the same as perceiving, either. For perception of exclusive objects is always true..., whereas discursive thinking (*dianoeisthai*) can also be false...[28]

The reader is likely to have doubts here. (1) Is Aristotle not comparing apples and oranges? Perception of exclusive objects is always true—but we have already learnt in *An.* II 6 and *An.* III 1 that there are other objects the perception of which need not be true;[29] and Aristotle is about to reaffirm that perception of incidental objects can be false, and that perception of common objects is even more likely to be so.[30] (2) Moreover, when we go on and read through *An.* III 4–5, we may easily end up wondering whether Aristotle can in fact explain errors of thinking any better than Empedocles. His core account of thinking starts from a parallel with perception of exclusive objects which is claimed to be always true: thinking seems to be a success term. So, it might easily seem that Aristotle's definitory account of *nous* in *An.* III 4–5[31] leaves no more room for errors of reason than the traditional LKL view did.

The second worry, I suggest, is one of the reasons why *An.* III 6 is indispensable. And this context also sheds light on the structure of the chapter. Yes, Aristotle will go on to admit in the final passage (430b26–31), there is a kind of thinking—indeed, thinking (*noein*) in the most proper sense, as analyzed in *An.* III 4–5—which cannot but be true, exactly like perception of exclusive objects.[32] But, crucially, this is *not* the only kind of thinking there is (as *An.* III 4–5 could make one falsely believe if Aristotle's discussion of *nous* stopped there). There is also "thinking" (*noein* in a broader sense) which consists in combining different things and "producing" a unity out of them: that is, roughly, what Aristotle called *dianoeisthai* in *An.* III 3. And this thinking can also be false, as explained in the opening passage of *An.* III 6. So, only in *An.* III 6 does Aristotle finally tell us how his account escapes the objection from *An.* III 3 and thereby surpasses Empedocles' account also in this respect.[33]

Indeed, it is only *An.* III 6 that makes us understand why Aristotle is entitled to draw the contrast between perception and thinking as quoted above, and why he is right to think that it reveals a superiority of his account vis-à-vis the traditional LKL

[28] *An.* III 3, 427b8–14.

[29] See *An.* II 6, 418a11–16 and *An.* III 1, 425a30–b4.

[30] *An.* III 3, 428b18–25.

[31] See *An.* III 3, 428a16–18, where *nous* is classed, together with *epistêmê*, under *aei alêtheuonta*, as at *Posterior Analytics* II 19, 100b5–17; cf. *EN* VI 6, 1141a3–6.

[32] Cf. *An.* III 10, 433a26.

[33] Aristotle's account of *phantasia* in the rest of *An.* III 3 (428a1–429a9) can hardly do so on its own, *pace* Caston 1996a. Not only is the falsity of *phantasia*, to a large extent, at least *prima facie* traced back to the falsity on the level of perception itself (428b17–30). More importantly, *phantasia* is equally indispensable for the false *and* for the true thinking (see 427b28, drawing apparently on *An.* I 1, 403a8–10; and more explicitly in *An.* III 7 and 8), so it can hardly contain Aristotle's answer to the question of falsity as raised in the opening section of *An.* III 3.

account. *An.* III 6 also allows us to resolve the first worry mentioned above, about the soundness of the contrast between the potential falsity of thinking and the essential truthfulness of perception drawn at *An.* III 3, 427b8–14. While each act of perceiving involves an act of perceiving exclusive objects, and so is necessarily true in some respect (despite being often false as far as common and incidental objects are concerned), most acts of thinking involve no grasp of any essence whatsoever, and so can be *utterly false*.[34] This utter falsity characteristic of thinking in contrast to perception, Aristotle thinks, is something the traditional LKL view is utterly unable to explain, whereas his definition of *nous*—despite first appearance—does enable us to account for it.

As a matter of fact, Aristotle mentions Empedocles at the beginning of *An.* III 6 for the first time after the opening passage of *An.* III 3. He compares propositional thinking to the workings of Love in Empedocles' colorful account of zoogony. When we form a proposition, it is like when Love joins a couple of free-floating organs and produces an organism.[35] The idea seems to be that just as some of the compositions spontaneously produced by Love are viable and others are not, so some of the propositions formed by us are true and others false.[36] Accordingly, propositional thinking has at least three important aspects in common with the workings of Empedoclean Love in contrast to the thinking of *An.* III 4–5: it is spontaneous, compositional, and can get it both right and wrong. On the face of it, this bizarre comparison may seem to provide nothing more than a baroque scenery for Aristotle's account. But in fact, one can discern a dialectical purpose behind this comparison, or that's at least what I want to suggest. Aristotle may be offering here a lesson in immanent criticism, very much like the one given, for example, in *Metaph.* I 10.[37] He may be suggesting how Empedocles *could have* arrived, from his own principles, at an account of *compositional* thinking which would have saved him from his inability to explain error.

If, according to Empedocles, Love is imperceptible by the senses and only *nous* can cognize Love, then it should follow from his LKL account of cognition that *nous* is like Love.[38] Had Empedocles realized this, he could have easily come to see the limits of the traditional LKL account and could have concluded, like Aristotle,

[34] Notice that this view does not imply *degrees* of truth and falsity. The point is rather that an act of perceiving which gets both the common and the incidental contents wrong will still be true as far as the modally specific contents are concerned, whereas an act of entertaining a wrong proposition will be true in no respect whatsoever.

[35] The same sentence from Empedocles (DK 31 B 57.1) is quoted at *Cael.* III 2, 300b30–31, and criticized as an implausible model of zoogony at *Cael.* III 2, 301a14–20.

[36] For this aspect of the comparison, see already Themistius, *In An.* 109.13–15.

[37] Cf. *Part. An.* I 1, 641a18–26, or *An.* I 4, 408a18–24 (for an excellent reconstruction on the role played by Empedocles in Aristotle's discussion of the view of the soul as *harmonia* in *An.* I 4, see Betegh 2021).

[38] This point is made by Delcomminette 2020: 162 who refers in this connection to DK 31 B 17.21: "And you, gaze on her [i.e., the Love] with your understanding (*noôi*) and do not sit with stunned eyes" (trans. B. Inwood). Cf. B 109.3 (= *An.* I 2, 404b15): "[We see] . . . Love by Love"; and B 133.

that there needs to be a spontaneous *compositional* activity of thinking consisting in combining thoughts in a way that can turn out both true and false. If Love and its workings are ever to be comprehended by our *nous*, then our *nous* must be capable of a spontaneous compositional activity, and this suggests that the LKL account cannot hold in the form in which Empedocles embraced it according to Aristotle. Empedocles, as interpreted by Aristotle, does not seem to have realized this, and so Aristotle's criticism from *An.* III 3 stands, while his own account is now shown to be immune to it. Unlike Empedocles' *nous*, Aristotle's *nous* can think things like the workings of the Empedoclean Love.[39]

Whatever we think about the justice of Aristotle's criticism, the point about truth and falsity made in *An.* III 6 is clearly important for his larger argument, not least because his final summary in *An.* III 8 will *resemble* very much the LKL view: "the soul is in a sense all beings," Aristotle will maintain.[40] So, he needs to make clear that his view is not susceptible to the difficulties with which the LKL view was confronted. And one of these was exactly the question of utter falsity on the level of thinking. The ability to explain how it is possible—or the lack of such explanation—was introduced in *An.* III 3 as a test for putative definitions of *nous*. So, it is no surprise that, after offering a definitory account of *nous* in *An.* III 4–5, Aristotle turns in *An.* III 6 to showing how his definition passes the test.

In the opening passage of the chapter, Aristotle goes out of his way to emphasize the compositional character of propositional thought:

> In those [cases] where both falsity and truth [can be found], [what occurs] is already a certain combination of thoughts as being one.... Falsity is always found in a combination.[41]

The notion of combination (*sunthesis*), as it is used here to characterize the compositional nature of propositional thought, is rather surprising for a reader coming from kindred texts, such as *Metaph.* VI 4 and *Metaph.* IX 10, where combination is the distinguishing feature of affirmations (*kataphaseis*) as contrasted with denials (*apophaseis*), and where the latter are analyzed in terms of *dividing* (*diairesis*) one thing from another. The same kind of shift in terminology, motivated by the aim of *An.* III 6 to capture the common characteristic of all propositional thinking, is encountered again in the final passage, where Aristotle introduces the structure "one thing of another" (*ti kata tinos*) as a common feature of propositional thought (430b26–27), whereas in *Int.* 6 or *Metaph.* VI 4 and *Metaph.* IX 10 this was

[39] For an interpretation of Empedocles' account of how we know love suggesting that Empedocles in fact came pretty close to this idea himself, see Kamtekar 2009: 226–236.

[40] *An.* III 8, 431b21. For a detailed discussion of the points in which Aristotle departs from the traditional LKL account, see Chapter 5.

[41] *An.* III 6, 430a27–28, 430b1–2.

a distinguishing feature of affirmations in contrast to denials (characterized by the structure of *ti apo tinos*).[42] In *An.* III 6 it is crucial to stress that even denials are compositional.[43]

What makes this contrast with kindred texts even more striking is that in the opening passage of *An.* III 6 Aristotle also uses the notion of division (*diairesis*), capturing elsewhere the specific nature of denials: "It is also possible, though, to say that all these are instances of division" (*An.* III 6, 430b3–4). Given the broad use of "combination" in what precedes, it is unlikely that Aristotle here means specifically denials or affirmations of a privative term.[44] Rather this seems to be a claim about all propositional thoughts.[45] Here is a suggestion on how to make sense of that claim. Up to this point Aristotle has been developing—in analogy with Empedocles' zoogony—a bottom-up approach to propositional thinking, starting with discrete (*kechôrismena*) thoughts and considering how these are combined. At *An.* III 6, 430b3–4, he seems to be suggesting a more holistic perspective on propositional thought: we can also conceive the object of a propositional thought as a single whole which, however, is not thought as an *adiaireton*, but by way of being divided (*diairesis*) or articulated into its elements. This holistic perspective does not contradict the compositional perspective; perhaps it rather serves as a reminder that the Empedoclean analogy has its limits, because even in propositional thoughts we are (standardly) trying to capture unities that already exist independently of our thinking, such as the immutable fact that the diagonal of a square is incommensurable with its side: we are starting from a whole which needs to be articulated.[46] So, the essential spontaneity and compositionality of propositional thinking does not (as the Empedoclean analogy could falsely suggest) exclude normativity pertaining to the unities produced in it.

2.4 An implicit presence of *adiaireta* in *An.* III 5

So far, I have yet to say anything about what seems to be the central notion of *An.* III 6: namely, *adiaireton*. One's understanding of it is obviously crucial for the way one interprets the argument of *An.* III 6 as a whole—if there is any overarching

[42] For more on the use of *ti kata tinos* in the final passage, see Sections 3.5 and 3.6 of this chapter.

[43] Aristotle's example at 430a2–3 ("even when [one thinks that] a white thing is not white, [one] has combined the not white [with it]") is *prima facie* somewhat misleading in that it may seem as if he had only affirmations of privative predicates in mind (e.g., Cleon is not-white) and not denials (e.g., Cleon isn't white), the logical value of both being elsewhere distinguished (see *Prior Analytics* I 46, especially 51b36–52a14, or *Int.* 10). But as is clear from the two quotes above, Aristotle commits himself to also analyzing denials as combinations—no matter whether he has or has not a denial in mind at 430a2–3.

[44] Also: what would the claim be? Aristotle would seem to be explicitly confusing what he elsewhere carefully distinguishes (see the preceding footnote).

[45] For the same interpretation, but spelled out in a different way, see Themistius, *In An.* 109.32–110.1 and in more detail Oehler 1962: 155–158; cf., e.g., Reeve 2017: 166n369.

[46] For a structurally similar use of *diairesis*, cf. *Phys.* I 1, 184a21–b14.

argument. Before addressing this question directly in Section 3 of this chapter, I want to make a preliminary comment on the context in which the notion of *adiaireton* first occurs in *An.* III 6.

Reading *An.* III 6 against the background of Aristotle's polemic with Empedocles in *An.* III 3 and *An.* I 5 sheds, arguably, some light on the notion of *sunthesis* as used in the opening passage of *An.* III 6 (430a26–b6). But any search for a similar context regarding the central notion of *adiaireton* in the preceding chapters of *De anima* is in vain.[47] Moreover, the other texts of the corpus that are usually considered as parallels to *An.* III 6 never mention any *adiaireton*: *Metaph.* VI 4 talks about "simples" (*hapla*), *Metaph.* IX 10 talks about "uncomposed" objects (*asuntheta*), and *De interpretatione* has no corresponding expression (unless *onoma* and *rhêma* are taken to have a similar role).[48]

Now, it is of course perfectly possible that there is no explanation for why Aristotle starts talking about *adiaireta* (rather than, say, *asuntheta* or *hapla*) at the outset of *An.* III 6.[49] But, as a matter of fact, there is one context, albeit only implicit, in *An.* III 5 which may help us understand Aristotle's motivation for introducing this particular notion. And not only that: it can also shed light on how *An.* III 6, and especially its central passage (430b6–26), is structured.

It is well known that the list of attributes ascribed to the eternally active *nous* in *An.* III 5 (whatever it is) corresponds neatly to what Aristotle says about *nous* (or *noêsis*) identified as the unmoved mover(s) of the heavens in *Metaph.* XII 7 and 9.[50] Now, the very last claim of *Metaph.* XII 9 (1075a5–11) is that this *nous* (or *noêsis*), as an object without matter, is *adiaireton.* Aristotle says this in response to a potential worry: "A difficulty remains as to whether what is being thought is composite (*suntheton*), for [if it were, then the *noêsis* in question] would be changing in passing from part to part of the whole."[51] His response is straightforward: "Or is it rather the case that everything which has no matter is *adiaireton*?"[52] The thought seems to be that since the *nous* (or *noêsis*) in question is *adiaireton*, we need not worry about its changing in passing from part to part while thinking itself. Aristotle can give such a straightforward answer here because he has already shown both that the heavenly unmoved movers are substances without matter

[47] The only passage in which the notion of *adiaireton* played an important role was *An.* III 2, 426b29–427a16, but I do not think this passage can help us understand why this notion becomes central in *An.* III 6. There are three other mentions of something being *adiaireton* in book I to which I refer below.

[48] At *Int.* 1, 16a13–14, Aristotle only says that these "resemble a thought without any combination (*synthesis*) and division (*diairesis*)." Cf. *Cat.* 2, 1a16–19, where he talks about *ta aneu sumplokês*, claiming at 4, 2a7–10, that these are neither true nor false; and the notion of *horos* at *Prior Analytics* I 1, 24b16–18.

[49] There are, of course, parallel texts, distinguishing different kinds of *adiaireta*, especially *Metaph.* V 6 and *Metaph.* X 1 exploring different meanings of the "one." The question is why this context becomes relevant at the beginning of *An.* III 6.

[50] The correspondences are nicely listed by Caston 1999: 211–212.

[51] *Metaph.* XII 9, 1075a5–7.

[52] *Metaph.* XII 9, 1075a7.

(*Metaph.* XII 6, 1071b20–22) and that such a substance is without magnitude, partless, and *adiairetos* (*Metaph.* XII 7, 1073a5–7), the latter claim being already the result of Aristotle's discussion in *Phys.* VIII 10: "It is thus clear that [the first mover] is *adiaireton*, partless and without any magnitude."[53]

With this context in mind it is not so surprising that immediately after *An.* III 5, Aristotle (using the transitional *men oun . . . de* construction) draws a distinction between thinking of "*adiaireta*" (rather than, say, *hapla* or *asuntheta*), on the one hand, and compositional thinking, on the other.[54] As a matter of fact, he has just discussed at length the thinking of an *adiaireton* in whose case it would indeed be hard to find any place for error; so it seems reasonable (especially given the context of *An.* III 3) to contrast in what follows this thinking with thinking which does allow for error.

What might come as a surprise, then, is the wide range of objects falling under the class of *adiaireta* in *An.* III 6. But Aristotle never says in *Metaph.* XII 9, *Metaph.* XII 7, or *Phys.* VIII 10 that the immaterial substances are the only *adiaireta*; they are perhaps *adiaireta par excellence*, but there may well be other *adiaireta* such that all these together need to be contrasted with objects thought compositionally. The central passage (430b6–26) provides, then, a classification of various *adiaireta* objects of thought, which helps us to distinguish between different cases of non-compositional thinking.

Some modern interpreters have been surprised by the fact that at the climax of this list (*An.* III 6, 430b24–26), Aristotle arrives at something which looks very much like the heavenly unmoved mover(s): he considers the case of there being a cause without any opposite and infers that it will cognize itself. Some readers have even tried to deny that this is what the text is about.[55] But once we have recognized the notion of *adiaireton* implicitly present in *An.* III 5, with which the opening sentence of *An.* III 6 seems to connect, this climax is not surprising at all: it is exactly what we should expect from the very beginning as the most genuine instantiation of the central notion.

3. The notion of *adiaireton* and the argument of *An.* III 6

Still, it is difficult to see how any coherent notion of *adiaireton* could unify the list presented in the central passage (*An.* III 6, 430b6–26), while, moreover, making good sense of what Aristotle says in the opening and final passages (430a26–b6, b26–31). How can a single coherent notion embrace the heavenly unmoved

[53] *Phys.* VIII 10, 267b26–27.

[54] We need not assume, rather drastically, that the stretch of text from *An.* III 4, 429b22, to *An.* III 5, 430a25, is a "digression" with no relevance for *An.* III 6, as Pritzl 1984: 143 claims (drawing attention to *oun* at *An.* III 6, 430a26). For *men oun . . . de*, see Denniston 1954: 470–473; cf. Bonitz 1870: 454.

[55] See especially Berti 1978: 146, Berti 1996: 398–401, and Polansky 2007: 477.

movers together with a point, and lengths together with things with a unitary form? And that is just a part of the problem: another question is how all these kinds of *adiaireta* distinguished in the central passage relate to the contrast between thinking of *adiaireta* and compositional thinking drawn in the opening passage (430a26–b6);[56] and then again, how the objects in whose case thinking can only be true according to the final passage (430b26–31) should be classified against the background of both the contrast from the opening passage, and the list introduced in the central passage.

As a first step toward addressing these questions, I wish to comment on one complication concerning the meaning of *adiaireton* which is manifested in the troubles experienced by translators endeavoring to find a single equivalent that could be used throughout the chapter.

3.1 The difficulties with translating the term *adiaireton*

As is well known, the verbal adjective *adiaireton* can mean both "indivisible" and "undivided." The first of these translations[57] feels very fitting when it comes to the third class of *adiaireta* (*An.* III 6, 430b20–24) exemplified by the point (*stigmê*). And this fits well with Aristotle's use of the adjective in *An.* I, referring twice to circular atoms constituting the soul according to Democritus (*An.* I 2, 405a8–13; *An.* I 3, 406b20–22) and once to the "place" of a *stigmê* (*An.* I 5, 409a24–25). But the translation of *adiaireton* as "indivisible" proves unsatisfactory and quite misleading when it comes to Aristotle's distinction at *An.* III 6, 430b6–9, between *adiaireton* "in potentiality" (*dunamei*) and *adiaireton* "in actuality" (*energeiai*). That distinction seems central to what Aristotle wants to say about the first kind of *adiaireta* (represented by lengths) at *An.* III 6, 430b6–14, and it plays, arguably, an important structuring role in the central passage as a whole.[58]

If *adiaireton* is translated as "indivisible," then Aristotle's distinction will seem, *prima facie*, to be between something that is actually indivisible (*adiaireton energeiai*), on the one hand, and something that *can* be indivisible, but is not (*adiaireton dunamei*), on the other. But then it becomes difficult to understand what Aristotle can mean when characterizing a length as being *adiaireton energeiai*, and, indeed, why he introduces such a distinction in the context of discussing continuous quantities at all. Not only are lengths (and other continuous

[56] This is already mentioned by Philoponus (*In An.* 543.17–28) as a difficulty recognized by interpreters.

[57] See, e.g., Oehler 1962: 151–169, Jannone and Barbotin 1966, De Koninck 1990 and 2008, Reeve 2017, and Judson 2020: 323.

[58] The passages which seem to come closest to this distinction are *Phys.* VIII 5, 258a32–b3, and *Gener. Corr.* I 2, 316b19–25. For more on the significance of this distinction for the central passage as a whole, see below.

quantities) obviously not "indivisible in actuality." It is not even *possible* for them to be indivisible.[59] The distinction seems entirely irrelevant to the objects Aristotle is discussing.

But the situation improves only slightly if we translate *adiaireton* as "undivided."[60] This works fine insofar as a length is indeed "undivided in actuality," and one can feel disposed to tolerate this translation also when a point is called *adiaireton* (*An.* III 6, 430b20–21), although saying that it is "undivided" sounds rather like an understatement. The main problem is that Aristotle's distinction at *An.* III 6, 430b6–9, between *adiaireton energeiai* and *adiaireton dunamei* still sounds awkward. *Prima facie* this will seem to be a distinction between an actually undivided, unified object (*adiaireton energeiai*), on the one hand, and a plurality of items that *could* be unified into a single undivided object, but are not (*adiaireton dunamei*), on the other. Now, in antiquity some commentators already understood the contrast along these lines; but it is difficult to see what function such a contrast should play in Aristotle's argument.[61] Why should Aristotle contrast a length as being actually undivided with something that can be, but is not undivided? It is true that at *An.* III 6, 430b11–14, he distinguishes between the case of two halves of a length being thought separately as two lengths, on the one hand, and the case of them being thought as two halves of a single composite length, on the other. But the latter is, crucially, *not* what Aristotle meant when he insisted at *An.* III 6, 430b6–9, that a length can be thought of as an *adiaireton* because it is *adiaireton energeiai*: what he meant was clearly the case of thinking a length without dividing it in any way at all.

Aristotle's claim seemed to be that thinking such an undivided length (in contrast to the length thought as the sum of two shorter lengths) can be analyzed as a case of thinking an *adiaireton* object of thought—but *adiaireton only* in the sense of *adiaireton energeiai*. An undivided length is surely *not adiaireton* in the sense that is perhaps most intuitive: it is not indivisible, for every length can be divided into shorter lengths. This is what Aristotle seems to mean by *adiaireton dunamei*: while an undivided length is not *adiaireton* in this sense (in which, e.g., a point is *adiaireton*), its undividedness (i.e., its being *adiaireton energeiai*) is enough for it to be an *adiaireton* object of thought. We will later come to why it

[59] In fact, *Metaph.* V 13 *defines* quantity as something "divisible (*diaireton*) into immanent parts" (1020a7).

[60] See, e.g., Hamlyn 1993[2] (insisting on this translation also in his commentary) or Corcilius 2017. Shields 2016 translates *adiaireton* as "undivided" throughout the whole chapter with the exception of its first occurrence at the very beginning (I am not sure I see the merits of this decision). Similarly to Hicks 1907, Miller 2018 opts for the strategy of deciding in each case *ad hoc* whether *adiaireton* should be translated as "indivisible" or "undivided."

[61] Philoponus offers this kind of interpretation in *De Int.* (71.18–72.25) and *In An.* (549.4–7), using in both cases the example of a certain quantity of water divided into several splashes and described as *adiaireton dunamei* insofar as it *can be joined* into one continuous ("undivided") quantity. But in neither of these two commentaries does Philoponus explain what such a notion of *adiaireton dunamei* could be good for in the present context.

is important for Aristotle to insist on this. For now, what matters is that the contrast intended at *An.* III 6, 430b6–9, is not correctly captured when we translate *adiaireton* either as "indivisible" or as "undivided."[62]

And there seems to be a very good reason for these difficulties with translating the text: by adding *dunamei* and *energeiai* to *adiaireton* Aristotle in fact disambiguates two meanings of the Greek adjective which do not coincide in any single English word. The ambiguity of *adiaireton* Aristotle is pointing to seems to consist in two possible understandings of the *diaireton* part of it: either we take this to mean "divided in potentiality" (i.e., "divisible") or we understand it as "divided in actuality" (i.e., "divided"). The adjective *adiaireton* (consisting of *diaireton* plus an *alpha privativum*) can then mean either "not (even) in potentiality divided" or "not divided in actuality." The former is what we call "indivisible;" the latter is what we call "undivided."[63] Given that each of these English words corresponds to the notion of *adiaireton already qualified as* either *dunamei* or *energeiai*, it is understandable that none of them can serve as a satisfying translation of *adiaireton unqualified*.

The least misleading solution I have been able to come up with is to translate *adiaireton* as "without division" and spell out *adiaireton dunamei* and *energeiai* as without potential and actual division, respectively.[64] This allows us to paraphrase Aristotle's thought at 430b6–8 as insisting that lengths are objects without actual division, and so can be thought without division, although they have (infinitely many) potential divisions. For the purposes of this chapter, however, I leave the word *adiaireton* untranslated. What really matters is the question whether it has an intelligible unitary meaning throughout *An.* III 6. I will now argue that it does.

[62] For this reason, I think the caution expressed by David Ross in his commentary is wise: "In dealing with this chapter in English, we must not use either the word 'undivided' or the word 'indivisible,' but rather some ambiguous word like 'unitary'" (Ross 1961: 300). But unfortunately, the adjective "unitary" is not a good candidate for a unitary translation of *adiaireton* in *An.* III 6, either. It has more or less the same downsides as "undivided": speaking of something as "potentially unitary" would sound as if we were referring, as Philoponus thought, to something which is not unitary as of yet—something which is unitary only in potentiality, unlike what is already unitary in actuality.

[63] Another example of a privative term qualified in such a way that the qualifications apply, strictly speaking, only to the positive core of it can be found at *Metaph.* XII 8, 1073a23–25 (I owe this reference to Hicks 1907: 516–517); cf. *Phys.* VIII 6, 259b22–26. The principle is here claimed to be *akinêton* both *per se* (*kath' hauto*) and accidentally (*kata sumbebêkos*): undoubtedly, by the second qualification Aristotle means that the principle is "not even accidentally movable," not that it is "immovable only accidentally" (whatever that would mean).

[64] A different solution is proposed by Hasper 2002: 248–253. He suggests that we should translate *adiaireton* as "indivisible" and paraphrase *dunamei* and *energeiai* as "across all possible situations" and "within the actual situation," respectively. Hasper argues on the basis of *Metaph.* VII 13, 1039a10–11, that Aristotle is ready to take on board a limited version of Democritus' Atomistic Principle, saying that *in the actual situation* it is impossible that something which is one turns into something which is two, or, in other words, he is accepting the claim that *in the actual situation* something which is one is *indivisible*. My worry is that Aristotle would be implicitly relying on rather sophisticated meanings of *dunamei* and *energeiai* in order to introduce a much simpler distinction between two senses of *adiaireton*.

3.2 "Thinking of *adiaireta*" in the opening passage (*An.* III 6, 430a25–b6)

The first complication met by any interpreter endeavoring to find a unitary meaning of *adiaireton* in *An.* III 6 is its very first sentence, which proves to be ambiguous in two important respects. Aristotle writes:

> Now thinking of *adiaireta* occurs in cases where falsity is not possible. But in those [cases] where both falsity and truth [can be found], [what occurs] is already a certain combination of thoughts as being one.[65]

It is not clear (1) what exactly Aristotle wants to say here about truth and falsity pertaining to the thinking of *adiaireta*. Is the idea that this thinking is neither true nor false, or that it is always true? Moreover, it is unclear (2) how the contrast between thinking of *adiaireta*, on the one hand, and thinking as a combination of thoughts, on the other, is intended: that is, how exactly the case of *adiaireta* here is supposed to differ from that of propositional contents. The way in which these two—closely related—questions are answered largely determines how the whole chapter is understood.

Most interpreters, not paying attention to the context of *An.* III 5, have understood the contrast in a straightforward way. By *adiaireta* Aristotle simply means the concepts from which propositions are composed.[66] In the next step these interpreters divide into those who think Aristotle wants to say (much like in *Int.* 1 and *Cat.* 4) that thinking of simple concepts is neither true nor false,[67] and those who think he is claiming that thinking of simple concepts is as such always true.[68] That the latter view is strange is masterfully shown by Antony Lloyd (which did not prevent him from ascribing it to Aristotle).[69] But even if we disregard the question of truth and falsity, the traditional understanding of the contrast (interpreting *adiaireta* as simple concepts) meets with serious difficulties as the chapter develops.

The list of four *adiaireta* provided in the central passage (*An.* III 6, 430b6–26)—lengths, things with a unitary form, geometrical divisions, causes without opposites—seems to be anything but a well-ordered list of simple concepts. And when in the final passage (*An.* III 6, 430b26–31) Aristotle talks about thinking of

65 *An.* III 6, 430a26–28.

66 For a thoughtful defense of this reading, see, e.g., Mignucci 1996.

67 For a list of interpreters embracing this view, see Harvey 1978, who argues, convincingly, against it (ending up himself with the second option: i.e., that the thinking of *adiaireta* is always true).

68 For a long list of interpreters who, on the basis of *An.* III 6 and *Metaph.* IX 10, ascribe to Aristotle the view that there is a non-propositional thought of simple concepts which is always true, see Crivelli 2004: 114n58.

69 See Lloyd 1970.

"what [something] is in virtue of [its] essence" he seems to have something considerably more advanced in mind than just the understanding of what a concept means. Rather, he seems to be talking about grasping of essences: that is, thinking in the technical sense of *An.* III 4–5.[70] The linguistic expression of this thinking is surely not a simple word, but rather a scientific definition, as was rightly emphasized by Richard Sorabji and Enrico Berti.[71]

But if we must abandon the idea that in the opening sentence Aristotle means by *adiaireta* simple concepts, how should we understand the contrast between *adiaireta* and propositional contents then? Berti provided a straightforward answer to this question. From the very beginning Aristotle is thinking of essences: these are the *adiaireta* he is contrasting with propositions in the opening sentence, and so he obviously wants to claim here, just like in the final passage, that thinking of *adiaireta* is always true.[72] However, while this robust understanding of *adiaireta* seems to prepare us well for the final passage, it proves even more helpless in the face of the central passage distinguishing between four different kinds of *adiaireta*, none of which is easily identifiable with essences.[73] Indeed, Aristotle's move from the opening passage to his discussion of lengths as the first class of *adiaireta* (*An.* III 6, 430b6–14) seems entirely unintelligible under Berti's interpretation. Moreover, it is hard to shake off the impression—motivating the majority view—that in the opening passage Aristotle is taking simple concepts, like the incommensurable and the diagonal, as examples of *adiaireta*.

But is there any sound alternative? That is: is there a way of understanding the contrast between thinking of *adiaireta* and propositional thinking in the opening passage, such that the thinking of "what [something] is in virtue of [its] essence" in the final passage would fall, together with the understanding of simple concepts, under the former, and that, moreover, the list of *adiaireta* in the central passage would make good sense?

[70] This is also why I do not think that Paolo Crivelli's alternative suggestion really works. According to him, when Aristotle talks about thinking of *adiaireta*, he has *existential statements* in mind. See Crivelli 2004: 100–125. But when I have a *nous* of "what something is in virtue of its essence" I seem to have significantly more than an awareness of the fact *that* (*hoti*) something exists: rather, I have a grasp of *what* (*ti*) something is which is the primary cause of *why* (*dioti*) it is.

[71] See Berti 1978, Sorabji 1980: 218, Sorabji 1981: 242, Sorabji 1982, Sorabji 1983: 139–142 and Berti 1996. Crivelli 2004: 115 traces this line of interpretation (which he himself rejects) back to Maurus 1668: IV 480–481. But the truth is that Themistius already finds it natural to spell out Aristotle's thought at 430b26–30 in terms of "contemplating the form [of something] and the definition (*ton logon*) of its essence (*tou ti ên einai*)" (*In An.* 112.14–15). And Philoponus (*De Int.* 87.45–59) offers a subtle criticism of this view with the upshot that Aristotle does not mean all definitions, but only definitions of immaterial forms. So, the allegedly modern "definitions-view" is in fact very traditional.

[72] See Berti 1978: 143 and Berti 1996: 393.

[73] Only in the case of the fourth kind of *adiaireta* does it make good sense to refer to them as essences (since in the case of these objects *X* and what it is to be *X* are identical; cf. *An.* III 4, 429b11–12), but such a claim would also be potentially misleading: they are introduced as causes, but certainly not causes in the sense of essences.

I believe there is. My diagnosis is that the two approaches sketched out above represent two extremes, both of which are too narrow.[74] As an alternative, I suggest that we should understand the contrast in the following broad terms: *adiaireta* in the sense relevant for *An.* III 6 are objects endowed with a kind of unity that allows one to think them in a non-compositional way (that is without dividing them into elements and putting these together). Objects which are *adiaireta* in this sense are contrasted with composite objects such that one can only think them compositionally (that is, by dividing them into their elements and putting these together in the right way). This is admittedly a very abstract contrast which is in need of some clarification.

I have suggested that a prominent example of *adiaireton* in the opening passage is the unmoved mover of *Phys.* VIII 10 and *Metaph.* XII 6, 7, and 9. And we have seen Aristotle's brief argument at the end of *Metaph.* XII 9, where the worry was that the thinking (*noêsis*) under consideration might turn out to be compositional, and so involve a transition from one part to another, which would be inadequate for something supposed to be changeless. Aristotle's response was that since the substance in question is immaterial, it is *adiaireton*, and so nothing prevents it from being thought non-compositionally. Indeed, it is *adiaireton* in such a sense that it is impossible for it to be thought in any compositional way at all.

For comparison we can take a very different example which has already been touched upon in the preceding section. An undivided length is an object without actual division (*adiaireton energeiai*) and this fact allows one to think without division (*to adiaireton noein*) when thinking a length: that is, it allows one to think a length without dividing it and putting the parts together—one thinks it non-compositionally. Here the implication is not that it is *impossible* to think the object in question compositionally: a length can surely be divided, for example, into two halves and be thought as the sum of these (*An.* III 6, 430b11–14). An immaterial substance and a length are objects as different as can be. And yet both fall under the category of *adiaireta*: that is, objects which can be thought without division or non-compositionally.

The category of compositional thinking seems to be correspondingly broad and to include, for example, the case of thinking a length as the sum of its parts. But the primary case of compositional thinking in *An.* III 6 is unquestionably propositional thinking. The entire opening passage is dedicated to the kind of compositionality involved in it, as we have already seen. One thing to be stressed here is that what

[74] For an attempt to find a middle way between understanding *adiaireta* as simple concepts grasped in a non-propositional way and understanding them as what is intended by definitions, see also Wedin 1988: 128–136: like Lloyd 1970, he thinks that all *adiaireta* are simple thoughts such as "flower" or "daffodil" and that Aristotle wants to say that there is a kind of "acquaintance" with these which is immune to error; in contrast to Lloyd, Wedin stresses that such an acquaintance "occurs only in contexts like c1": i.e., contexts of predicative sentences such as "the flower in the vase is a daffodil" (Wedin 1988: 131). I think that Wedin's suggestion remains too close to Lloyd's interpretation and that it does not allow him to provide a satisfactory explanation of the final passage.

Aristotle means by composition is a composition of discrete units (*kechôrismena*; *An.* III 6, 430a30), such as the notion of diagonal and the notion of incommensurable (or, for that matter, two parts of a line after a division has been drawn).[75]

I want to suggest now that this broad contrast between compositional thinking and thinking of *adiaireta* can be better appreciated against the background of an idea that was around in Aristotle's time. Roughly put, the idea is that all thinking, or at least all knowledgeable thinking, is necessarily compositional. The best-known instance of this idea is the so-called Dream Theory in Plato's *Theaetetus*, which implies that the object of knowledge is always composite and one can only think it (or account for it) by dividing it into its elements and combining these in the right way; these elements themselves, in contrast, can never be thought, but at most perceived, due to their non-composite nature.[76] When Aristotle contrasts compositional thinking with thinking of *adiaireta* in *An.* III 6, he can be understood as setting out to demarcate the limits of such a compositional account of thinking.

If the contrast drawn at the outset of *An.* III 6 is interpreted in the suggested way, then it seems plausible to assume with the majority of interpreters that the basic components or structural elements of propositional thinking—that is, the objects which can play the role of subjects or predicates of propositions (e.g., the incommensurable and the diagonal)—fall under the notion of *adiaireta* as intended by Aristotle. Without there being some such *adiaireta*, propositional thinking would not be possible at all.

But, if the contrast is interpreted in the suggested broad terms, it seems unlikely that this could be the only kind of *adiaireta* Aristotle has in mind. After all, the thinking of an immaterial substance is surely not (or not primarily) a case of thinking an *adiaireton* in the sense of an actual or potential *component* of propositions: unlike, for example, the thought of the diagonal, this is a self-standing act of thinking, independent of propositional context. It seems likely that when Aristotle introduces the notion of "thinking of *adiaireta*," he has more kinds of possible "dividing" of propositional contents in mind than just identifying their components or structural elements. In fact, Aristotle is fond of imagining propositions as a sort of interval delimited by the subject and the predicate. And these intervals can be "divided" by means of the *why* (*dia ti*) question. This question is asking for a middle term which would "divide" the interval between the subject and the predicate and so mediate their relation, as when, for example, the observed

[75] Not any thought concerned with a manifold object is thus compositional. That seems to be the point of Aristotle's discussion of lengths at *An.* III 6, 430b6–14: it is possible to think a length non-compositionally—i.e., as an *adiaireton*—despite its infinite divisibility. More on the relevance of this claim below.

[76] See *Theaet.* 201 C–208 B. "Thus, the elements are unaccountable and unknowable, but they are perceivable, whereas the complexes are both knowable and expressible and can be the objects of true judgment" (202 B, trans. M. J. Levett).

fact that the part of the moon that is lit is turned toward the sun is divided, by means of the notion of receiving light from something else, into the assertions that whatever receives light from something else has the part turned toward it lit and that the moon receives its light from the sun.[77]

This consideration opens the possibility that thinking of *adiaireta* can also be contrasted with propositional thinking in quite a different way than the one described above. Thinking of *adiaireta* occurs not only when it comes to thinking the components of a proposition, but also when the ultimate answer to the *why* question about some proposition(s) is found. As a matter of fact, once the contrast at the outset of *An.* III 6 is interpreted along these lines, Aristotle is committed to insisting that there is, indeed, thinking of *adiaireta* in this other sense, too. If there were not, there would only be beliefs (*doxai*) and doxastic thinking, but no scientific knowledge (*epistêmê*) and epistemic thinking.[78] If scientific knowledge is to be possible, there must also be *adiaireta* that are not components, but ultimate *explanatory grounds* of propositions—the principles from which these are explained and which themselves cannot be explained by anything else.[79]

The truth is that while Aristotle never uses the notion of *adiaireton* to refer to structural elements of propositions, he describes the ultimate explanatory grounds of propositions as *adiaireta* in *Posterior Analytics*. He does so in I 22 and 23, which conclude Aristotle's polemic against anonymous thinkers (introduced in I 3) who—like the Dream Theory, but from a different perspective—entertain the view that all knowledgeable thinking is compositional. Roughly, their idea is that every propositional thought can be referred to other propositional thoughts that are supposed to explain it; the result is that all demonstrations are either circular or go on *ad infinitum*. Aristotle opposes this idea and insists that the "dividing" of propositions by means of the *why* question must have a natural limit: there must be indivisible (*adiaireta*) intervals representing the so-called immediate propositions (*protaseis amesoi*): that is, propositions without any available middle term which are the explanatory grounds for other propositions.[80]

[77] Cf. *Posterior Analytics* I 34, 89b15–20. For this kind of division underlying Aristotle's idea of immediate propositions as elements and material causes of the conclusion, see Malink 2017.

[78] For the contrast, see *An.* III 3, 427b9–10 and 427b24–27.

[79] Even though they may be endowed with a certain complexity, as the essences of physical things arguably are, unlike immaterial substances.

[80] "For if there are principles, it is not the case that everything is demonstrable, nor is it possible to continue *ad infinitum*: for either of these things to be the case is simply for there to be no immediate and indivisible (*adiaireton*) intervals but for all of them to be divisible (*diaireta*)" (*Posterior Analytics* I 22, 84a32–35, trans. J. Barnes). "When you have to prove something, you should assume what is predicated primitively of *B*. Let it be *C*; and let *D* be similarly predicated of *C*. If you always continue in this way, no proposition and no term holding outside *A* will ever be assumed in the proof. Rather, the middle terms will always be thickened until they become indivisible (*adiaireta*) and single (*hen*).... So too in deduction (*sullogismos*) the unit (*to hen*) is the immediate proposition (*protasis amesos*), and in demonstration (*apodeixis*) and understanding (*epistêmê*) it is comprehension (*nous*)" (*Posterior Analytics* I 23, 84b31–35, 84b39–85a1, trans. J. Barnes). For a systematic reconstruction of Aristotle's argument in *Posterior Analytics* I 3 and I 19–23, see Crager (forthcoming).

To illustrate the difference between the two kinds of "dividing" of propositions, we can take the claim "all humans are capable of perception." The components or structural elements of it are the concepts "human" and "capable of perception." Its explanatory grounds are the immediate or "indivisible" propositions "every human is animal" and "every animal is capable of perception."[81] These propositions are in fact just partial expressions of the respective scientific *definitions* of "human" and "animal." And that partly explains their special status: unlike in all other propositions, here the predicate does not express something that simply *holds of* the subject; rather, it explicates a part of the *very essence* of that subject. Aristotle says that these *adiaireta* (i.e., immediate propositions) stand to deduction as *nous* (i.e., a grasp of an essence) stands to demonstration and scientific knowledge.[82] This does not mean that grasping an essence, as analyzed in *An.* III 4–5, should be *identified* with entertaining immediate propositions or with predicating the whole *definiens* of the *definiendum*.[83] We will return below to the question of how these predicational acts might depend on the grasping of essences in terms of *An.* III 4–5 without the latter being reducible to the former. What matters for now is that once we adopt the perspective of dividing propositions by means of the *why* question, this points us to a very different kind of thinking of *adiaireta*, be it conceived as the entertaining of immediate propositions or as a non-propositional grasping of essences on which immediate propositions are grounded.

To sum up, I suggest that the notion of "thinking of *adiaireta*" in the opening passage of *An.* III 6 should be understood broadly in terms of non-compositional thinking: that is, thinking something without dividing it into elements and putting these together. Contrasting it with propositional thinking, this notion can be spelled out in two quite different ways, either as thinking of objects that can become subjects or predicates of propositions, or as thinking of the ultimate explanatory grounds on which any epistemic propositional thinking needs to be based. If this is true, it shows that the agenda of *An.* III 6 is more complex than it might first appear. The task of introducing propositional thinking as explanatorily dependent

[81] Notice that the only correct middle term here is animal, and not, e.g., mammal, which would produce an explanatory syllogism, but such that it would only be doxastic, and not epistemic, due to the failure to identify the commensurate universal. See *Posterior Analytics* I 33 on this contrast and a helpful discussion of it in Angioni 2013 and Angioni 2019.

[82] See the last sentence quoted in footnote 80.

[83] Not even in the *Posterior Analytics* does Aristotle really *identify nous* with entertaining an immediate proposition, although this claim is not uncontroversial, for recent interpreters have assumed that such an identification is *intended* in what Aristotle says. He (i) describes *nous* as "the principle of scientific knowledge" (I 33, 88b36; II 19, 100b15); he (ii) introduces the notion of "indemonstrable scientific knowledge" which consists exactly in "entertaining (*hupolêpsis*) an immediate proposition" (I 3, 72b18–20; I 33, 88b36–37); and he (iii) *closely associates* "the principle of scientific knowledge" (i.e., *nous*) with "indemonstrable scientific knowledge" (I 3, 72b18–25; I 33, 88b35–37). I would resist, though, the idea (for which, see Morison 2019: 14–17; cf. Bronstein 2016: 51–52) that Aristotle's association is meant as identification (Aristotle never, to my knowledge, describes *nous* as a kind of *hupolêpsis*; and I have not been persuaded that the second *oude* at *Posterior Analytics* I 33, 88b36, should be interpreted as epexegetic).

on the grasping of essences with respect to which *nous* was defined in *An.* III 4–5 turns out to be intimately connected with the task of disambiguating the kinds of objects that can become components of propositional thoughts from the ultimate explanatory grounds of propositions.

If this interpretation of the contrast between thinking of *adiaireta* and compositional thinking drawn at the outset of *An.* III 6 is correct, it also sheds light on the other issue raised above, concerning Aristotle's ambiguous claim that thinking of *adiaireta* "occurs in cases where falsity is not possible." *Prima facie* this can be read either in the light of *Int.* 1 (and *Cat.* 4), where cognitive acts relating to simple concepts are said to be neither true nor false, or in the light of *Metaph.* IX 10, where thinking of *asuntheta* is said to be always true (much like the thinking of "what [something] is in virtue of [its] essence" in the final passage of *An.* III 6). Since antiquity, interpreters have felt obliged to decide between these two options.[84] But once we realize that there are two quite different kinds of thinking of *adiaireta* in play here, we can understand why Aristotle's expression is ambiguous.[85] Thinking of something as a component of propositions is on its own neither true nor false. But thinking of something as the ultimate explanatory ground of propositional thoughts—that is, understanding "what [something] is in virtue of [its] essence"—cannot but be true.

In what follows I attempt to show that the suggested interpretation of the opening sentence has significant advantages over competing interpretations when it comes to understanding how the chapter develops further and how the central and the final passage contribute to Aristotle's overall argument. Roughly, in the central passage Aristotle analyzes different ways of being *adiaireton* on the side of the object that allows it to be thought without division. In most cases the relevant kind of "thinking of *adiaireta*" is thinking of something as a potential or actual *component* of a proposition which is as such neither true nor false. But the list is structured in such a way that it naturally leads to the kind of thinking that cannot but be true: namely, "thinking of *adiaireta*" in the sense of understanding the ultimate explanatory grounds of propositions—the topic of the final passage. In the following section I start with the first item on Aristotle's list (i.e., lengths) and explain how their discussion fits into the larger argument. Then, I briefly discuss the other three items and offer a reconstruction of the logic behind the list. In Section 3.5,

84 Cf., e.g., Philoponus (*In An.* 544.18–545.6), who opts for the latter, after alleging that the accounts of *Int.* 1 and *Metaph.* IX 10 are incompatible. This idea seems to be in line with the view that *Int.* 1 is incompatible with the account of *De anima* that seems to go back to Andronicus of Rhodes (thanks to Andrea Falcon for this observation).

85 Another candidate for such an intentionally ambiguous formulation is *Metaph.* VI 4, 1027b27–29. That Aristotle's expression at *An.* III 6, 430a26–27, is intentionally ambiguous is also claimed by Delcomminette 2020: 161. But I do not agree with how Delcomminette fleshes out this promising suggestion, claiming that "*certains noêmata au sens du De Interpretatione peuvent admettre la verité*." I see no indication of this in *Int.* and no need for this being so in *An.* III 6.

then, I turn to Aristotle's claim in the final passage that the thinking of "what [something] is in virtue of [its] essence" is always true.

3.3 Why lengths? (*An.* III 6, 430b6–14)

The relation between the passage on lengths as *adiaireta* (*An.* III 6, 430b6–14) and the opening passage of the chapter has been the main stumbling block for most interpretations of *An.* III 6. It has seemed difficult to find much coherence, let alone continuity, between the notion of *adiaireton* introduced in the opening passage by way of contrast with propositional thinking and the notion of *adiaireton* as it is applied here to undivided lengths. It is unclear why Aristotle begins to talk about lengths in a way which suggests that he has neither a universal concept nor an essence in mind.

I have explained how I think the unity of the notion of *adiaireton* should be understood: *adiaireton* is any object such that one can think it without dividing it into elements and putting these together. It makes perfect sense to ask whether a length falls under this category. What remains to be explained is why Aristotle should be interested in emphasizing that it can. There are, I believe, two interconnected reasons: (1) what is at stake at *An.* III 6, 430b6–14, is in fact a much larger domain of thinking than it may *prima facie* appear, and (2) there is a potential *aporia* concerning the possibility of this kind of thinking directly connected to the overarching topic of *An.* III 6.

(1) Lengths seem to stand as *pars pro toto* here for all continuous quantities: they are the most primitive, unidimensional continuous quantities, and what Aristotle says about them can easily be extended, *mutatis mutandis*, to any continuous quantity. The question of how we can think lengths, thus, directly concerns the possibility of geometry: if it were impossible to think continuous quantities, no one could ever entertain, say, the thought that something is incommensurable with something else (not to mention the possibility of proving some such proposition).

In fact, the domain concerned here may be even larger. Aristotle believes that continuous quantities are, in one way or another, involved in a great majority of, if not all, our thinking acts. They are certainly involved also in thinking which is not concerned with continuous quantities as such. This is something Aristotle says explicitly in *Mem.* 1: "... and in the same way [as in diagrams] the one who thinks (*ho noôn*), even when he does not think (*noêi*) a quantity, he posits a quantity before his eyes, but thinks (*noei*) it not *qua* quantity ..."[86] Aristotle is here concerned with the way in which thinking depends on *phantasia*, as in *An.* III 7 and *An.* III 8.[87] In

[86] *Mem.* 1, 450a4–5.

[87] See *An.* III 7, 431a16–17, 431b2–4 (with Chapter 4); *An.* III 8, 432a3–10 (with Chapter 5); cf. *An.* III 4, 429b13–16, and Chapter 6.

the quoted passage, "quantity" seems to fall primarily on the side of *phantasia* (we are "positing it before our eyes"[88]), but the person needs to be capable of *thinking it* somehow: namely, *qua* something else. Although the quantity is not thought *qua* such here, one could ask whether thinking it *qua* something else would ever be possible if it could not be thought on its own in the first place. If the answer is no, then there is even more at stake in the passage discussing lengths (*An.* III 6, 430b6–14) than the possibility of geometry.

(2) Be that as it may, Aristotle seems to recognize an *aporia* about how thinking of continuous quantities, such as lengths, takes place—an *aporia* which is intimately connected to the distinction between compositional thinking and thinking of *adiaireta*, introduced in broad terms (as I argued) in the opening passage. One might be inclined to believe that thinking of a continuous quantity must be a case of compositional thinking—perhaps because one believes that all thinking is compositional (like all accounting, knowing, and judging according to the Dream Theory) and that undivided objects can only be perceived; or because one specifically thinks that quantities can only be thought, if at all, by way of summing their parts. If some such assumption is made and it is combined with the view endorsed by Aristotle that all continuous quantities are infinitely divisible, one is immediately faced with an epistemological variation on Zeno's paradoxes:[89] since every chosen continuous quantity can be further divided, we will never come to any *basic* quantities from which the summing could begin, and so we will never be able to think any continuous quantity whatsoever.[90]

Aristotle's response to this kind of worry is prepared by the very distinction drawn in the opening passage between compositional thinking and thinking of *adiaireta*. And this response is announced at the very beginning of the passage on lengths (*An.* III 6, 430b6–14). Nothing prevents lengths from being *adiaireta* objects of thought (i.e., objects thought without division)—not even their infinite divisibility (i.e., the fact that they are not *adiaireta dunamei*, objects without potential division): it is enough for the length in question to be actually undivided (i.e., without actual division) and to be thought as such.

It makes perfect sense for Aristotle to start with continuous quantities not only because the question of how they are thought may have a more general relevance for his account of thinking, but also because continuous quantities are *adiaireta* objects of thought in the weakest possible sense due to their infinite *per se* divisibility, which also allows them to be thought compositionally. In a way, lengths are the most rudimentary kind of *adiaireta* and it is important to stress that a

[88] Cf. *An.* III 3, 427b18–20.

[89] Besides the first two paradoxes of motion (DK 29 A 25–26), it is above all the proof that if something has a magnitude it is both infinitely large and infinitely small in DK 29 B 1 that comes to mind.

[90] The worries Aristotle is implicitly addressing here seem, thus, close to the ones spelled out, in a more sophisticated way, by Sextus Empiricus in *M* IX 380–388.

distinction between compositional thinking and thinking of *adiaireta* is already indispensable here.[91]

From this perspective, Aristotle's division at *An.* III 6, 430b6–14, into three cases of thinking lengths makes good sense, too. After formulating and commenting on the key claim that even a divisible but undivided length can be an *adiaireton* object of thought at 430b6–10, Aristotle turns at *An.* III 6, 430b11–13, to the case where the length is divided (and with it also the time in which it is thought). This could be conceived as a candidate for how the original length is thought compositionally—but, Aristotle says, it is, strictly speaking, not the original length (*AC*) which is thought; indeed, it is no single length at all, but rather two different lengths (*AB*, *BC*).[92] In order to think the original length, one would have to put the two shorter lengths together and think the original one as composed out of these, so that the time of thinking the whole length (*AC*) would also be composed out of the two shorter times, as suggested at *An.* III 6, 430b13–14. This third case represents a kind of thinking of the original length *AC* different from the first case: *AC* can be thought either compositionally or as an *adiaireton*. The implicit point seems to be that *some* thinking of an *adiaireton* is in any case indispensable, since, of course, *AC* can only be thought compositionally if *AB* and *BC* (or their parts) are thought of as *adiaireta*. So, no length (and no continuous quantity in general) can ever be thought without involving a thinking of an *adiaireton* at some level.[93]

[91] It is worth noting that while the *problem* that arises for scientific explanations (cf. *Posterior Analytics* I 3) and for lengths is structurally similar (if there is no *adiaireton*, nothing will be thought, for one would need to pass through an infinite number of steps), Aristotle's *solution* is entirely different in the two cases. In the former case, it consists in denying infinite divisibility and accepting explanatory factors which themselves cannot be further "divided" and so explained. In the latter case, it consists in affirming infinite divisibility, but denying that thinking of divisible items would need to have the form of combining that into which they can be divided.

[92] For this understanding of the short sentence at 430b12–13 (*tote hoionei mêkê*), see already Themistius, *In An.* 110.13–14: "for in this way one would think two lengths (*duo mêkê*), and not a [single] length (*mêkos*). Cf. *Metaph.* VII 10, 1035a17–21.

[93] One issue I left aside concerns the kind of temporality Aristotle ascribes in this passage to the thought of an undivided length. There are two basic options on the table in the secondary literature. One possibility is that the temporality is of the same kind as, say, the temporality of perceiving a color or indeed of grasping an essence: the thought is complete in every part of its duration (this is, e.g., Philoponus' understanding: see *In An.* 549.10–11; cf., e.g., De Koninck 1990: 218–219 and 2008: 102). This has recently been called into question by Delcomminette 2020: 168, who argues that the parallelism between the divisibility of a length and of the time in which it is thought at 430b9–10 suggests that each thought of a length takes some time in the sense that the thought needs to literally "run through" ("*parcourir*") the length, so that it is *not* complete in every part of its duration. I find this idea too awkward to be what Aristotle means, but I agree that he wants to contrast the temporality of thinking a length with the temporality of grasping an essence and with the temporality of thinking an *adiaireton* in form introduced in what follows (430b14–20). When Aristotle says that the time in which a length is thought is divisible in the same way as the length itself, what he means, I suggest, is not that the thought needs to "run through" the length, which takes a determinate amount of time, but rather that the time of thinking the length *could* be divided into times corresponding to various parts of the length and still be the time of thinking the same length (albeit now thinking it compositionally). This does not commit Aristotle to any dubious assumption, while providing a robust enough contrast between the temporality of thinking lengths and that of thinking *adiaireta* in form (more on the contrast in footnote 102).

3.4 The logic behind the central passage (*An.* III 6, 430b6–26)

If it is true that Aristotle starts discussing lengths at 430b6 as the most rudimentary kind of *adiaireta* objects of thought (essential for geometry, but indirectly perhaps involved in many other kinds of human thinking), how can we understand the way in which he then proceeds with the three other kinds of *adiaireta*? The first thing worth stressing is that Aristotle does indeed distinguish at *An.* III 6, 430b6–26 *four* kinds of *adiaireta*, as the Greek commentators known to us unanimously agreed: quantitative *adiaireta* (b6–14), *adiaireta tôi eidei* (b14–20), divisions (b20–24), and causes without opposites (b24–26). By contrast, some modern interpreters have thought that only three kinds of *adiaireta* are distinguished here;[94] and quite a few modern scholars have believed that the first kind is treated throughout 430b6–20, while the second kind is then only mentioned in one short sentence.[95]

These tendencies are motivated by genuine difficulties encountered when we try to understand how exactly the four kinds of *adiaireta* are distinguished from each other. Another related tendency already mentioned above is to treat Aristotle's list (or indeed *An.* III 6 in its entirety) as if it were an entry from Borges' Chinese encyclopedia. In contrast to these approaches, I suggest that there is an overarching ascending logic at work here. Each newly introduced kind of *adiaireton* is *adiaireton* in a stronger sense than the preceding one, and so starting from the most rudimentary case of *adiaireta* objects of thought (i.e., lengths) we arrive at the *adiaireton par excellence*—the *adiaireton* of *An.* III 5 (and *Phys.* VIII 10 and *Metaph.* XII 7 and 9). The way Aristotle proceeds is, I propose, governed by two main criteria according to which different kinds of *adiaireta* are distinguished from one another.

(1) The first criterion concerns their spatial *divisibility*: the first kind of *adiaireta* (quantitative *adiaireta*), such as a length, differ from the second kind (*adiaireta tôi eidei*) because the former are divisible *per se*, while the latter are only divisible *per accidens*.[96] An *adiaireton tôi eidei*, I take it, is an object with a unitary form

[94] So, e.g., De Koninck 1990 and De Koninck 2008 (collapsing the last two kinds into a single class), or Berti 1978 and Berti 1996, or Polansky 2007 (identifying *de facto* the second and the fourth kind). See also Hasper 2002: 248–253, who argues that the quantitative *adiaireta* and the *adiaireta tôi eidei* in fact refer to the same kind of entities. I agree that when talking about a quantitative *adiaireton* and an *adiaireton tôi eidei* we may in fact be referring to a numerically identical object; indeed, this observation can be extended to the third class of *adiaireta*, the divisions: a single line *AC* may be thought as a certain length, or as a straight line (rather than a circle or semicircle), or, again, as the division of, say, two triangles *ABC* and *ACD*. It seems important for Aristotle, though, to stress that these are three different kinds of *adiaireta* (while they can be numerically identical, they differ in being).

[95] This view is shared by all the interpreters accepting Bywater's (arbitrary) transposition of lines *An.* III 6, 430b14–15, after 430b20 (e.g., Ross 1961, Hamlyn 1993^2, and Trentini 2016; cf. also Shields 2016: 77n52).

[96] I take this contrast to be implied in the difficult sentence at *An.* III 6, 430b16–17. If *ekeina* refers here to the quantitative *adiaireta* from 430b6–14, then Aristotle is contrasting their divisibility with the divisibility of the time in which and "that by which" *adiaireta* in form are thought. But we know from *An.* III 6, 430b9–10, that the time in which these are thought is "divisible and without division

(hence "*adiaireton* in form"), such as an elephant.[97] And the point of Aristotle's contrast is the following: while a quantitative *adiaireton* can be divided *qua* such into material parts (of the same kind) and can be thought as a sum of these parts,[98] something *adiaireton* in form cannot be divided *qua* such,[99] but only *qua* being an object of a certain quantity, and it can never be thought as a sum of its parts.

To illustrate the contrast between the first two kinds of *adiaireta*, we can use Aristotle's example from *Metaph.* V 6 of what is one (and *adiaireton*)[100] in form in contrast to what is one (and *adiaireton*) only in quantity:

> Further on, there is a sense in which we call anything one (*hen*) as long as it is a [unitary] quantity (*poson*) and is continuous (*suneches*), but there is a sense in which we don't unless it is a whole (*holon*): that is, unless it has one form (*eidos hen*). For instance, if we saw the parts of a shoe put together in any way whatsoever, we would not call them one all the same, unless on account of [their] continuity; but we would do so [properly speaking] only when they are put together in such a way as to be a shoe: that is, to have a single form (*eidos ti hen*).[101]

The point of Aristotle's example, I take it, is that the same object (here a shoe) can be thought either as a quantitative *adiaireton* or as an *adiaireton* in form. In the first case, the arrangement of parts does not matter. In fact, the shoe can remain the very same quantitative *adiaireton* (the same continuous three-dimensional magnitude) even when its parts are rearranged. In the second case, in contrast, changing the arrangement of parts means abandoning the original *adiaireton* in form because the thing loses the unitary form that made it what it was. Indeed, it is not

in the same way" as the objects. And it is to be expected that a similar correspondence will also hold for *adiaireta* in form. See footnote 102 below on how it pertains to the time in which the two kinds of *adiaireta* are thought, respectively. In footnote 114 I say more about the final words of this difficult sentence (*all' hêi adiaireta*). For the notion of accidental divisibility, see, e.g., *Cael.* III 1, 299a21–25.

[97] Since antiquity interpreters have disagreed as to whether *adiaireta tôi eidei* are *infimae species* (not divisible into *species*) or material objects with a unitary *form*. The former, more popular, option goes back to Themistius (*In An.* 110.15–27; cf. e.g., Rodier 1900, Hicks 1907, Ross 1961, Berti 1996: 397, Trentini 2016: 180, and Delcomminette 2020: 172–173). The latter option was adopted and defended by Philoponus, *De Int.* 65.63–67 (cf. De Koninck 1990: 220 and 2008: 103–104). There are at least two reasons that speak against the first option. First, it would be strange for Aristotle to define one category of *adiaireta* in such a way that it would include "man," but exclude "animal" (what would this category be useful for in the present context, other than adding one more possible meaning of indivisibility?). Second, it would be strange for Aristotle to say that *infimae species* are *accidentally* divisible: what he would apparently mean is their divisibility into *genera* and *differentiae specificae* (see Berti 1996: 397 or Oehler 1962: 161), but this divisibility seems anything but accidental for them.

[98] See *An.* III 6, 430b13–14.

[99] If you divide an elephant into parts, these will not be elephants (unlike parts of a length which are themselves lengths) and, less trivially, they will not even be parts of an elephant (for a tusk cut off an elephant is a tusk only in name).

[100] What is one is also *adiaireton* and vice versa: see *Metaph.* V 6, 1016b3–6 and 23–24, and already *Metaph.* III 3, 999a1–6, and again *Metaph.* X 1, 1052b15–17, 1053a20–21, 1053b4–8.

[101] *Metaph.* V 6, 1016b11–16.

possible at all to think it as what it is by starting from parts and combining these (even in the right way)—unlike in the case of a quantitative *adiaireton* (where the parts can be combined in any way whatsoever).[102]

So, the quantitative *adiaireta* and *adiaireta* in form differ in how spatial divisibility pertains to them (*per se* or accidentally).[103] What they have in common is the fact that they are both spatially divisible. That qualifies the sense in which they are *adiareta*: both are *adiaireta energeiai*—that is, without actual division—but none of them is *adiaireton dunamei*: that is, without potential division, indivisible. In this way they can be together contrasted with the third and the fourth kind of *aidaireta* which are both *adiaireta dunamei*: that is, not even in potentiality divisible. What these latter two kinds of *adiaireta* have in common is that they are not divisible at all—neither *per se*, nor accidentally.[104] But how are they distinguished from one another?

(2) The second main criterion behind Aristotle's list, I suggest, concerns *that by which* each *adiaireton* is known and thought, or in other words, what the *knowledge* of each *adiaireton* is like. While there already seems to be a distinction between the first and the second kind in this respect,[105] it becomes crucial especially for distinguishing the third and the fourth kind: that is, the two kinds of objects which are indivisible. While in the case of the former the knowledge is always necessarily *a potentiality* for two opposite acts (acts relating to two opposites), in the case of the latter the knowledge is simple; moreover, nothing prevents it from existing—apart from any subject—as a *pure actuality*, identical to what it is knowledge of.

[102] This, I think, also explains how the divisibility of the time in which quantitative *adiaireta* are thought and the time in which *adiaireta* in form are thought differ. Unlike in the case of quantitative *adiaireta* (see footnote 96 above), the time of thinking an *adiaireton* in form cannot be divided into times of thinking the parts of this object in such a way that the whole time would still be the time of thinking—now compositionally—the same object.

[103] For a similar distinction, cf. *Metaph.* V 13, 1020a14–32: some things are said to be (continuous) quantities *per se*, others *per accidens*.

[104] I thus think it is wrong to identify being *diaireton per accidens* with being *adiaireton dunamei*: i.e., being indivisible (as Rodier 1900: 481–482 does, followed by Delcomminette 2020: 171–173).

[105] At *An.* III 6, 430b14–15, Aristotle introduces *adiaireta* in form in contrast to quantitative *adiaireta* by saying that they are not only thought *en adiairetôi chronôi* (as the quantitative *adiaireta*: see 430b8–10), but also by an *adiaireton tês psuchês*. What does Aristotle mean by *adiaireton tês psuchês*? Some interpreters (see, Themistius, *In An.* 110.19, 24, Rodier 1900, Tricot 1934, Jannone and Barbotin 1966, Bodéüs 1993, Thillet 2005, and Delcomminette 2020: 173) assume it is an *act* of the soul, but then it is not clear how being thought by an *adiaireton tês psuchês* differs from being thought *en adiairetôi chronôi*. Other interpreters (see Philoponus, *In An.* 550.20–21, 31–32, and *De Int.* 75.99–9, cf. Ross 1961, Hamlyn 1993^2, Polansky 2007, Shields 2016, Corcilius 2017, Reeve 2017, and Miller 2018) assume that Aristotle has a *capacity* of the soul in mind like at *An.* III 4, 429b10–22; but there does not seem to be any relevant contrast between quantitative *adiaireta* and *adiaireta* in form in this respect. There is, however, a third option: *adiaireton tês psuchês* may refer to *an acquired aspect* (a dispositional cognitive achievement) of the soul which can be identified as the form of the object in question present in the soul: i.e., an understanding of the respective concept, on the basis of which one can think the respective object (e.g., an elephant) as an *adiaireton* in form. If this is what Aristotle means, the implication would seem to be that the quantitative *adiaireta* can be thought without any such preceding achievement (concept formation).

Aristotle prepares this contrast while discussing the third kind of *adiaireton* at *An.* III 6, 430b20–24. The model example of this kind of *adiaireton* is a point which is indivisible in all three dimensions. The notion may well apply to the now (*nun*), too.[106] And Aristotle extends it to any kind of geometrical division: a line dividing two plane figures or a plane figure dividing two solids, the former being indivisible in two dimensions, the latter in one. Most of Aristotle's attention at 430b20–24 goes to how one cognizes this kind of *adiaireton*. And the answer is given by way of subordinating this case under a larger class containing explicit privations (e.g., not-white) and privative terms like the bad or the black. One important implication seems to be that this larger class will also include privations of forms determining the second kind of *adiaireta* (e.g., not-elephant). The account of how all these are cognized offered by Aristotle seems closely related to his account in *Metaph.* IX 2 and 5 of rational capacities as capacities for opposites.[107] The difference is that in *An.* III 6 the reasoning proceeds, so to speak, the other way round: that is, from the object to the capacity. Privations and privative terms (e.g., the not-white or the bad) can only be cognized by means of their opposites (e.g., the white or the good); and that which cognizes them needs to be endowed with a *capacity*—a *single* capacity that, as it were, encompasses both opposites.[108]

To understand the way Aristotle introduces the fourth kind of *adiaireton* at *An.* III 6, 430b24–26, it is important to realize that the account of the cognition of privative terms at *An.* III 6, 430b20–24, also says something important about the cognition of their positive counterparts. While these are surely not cognized by their opposites, it is no less true about them that what cognizes them must be endowed with a capacity which is at the same time the capacity for cognizing the respective privation.[109] That might sound trivial, but only until we realize that according to Aristotle the primary cosmic principle has nothing opposite to it, as he emphasizes

[106] Thanks to Michel Crubellier for this observation.

[107] "And the rational (*meta logou*) capacities are all such that the same capacity is a capacity for opposites" (*Metaph.* IX 2, 1046b4–5).

[108] Cf. *Metaph.* IX 2, 1046b24: the opposites "are contained in a single principle (*miai archêi periechetai*)—a *logos*." In contrast to Trentini 2016: 195–209, I do not think Aristotle's point is that the thought of a privative term *involves* a thought of an *adiaireton*, which would be the thought of its positive counterpart. Rather, Aristotle wants to insist that a privative term can *itself* be thought without division, in line with *Int.* 10 where Aristotle insists that "also the indefinite expression [such as not-man] signifies in a way one thing (*hen*)" (*Int.* 10, 19b8–9), and so it can serve as a noun, albeit an indefinite noun, which still "resembles a thought devoid of any combination and division" (*Int.* 1, 16a13–14). This seems necessary for distinguishing between denials of the form "*S* isn't *P*" (where negation characterizes the way in which *S* and *P* are combined) and affirmations of the form "*S* is not-*P*" (where negation belongs to a single, undivided predicate): see *Prior Analytics* I 46, especially 51b36–52a14. And this distinction seems important for action: the judgement "*S* isn't good" has no immediate practical consequence, for it allows for the case of *S* not existing at all; it is only the judgement "*S* is bad" which immediately leads to avoiding *S*.

[109] The difference comes from the fact that the capacity does not relate to the two opposites in the same way: it is primarily the capacity for thinking the positive term, and only derivatively the capacity for thinking the respective privation.

in *Metaph.* XII 10, and so there is nothing opposite to the act of cognizing it.[110] This seems to be the sense in which Aristotle asks at *An.* III 6, 430b24–25, whether there is some cause "such that it has nothing opposite to it." Now the form that makes an *adiaireton* in form, like an elephant, be what it is does have an opposite in the relevant sense, for its effect is material and capable of not-being. Accordingly, the knowledge of a form will be a capacity for thinking both the form and its privation (e.g., an elephant corpse).[111] Aristotle's point at *An.* III 6, 430b24–26, I suggest, is that if there is a cause with no opposite whatsoever (which would have to be the cause of an eternal effect), it does *not* follow that what cognizes it is in capacity. Unlike in all the preceding cases, its cognition does not need to involve any capacity at all: it does not need to be the fulfilment of a capacity but can exist as a pure self-standing actuality or activity (*energeia*). And this activity of cognition would be nothing other than the cognized object itself. If that is indeed what Aristotle has in mind when inferring at 430b24–26 that a cause without any opposite would cognize itself, then this inference is intimately related to his argument at *An.* III 4, 430a3–6 (and *An.* III 5), according to which nothing prevents an immaterial object of thought from being itself a self-thinking *nous*. Indeed, Aristotle's telegraphic remark at the climax of his list of *adiaireta* seems to presuppose that we are already familiar from An. III 4–5 with this peculiar class of objects of thought.[112]

Schematically, my understanding of the logic behind the list provided by the central passage is expressed in Table 3.1. If this is right, the central passage provides a well-ordered list of *adiaireta*: that is, objects endowed with such a kind of unity that they can be thought without division, and so non-compositionally. Only the fourth class represents objects that are *adiaireta par excellence*. The remaining three kinds of *adiaireta* fail on at least one of the two criteria. The first two kinds are spatially divisible, and so are *adiaireta* only *energeiai*. The point, in contrast, is indivisible; but there is necessarily a certain complexity on the side of that which

[110] See *Metaph.* XII 10, 1075b20–24: "And for all other thinkers there is necessarily something opposite to wisdom—i.e., to the most honorable knowledge—but not for us. For there is nothing opposite to the first, since all opposites have matter and are in potentiality the same. And the ignorance which is opposite [to wisdom] would be concerned with the opposite, but there is nothing opposite to the first."

[111] And with a more advanced knowledge, also the ways in which the living body can be efficiently turned into a corpse.

[112] The proposed interpretation is close to how Philoponus read the argument of 430b24–26 (see *De Int.* 84.60–81; *In An.* 552.27–553.16). But most interpreters have approached the passage differently. Some modern scholars found the claim expressed here too bizarre to be ascribed to Aristotle, so they tried to show that the passage talks in fact about how forms are thought by human *nous* (see Berti 1978: 146, Berti 1996: 398–401, relying on Codex Laurentianus 81,1 (S), and Polansky 2007: 477). Other interpreters duly recognize in these lines a reference to the unmoved mover(s) of *Metaph.* XII 6–10, but it is much less clear how they take Aristotle's inference to proceed. Most modern interpreters seem to follow, explicitly or implicitly, Themistius' understanding (*In An.* 111.34–112.8), which takes Aristotle to be reasoning, roughly, in the following way: if there is *a cognizing subject* which has nothing opposite to it, then this subject will be cognizing itself. But it is not clear what consideration should lead one to believe that there is such a subject in the first place, and it is embarrassing for this interpretation that the words *tôn aitiôn* seem to be doing no job at all (some interpreters even delete them in the wake of Zeller's suggestion: see Bywater 1888: 60, Ross 1961, Hicks 1907, Hamlyn 1993², and Shields 2016).

Table 3.1 Types of *adiaireta* in *An.* III 6

Adiaireta	**Spatial divisibility**	**"By what" (knowledge)**
(1) quantitative	*per se* → *adiaireton energeiai*	no *adiaireton* [potentiality for opposites]
(2) in form	*per accidens* → *adiaireton energeiai*	an *adiaireton* [potentiality for opposites]
(3) divisions	none → *adiaireton dunamei*	potentiality for opposites [no *adiaireton*]
(4) cause(s) without opposite(s) = *adiaireton par excellence*	none → *adiaireton dunamei*	simple → existing as a pure actuality

cognizes it: thinking of *adiaireta* here presupposes a capacity (which is the capacity for two opposite acts). This last point, in fact, seems to hold about all *adiaireta* except for the fourth kind. The exceptional status of it is emphasized at the climax of the central passage.

In what precedes this climax, the role played by forms is worth noticing. Aristotle does not talk about thinking of forms as such, but forms are obviously crucial for distinguishing between the first and the second kind of *adiaireta*. As suggested above, these do not need to be two numerically distinct objects.[113] Rather, a single object can be conceived both as a quantitative *adiaireton* when we think it as a certain quantity (e.g., a solid of such and such an extension) and as an *adiaireton* in form when we think it as unified by a single form (e.g., an elephant). In fact, this point can be extended to the third kind of *adiaireta*: a numerically identical object can be considered as a length, as a straight line, or as a division of two plane figures. What makes my thought a thought of an *adiaireton* in form is exactly that I conceive it as unified by a single form—although I usually don't have a proper grasp of this form as such: that is, I understand *that* it is, for example, an elephant, but not *why* it is an elephant (i.e., what makes it an elephant, or, in a word, the essence of elephant).[114]

[113] See footnote 94.

[114] I only seem to have a provisional understanding of the form—a concept (cf. footnote 105 above on the expression *adiaireton tês psuchês*), which can perhaps be spelled out, in line with *Posterior Analytics* II 1–2, as an understanding *that* there is a middle term: i.e., *something* which makes the thing be what it is. More speculatively, Aristotle may be implying that forms are the ultimate causes not only of *adiaireta* in form, but also of quantitative *adiaireta*. When he says that "in them [i.e., the quantitative *adiaireta*] too there is something without division, but presumably not separable (*chôriston*) which makes the time and the length one" (*An.* III 6, 430b17–19), he may be making forms responsible for the unity of quantitative *adiaireta*. The idea would roughly be that a quantitative *adiaireton* always exists parasitically on an *adiaireton* in form: e.g., a length is always the length *of* something, be it a straight line, or a circle, or something else. That may be what Aristotle means when he says that the *adiaireton* in length or time is not separable: a length is *adiaireton* only *qua* being something else (*allo ti on*) or

3.5 Thinking of "what [something] is in virtue of [its] essence" is always true (*An.* III 6, 430b26–30)

Aristotle's consideration of the fourth kind of *adiaireta* leads naturally to the topic of the final passage where propositional thinking, as potentially both true and false, is contrasted with grasping of essences, which is always true and never false. To see the connection, we only need to recall Aristotle's distinctions from *An.* III 4. Among the primary objects of thought there are those which have no matter[115] and for which there is no difference between *X* and what it is to be *X*.[116] These seem to be nothing other than the cause(s) without opposite(s) from *An.* III 6, 430b24–26, and so thinking this kind of object just means thinking an essence.

But the subject of Aristotle's final comments at *An.* III 6, 430b26–30, is clearly broader: what he claims to be always true is *nous* of any essence whatsoever—not necessarily of a cause without any opposite. Geometrical divisions and privations do not seem to have proper essences, but *adiaireta* in form certainly do: to grasp the essence of such an object, I take it, means to acquire the proper understanding of its form as being responsible for what the object is like. Such a grasp, Aristotle insists at the end of *An.* III 6, cannot but be true—just like a grasp of a cause without any opposite.

In this way Aristotle's ascending list of *adiaireta* in the central passage provides the foil against which he can effectively disambiguate the claim made in the opening passage according to which thinking of *adiaireta* "is among the things concerning which falsity is not possible." The first three kinds of *adiaireta* are objects endowed with such a kind of unity that they can be thought without division—as potential or actual components of propositional thoughts. In their cases the thinking of *adiaireta* seems neither true nor false. But the *adiaireton* of the fourth kind, *adiaireton par excellence*, can be thought without division in a very different sense: this is a self-standing kind of thinking, independent from propositional thinking. And the case of thinking the fourth kind of *adiaireton* is just a very special instance of a larger

of something else—namely, as being the length *of* a certain kind of line, such as a circle, unified by its form. And this may also be what Aristotle meant by the last words of the difficult sentence at 430b16–17: *all' hêi adiaireta* (this phrase is difficult on any reading and was bracketed by Torstrik and several editors and interpreters following him, including Förster). What Aristotle seems to be saying here is that the *adiaireta* in form are *diaireta* in the way in which the quantitative *adiaireta* are divisible: i.e., accidentally. In other words: *adiaireta* in form are only divisible *qua* being something else—namely, three-dimensional continuous quantities—just as quantitative *adiaireta* are only *adiaireta qua* being quantities *of* certain *adiaireta* in form. Cf. Christian Pfeiffer's insightful discussion of the matter and the form of magnitudes, and especially his explanation (in Pfeiffer 2018: 125–128) of how to understand the claim of *Phys.* IV 2 that "extension" (i.e., the matter of the magnitudes) is indeterminate (cf. also Morison 2002: 109). It is exactly such an indeterminate extension (ontologically dependent on a definite shape) that Aristotle is, I take it, focusing on at *An.* III 6, 430b6–14.

115 *An.* III 4, 430a3–5.

116 *An.* III 4, 429b11–12.

class: it happens to be a case of grasping an essence because for the object in question there is no difference between *X* and what it is to be *X*. There clearly is such a difference in the case of *adiaireta* in form, and so from thinking such an object without division (as a potential or actual constituent of propositions) one can arrive at thinking *what it is to be* such an object: that is, I take it, at grasping its form as the cause of its being this or that. In the final passage Aristotle focuses again on this larger class of grasping of essences—with respect to which *nous* was defined in *An.* III 4–5—and contrasts it, now unambiguously, with propositional thinking as being always true. This disambiguation was facilitated by the central passage which analyzed different kinds of objects that can be thought without division in the sense of being potential or actual components of propositions, and which showed how different this thinking is from the most exalted kind of grasping of essences, while also implicitly pointing to a contrast with the grasping of matter-involving essences. Unlike undivided continuous quantities, objects of unitary forms, or geometrical divisions, essences do not primarily relate to propositional thinking as its (actual or potential) constituents, but as its ultimate explanatory grounds.[117]

In the final passage, Aristotle draws the following contrast:

> A statement (*phasis*) is [predicating] one thing of another (*ti kata tinos*), just as is the case with an affirmation, and it is in all cases true or false. But this is not so with all thought (*nous*); rather, the thought (*nous*) of what [something] is in virtue of [its] essence (*tou ti esti kata to ti ên einai*) is [always] true, and it is not [predicating] one thing of another (*ti kata tinos*).[118]

"Statement" (*phasis*) here seems to be picking up on both affirmations and denials as discussed in the opening passage, just as is the claim that a statement is in all cases true or false.[119] Its characterization as predicating one thing of another

[117] To the extent to which the essence coincides with the *definiens*, it can become a constituent of a proposition (thanks to David Bronstein for this observation). But the grasping of that essence consists neither in predicating it of the *definiendum*, nor just in it providing an element for such a predication.

[118] *An.* III 6, 430b26–29.

[119] Interpreters found the meaning of *phasis* at *An.* III 6, 430b26–27 puzzling. At *Metaph.* IX 10, 1051b23–25, *phasis* is contrasted with propositions and claimed to be always true. A few lines below in *An.* III 7 the verb *phanai* seems to mean pronouncing a simple concept (*An.* III 7, 431a8; cf. e.g., *Int.* 4, 16b26–28). But none of these contexts seems fitting here. That is why most modern interpreters concluded that *phasis* can only mean affirmation—the sense in which *phanai* was used at *An.* III 6, 430b4, and will be used again at *An.* III 7, 431a15, and indeed in which *phasis* is very often used by Aristotle (see Bonitz 1870: 813). But this understanding makes the phrase *hôsper hê kataphasis* (*An.* III 6, 430b26–27) meaningless, which is why Torstrik 1862: 196–198 (followed, e.g., by Ross 1961, Hamlyn 1993², Shields 2016, and Reeve 2017; cf. Mignucci 1996: 412 and Crivelli 2004: 102) suggested—without any support in the manuscript tradition—changing *kataphasis* into *apophasis* (while adopting the reading of W: *hôsper kai hê*). Another approach was proposed by Philoponus, *De Int.* 86.34–44, who took the relation of *phasis* to *kataphasis* to be that of an inner to an outer speech, which, however, seems unlikely. A different kind of solution was suggested by Wedin 1988: 125, who proposed to understand *phasis* in very broad terms as covering both the *phasis* of *Metaph.* IX 10 and any kind of proposition, and to interpret *ti kata tinos* attributively rather than predicatively, so that Aristotle would be narrowing

(*ti kata tinos*) replaces the notion of combination (*sunthesis*),[120] apparently because it allows Aristotle to draw more sharply the intended contrast with thinking of "what [something] is in virtue of [its] essence." This kind of thinking refers undeniably back to the activity of grasping essences as analyzed in *An.* III 4–5. But in the present passage Aristotle seems to be putting it into the context of propositional thought, which has been the main topic of *An.* III 6. One way to understand the move is as follows. Thinking of what something is (*ti esti*) seems to have a structure that *prima facie* resembles the structure of a statement. A statement predicates something of something, *ti kata tinos*, and in this sense it also says what (*ti*) something is (e.g., S *esti* P). The point would then be that the thinking contrasted with statements here is of what something is *with respect to its very essence*.[121] What appears to be a predicate (*ti*) of something else (*tinos*) is in fact expressing the very essence of that thing, and so the thinking in question does *not* have, strictly speaking, the structure of *ti kata tinos* (i.e., predicating one thing *of another*).[122]

If this is how the contrast is intended, it does not imply that the quasi-propositional structure of a *definiens* being predicated of its *definiendum* is essential to the activity of grasping essences. No such structure was mentioned in the definitory account of *An.* III 4–5. Moreover, Aristotle seems to have good reasons to allow for the possibility of there being essences that can only be grasped but not *defined* scientifically.[123] The point may then be that in order to properly understand the quasi-propositional relation of a *definiens* to its *definiendum*, one needs to have a non-propositional grasp of the respective essence, whatever that grasp amounts to.[124] It may well be that humans cannot grasp any essence (of a material

the focus down to a specific kind of *phasis* (for a similar approach, see already Ps.-Simplicius, *In An.* 260.3–14, who takes Aristotle to speak of a simple thought used in a synthetic context). But this very broad understanding of *phasis* is unprecedented. The solution of this "textual problem" is, in fact, very simple. In all likelihood, *phasis* at 430b26 is used in the sense of *apophansis*: i.e., statement or proposition (this solution may have already been proposed by Alexander in his lost commentary—at least if in Ps.-Simplicius' report at *In DA* 260.2 we must read *apophansis* instead of *apophasis*, where the latter makes little sense in the context). This is less frequent than the meaning corresponding to affirmation, but there are a fair number of passages documenting it (see Bonitz 1870: 813, who lists this as one of the three standard meanings and gives a number of references). Now, Torstrik was aware of this possibility, but thought it is excluded because *hôsper* cannot have the requested meaning of "*ex genere descendere ad species*" (this would allegedly demand a *hoion*): see Torstrik 1862: 196–197. In response to this worry it should be stressed that *kataphasis* is not introduced simply as one arbitrary species of the genus *phasis*; rather, it is the exemplary case of it, the model example of the structure *ti kata tinos* from which this structure is here effectively extended to other statements (i.e., *apophaseis*). For this function of *hôsper* one easily finds parallels: e.g., at *An.* I 1, 402b16–21; *An.* II 10, 422b6–10; and *An.* II 11, 424a10–15. In fact, this is exactly the role that I take *hôsper* to play at *An.* III 5, 430a10, as well (in contrast to *hoion* at 430a12); see Chapter 6 (Section 3).

[120] On the surprisingly broad extension of these two notions, see Section 2.3 in this chapter.

[121] Cf. Chiba 2010 for an analysis of the phrase *to ti ên einai* as directing the *ti esti* question to the very essence of the thing.

[122] Cf. Berti's and Sorabji's reading of the final passage (the references are given above in footnote 71).

[123] I.e., the immaterial substances. Thanks to Klaus Corcilius for this observation.

[124] In the case of material substances, it may consist in understanding how the form in question makes the respective matter be this or that (cf. *Metaph.* VII 17, 1041b2–33): i.e., how the respective matter and form are one. No such complexity can, of course, pertain to immaterial substances.

thing) without forming the respective definition in their minds, but that wouldn't mean the former is reducible to the latter.

Alternatively, the notion of *nous tou ti esti kata to ti ên einai* could be putting the activity of grasping essences into the context of propositional thought in the following way. It could mean grasping *what something is* with respect to the essential core of it (*to ti ên einai*), just as one grasps, say, what thunder is by capturing *extinguishing of fire* as the explanatorily basic element of thunder.[125] In this case what is grasped can surely become an element of propositions—indeed, of the immediate propositions "extinguishing of fire belongs to clouds" and "noise (thunder) belongs to extinguishing of fire"; but this status belongs to what is grasped here only instrumentally, as a way of carrying out its primary role as the ultimate explanatory ground (*archê*) for the respective set of propositions.

Be that as it may, the least probable appears to be the idea that by *nous* of "what [something] is in virtue of [its] essence" Aristotle means a thought of an isolated concept (e.g., the diagonal or the incommensurable).[126] In fact the *nous* in question resembles such a thought *even less* than it resembles a propositional thought of *ti kata tinos*. The thought of an isolated concept *falls short of* propositional thinking because it does not on its own reach the sphere of truth and falsity at all (it is nothing more than a building block for propositional thoughts that can be true or false). A *nous* of "what [something] is in virtue of [its] essence," in contrast, *surpasses* propositional thought because it not only reaches the sphere but, in addition, excludes falsity: it achieves what no propositional thought can ever achieve on its own: namely, being *unquestionably* true (whereas all propositions can either be further questioned as to *why* they are true or are, as immediate propositions, directly based on such a *nous*). While the claim, ascribed to Aristotle by numerous readers, that the understanding of an isolated concept is always true, sounds pointless and extravagant, the insistence that grasping of essences cannot but be true is perfectly understandable. If the essence I grasp explains why a certain true proposition holds, it would be strange, to say the least, if this grasp were not itself true.[127]

[125] In the case of immaterial substances *to ti esti* would simply coincide with *to ti ên einai*. I owe this suggestion to David Bronstein. Cf. Bronstein (forthcoming) for an account of understanding of definitions in *Posterior Analytics* as non-propositional acts.

[126] One could think that this is suggested by the comparison at the very end of *An.* III 6 (430b29–31) between the *nous* in question, on the one hand, and perception of exclusive objects, on the other. But we must bear in mind that while essences play the role of primary objects for thinking as the exclusive objects do for perception (that seems to be the basis of the parallel at *An.* III 6, 430b29–31), there is an important disanalogy in the way they relate to other objects of thought and perception, respectively. See Section 2.1 in this chapter. I return to the disanalogy in the following section.

[127] Cf. *Posterior Analytics* II 19, 100b5–17, and especially the claim at b11–12 that nothing can be truer (*alêthesteron*) than scientific knowledge besides *nous*. I take *Metaph.* IX 10, 1051b17–26 to be making a similar point.

It should be mentioned that there is a popular objection to the idea of associating the *nous* of "what [something] is in virtue of [its] essence" with scientific definitions: surely, Aristotle does not want to deny that my search for a definition can go wrong and that I can be offered, and even accept, something as a definition of *X* which in fact is only an assertion of a necessary (or even accidental) attribute of it.[128] But this objection, I think, misses the target, for when Aristotle talks about *nous* of "what [something] is in virtue of [its] essence" he can only have in mind what happens in, or is presupposed by, a *successful* definition: as long as my attempts at defining *X* go wrong, he would not say that I have a *false nous* of what it is with respect to its essence, but rather that I do not yet have *any* such *nous*, properly speaking. I do not have a wrong grasp of the essence; rather, I am ignorant of it as such, as Aristotle famously puts it at *Metaph.* IX 10, 1052a1–2.[129]

3.6 How propositional thinking depends on the grasping of essences

We are now in a position to take up the question raised at the outset of this chapter concerning the nature of the expansion undertaken in *An.* III 6. That question, in fact, becomes almost explicit at the end of the chapter: how exactly does propositional thinking relate to the grasping of the essences, and in what sense, if any, can the former be described as secondary to, or grounded in, the latter? We have seen why this question is important: if it turned out that propositional thinking is in no way grounded in the activity of grasping essences, then Aristotle's definitory account of *nous* in *An.* III 4–5 would be a failure, for what it can explain is at most a very specific and rare phenomenon; there would, apparently, have to be another capacity of the soul defined with reference to propositions as its primary objects. But that is not how Aristotle thinks about the matter. Rather, he rather believes that the same capacity of the soul that was defined in *An.* III 4–5 with respect to essences is also responsible for propositional thinking: it is the *nous* as defined in *An.* III 4–5 that, according to *An.* III 6, produces the unity of every propositional thought. The question is whether Aristotle is justified in making this claim.

[128] See, e.g., Mignucci 1996: 410 or the more elaborate argument developed by Butler and Rubenstein 2004.

[129] My error, strictly speaking, is not *about* the essence, but *about* my cognitive state, since I believe I have found the proper necessary principle of the thing in question, while this is not the case. Most likely, I am simply predicating one thing of another, while falsely believing that I am in fact expressing the essence of the subject. See in this connection *Posterior Analytics* I 9, 76a26–27: "It is difficult to know whether we know something or not. For it is difficult to know whether or not our knowledge of something proceeds from its proper principles..." (trans. J. Barnes, slightly mod.). It is also worth stressing that being ignorant of the essence as such does not mean that there is no epistemic connection at all: I may very well know some facts for which the essence is the ultimate *explanans*, and even know *that* there is such an *explanans*, without yet knowing *what* it is.

The structural parallel between *An.* III 6 and *An.* III 1 is helpful in various respects, but it cannot settle the question on its own. That is because, as already observed above, we are confronted with an obvious dissimilarity. In *An.* III 1 perceiving of common and incidental objects is explained as grounded in perceiving of exclusive objects in the straightforward sense that the former cannot take place without the latter.[130] It seems plausible, then, to insist that the acts of cognizing the common and the incidental objects are secondary acts of the same capacity as was defined in *An.* II 5 and *An.* II 12 with respect to exclusive objects. But the situation is clearly different in the case of propositional thought, which can perfectly well take place *without any proper grasp* of an essence (in terms of *An.* III 4–5). Indeed, this seems to be what happens in the great majority of cases and what almost all human thinking consists in. Does it still make sense, then, to insist that Aristotle's account of propositional thinking is grounded in his account of grasping of essences, and that the former can, thus, be traced back to the same part of the soul which was defined with respect to the latter? As noted above, this grounding would seem to be primarily teleological. Our *nous* is defined as the capacity for grasping essences, just as our sight is defined as the capacity for seeing colors. But since *nous* is not a part of our nature, it only rarely attains its proper fulfilment. Nevertheless, Aristotle seems committed to the claim that all activities for which *nous* is responsible, even at its "embryonic" stage, are directed at grasping of essences as their final goal. Can we make better sense of that claim now? There are, I believe, at least two clues contained in the argument of *An.* III 6 as reconstructed in this chapter.

(1) Propositional thought is always potentially both true and false. There is an irreducible potential of falsity embedded in propositional thought. It can never on its own exclude falsity. The only way to achieve this is by a grasp of an essence which cannot but be true and which can as such ground the truth of certain propositions, primarily the immediate ones and secondarily many others. This analysis of the relation between propositional thinking and grasping of essences provides the first clue toward better understanding the teleological dependence of the former on the latter that seems to structure Aristotle's way of proceeding in *An.* III 4–8. It seems *prima facie* more plausible to say that all our thoughts are directed at truth than to say that they are directed at grasping of essences. And *An.* III 6 makes a strong case for the directedness at truth being, ultimately, nothing other than directedness at grasping of essences. While thinking of structural elements on its own does not reach the sphere of truth and falsity at all, propositional thoughts *can* be true; but they can never ground their own truth. It is always possible to ask *why* such and such proposition is true, and no ultimate answer to this question can be given without the grasp of an essence. So, if all our thoughts are directed at truth, then all our thoughts teleologically relate to grasping of essences, which alone can provide

130 Similarly, it would seem, growth and reproduction cannot take place without nutrition.

the ultimate ground for the truth of some (i.e., demonstrable) propositions.[131] If that is so, then it seems sound to define *nous*—the principle of human intellectual life—with reference to essences as its primary objects.

(2) Another, complementary, perspective on the relation between propositional thinking and the grasping of essences offered by *An.* III 6 emerges if we reflect on *the unity* of thought. The notion of unity comes twice to the foreground in the opening passage of the chapter. Propositional thought is "a combination of thoughts as being one (*hôsper hen ontôn*)" (*An.* III 6, 430a27–28) and *nous* is what "produces the unity (*hen poioun*) in each case" (*An.* III 6, 430b5–6). What is important about this kind of unity is that it is compositional, and that *nous* is, in some sense, its originator or producer (*to poioun*). This can be contrasted in two respects with the unity of essences as the primary objects of thinking: the latter unity is not compositional, and *nous* is not its producer but receiver—it is *to paschon* rather than *to poioun* with respect to its primary objects. The notion of *adiaireta* in the sense of ultimate explanatory grounds of propositions offers, then, a clue for better understanding how the compositional unity of propositional thought is derivative from the non-compositional unity of the activity of grasping essences. While a thought of a structural element does not as such constitute any self-standing unity at all, but only a (potential or actual) *part* of a propositional thought, propositional thought is already a self-standing unity; but it has not, so to speak, the source of its unity in itself. The compositional unity of propositional thoughts (predicating *ti kata tinos*) is imperfect in the sense that it could be mediated by a middle term. Again, one can always ask *why P* holds of *S*. There are, of course, propositions in whose case any search for a middle term would be in vain (because they describe an accidental connection or because they are false). But that does not mean that the unity is more perfect here than in the case of demonstrable propositions. On the contrary, in these cases the unity is even weaker because not only is it not unmediated, but, in addition to that, no mediation is possible at all.[132] If one grants Aristotle that thinking always aims at unity, he is thereby entitled to infer that all thinking teleologically relates to grasping of essences, because only essences are genuinely unitary objects of thought.[133]

Either way, as soon as we agree that each act of thinking aims at truth or at unity, it will turn out that all our thinking acts are, ultimately, directed at grasping of essences—whether we are aware of it or not, and whether we even believe in essences or not. In this way *An.* III 6 helps justify one of the most important assumptions behind the architecture of *An.* III 4–8.

[131] Indemonstrable (because accidental) propositions can, of course, also be true, but only temporarily: they, so to speak, only happen to be true; their truth is unstable and cannot be properly grounded.

[132] Cf. *Posterior Analytics* I 33, 89a3–4, where *protasis amesos* seems to be used, non-standardly, in something like the latter sense, referring to an object of opinion.

[133] The unity of immediate propositions, although not mediated, is, I take it, dependent on the unity of definitions, which in turn is grounded in the unity of essences.

4. Conclusion

I conclude by summing up the main points reached in this chapter.

An. III 6 does play an important role in the larger argument of *De anima*, and this role is prefigured most clearly by the role played by *An.* III 1 (425a13–b11) in Aristotle's account of perception. This parallel shows that Aristotle's inquiry into thinking is perfectly in line with the methodological prescription he lays down in *An.* II 4. More specifically, *An.* III 6 is important for Aristotle's larger argument, first, because it demarcates where errors of reason are possible and where they are not. As such, it allows Aristotle to maintain that the grasping of essences cannot but be true, without falling prey to his own objections to the traditional LKL view: despite the impression that *An.* III 4–5 could make on its own, Aristotle is capable of explaining how utter falsity is possible on the level of thinking. Indeed, *An.* III 6 is an indispensable part of Aristotle's polemic against the LKL view. Second, one can understand the importance of *An.* III 6 also independently from this dialectical context. By expanding the account of *An.* III 4–5, Aristotle shows how all kinds of phenomena of human intellectual life can be traced back to the same basic capacity or part of the soul: namely, *nous* defined narrowly with respect to essences as its primary objects. In this way Aristotle displays the explanatory power of his definitory account. And he also lays the groundwork here for his subsequent inquiry into the cognitive soul in *An.* III 7, for his summary of the findings about it offered in *An.* III 8, as well as for the account of practical thought developed in *An.* III 9–11.

The argument of *An.* III 6 is built around a unitary notion of *adiaireton*. An *adiaireton* is any object such that it can be thought non-compositionally. And so, both the structural elements (components) of propositions and their ultimate explanatory grounds fall under this notion. While the thinking of an ultimate explanatory ground cannot but be true, the thinking of a component falls short of being either true or false. Both kinds of thinking together can be contrasted with the propositional thought, which can as such be both true and false. This broad notion of *adiaireton* also helps us understand why Aristotle discusses lengths (as the most basic continuous quantities) in *An.* III 6. These are neither concepts nor essences, but it is important to insist that they can be thought and not just perceived (otherwise geometry, and perhaps also other kinds of human thinking, would turn out to be impossible). And they can only be thought if they either are or break down into *adiaireta* which can be thought non-compositionally. Finally, the proposed interpretation of *adiaireta* sheds light on the central passage (430b6–26) as a whole: its internal logic and its role in *An.* III 6. The ascending list of four *adiaireta*, governed by two main criteria, helps to disambiguate the components of propositions from their ultimate explanatory grounds, and hence also the opening claim that thinking of *adiaireta* is never false.

As a whole, I suggest, the chapter points to at least two ways in which the key assumption behind the architecture of *An.* III 4–8—namely, that propositional thinking teleologically depends on the activity of grasping essences—can be made more palatable. It is enough to assume that all human thinking aims at truth and/or at unity, for none of these strivings can ever be truly satisfied without grasping an essence.

4

The cognitive soul and how embodied thinking comes about

The practical embeddedness of human thought

1. Introduction

There are at least two exegetical questions that any interpreter of *An.* III 7 is expected to answer. The first is whether there is a single and coherent argument unfolding in the chapter. An affirmative answer to this question is far from a foregone conclusion. On the contrary, scholars have often judged *An.* III 7 to be a mere collection of loosely connected, if not even disconnected, fragments. This judgement goes back at least to the German scholar Adolf Torstrik.[1] It is accepted by David Ross in the *apparatus criticus* of his *editio minor*, who also adopts the editorial convention of inserting several em dashes ("—") into the Greek text to mark the various fragments that in his view compose the chapter.[2] Most interpreters of *De anima* have accepted Torstrik's verdict (via Ross).[3] For instance, in his Clarendon translation and commentary on *De anima*, Christopher Shields claims that "the chapter is a collection of fragments conspicuously lacking the kind of connection and inferential particles characteristic of Aristotle's prose style."[4] Leaving

Special thanks go to Klaus Corcilius, Michel Crubellier, and Robert Roreitner, who read multiple versions of this chapter and offered many helpful comments and suggestions for improvement. I have done my best to take on board their generous feedback. I benefited immensely from reading Corcilius 2020a, but I also departed from the results reached in that essay in a few crucial places. They are clearly indicated in the pages to follow. This chapter is not an attempt to update, let alone replace, Corcilius 2020a; rather, it is an entirely independent piece of work meant to enhance our understanding of how *An.* III 7 contributes to the argument offered in the stretch of text known as *An.* III 4–8.

[1] Torstrik 1862: xxv.

[2] Ross 1956: "*hoc caput has partes, sine cura scriptas et sine connexu sensus conglutinatas, continere arguit Torstrik*: 431a1–4, 4–7, 8–16, 16–17, 17–20, 20–b1, b22–12, 12–17, 17–19. *Melius sic dividitur*: 431a1–4, 4–7, 8–17, 17–20, 20–b1, b2–12, 12–19." These words are omitted in the *apparatus criticus* of his *editio maior* of the Greek text of Aristotle's *De anima* (Ross 1961). Did Ross change his mind between the two editions? Not quite: he still adopts the editorial practice of marking em dashes in the Greek text to highlight the putative fragments; furthermore, in the endnotes to his *editio maior*, Ross endorses Torstrik's thesis and argues that the chapter is just "a series of scraps." By his lights, these "scraps" were put together by an early editor rather than by Aristotle (Ross 1961: 310).

[3] Wisely to my mind, no recent editor of the *De anima* has followed Ross in marking up the putative fragments with an em dash even though they all seem to accept some version of Torstrik's verdict. Among the editors who explicitly recall Torstrik's verdict but do not follow Ross' editorial practice, I single out Siwek 1965: 339, endnote 703 ("*in capite praesenti deest perfecta unitas*").

[4] Shields 2016: 335. On this front, Shields' new and expanded Clarendon translation and commentary of Aristotle's *De anima* is no improvement over the old one. Cf. Hamlyn 1993[2]: "This chapter is a

Aristotle on the Essence of Human Thought. Klaus Corcilius, Andrea Falcon, and Robert Roreitner, Oxford University Press.
 DOI: 10.1093/9780198921820.003.0004

considerations of style aside, the question is whether there is a coherent train of thought in the chapter as a whole, and whether this train of thought amounts to a *bona fide* argument. I will answer this question in the affirmative by building on the results that Klaus Corcilius has recently achieved in an essay devoted to defending the unity of *An.* III 7.[5]

The second interpretative question, distinct but connected to the first, is how *An.* III 7 contributes to Aristotle's account of human thought and human thinking. This is an especially important question for this book given that we (the three co-authors) have the ambition of recovering and elucidating the original train of thought in Aristotle's treatment of *nous* (*An.* III 4–8). So let me elaborate on this front by recalling what Aristotle has achieved so far. In *An.* III 4–5 Aristotle supplied all the ingredients for a complete definition of *nous* as the principle (*archê*) of human thought. Aristotle has reached this important result by focusing on what he regards as the core case of thinking: namely, our grasping the essences. This is not only a highly specialized but also a very narrow form of *theoretical* thinking. As a matter of fact, not all human thinking which does not involve action requires grasping the essences as a precondition. Moreover, there is *practical* thinking in addition to non-practical thinking (*alias* thinking without action).[6] If Aristotle is trying to provide us with at least an outline of an account of human thinking, he is expected to deal with thinking that results in action in addition to dealing with thinking that does not involve action. When we take all the above into account, we immediately see that *An.* III 6 is only a first, limited step toward a fuller explanation of human thinking. *This chapter is a first expansion of the core model of thinking outlined in An. III 4–5.* In *An.* III 6 Aristotle considers kinds of thinking which go beyond the case of grasping essences since he explains how complex thoughts and their constituents are possible. But more work is needed on this front because the results of Aristotle's investigation to this point are still a far cry from even the bare outline of an account of human thinking.

So how exactly does *An.* III 7 fit into Aristotle's treatment of *nous*? To begin with, the chapter builds on some of the results reached in *An.* III 6. The equation of thinking to saying, introduced in *An.* III 6 to explain how one can combine thoughts, and how their combination amounts to saying something of something

collection of fragments" (145). A similar judgment is passed in Theiler 1979[3]: "the chapter contains a number of individual considerations (*Einzelüberlegungen*), [only] loosely associated with one another" (146). Unsurprisingly, this judgment is also found in the Italian scholarly tradition. For this branch of the scholarly tradition, I single out Zucca 2015: "*An.* III 7 is a highly disorganized chapter (*fortemente disorganico*)" (10).

[5] Corcilius 2020a: 185–219.

[6] Admittedly, the expression "thinking without action" is a bit cumbersome. But I am following Aristotle here, who adopts this expression in *An.* III 7, 431b10. We can only guess at his reason for this choice of words. To me it seems obvious that thinking without action need not be identical with theoretical thinking. There is plenty of thinking that does not result in action and yet does not amount to theoretical thinking.

else, resurfaces in the first part of *An.* III 7, where it is invoked to explain how the soul pursues or avoids something.[7] But there is a less obvious, yet deeper, and ultimately more important, strand of unity binding *An.* III 7 together with the previous chapters concerned with *nous* and its distinctive activity: that is, *noein*. Let me recall how Aristotle's treatment of *nous* begins in *An.* III 4:

> Regarding the part of the soul by which the soul knows and understands—be it separate or separate not in extension but [only] in account—we must examine what its distinguishing mark is and how (*pôs pote*) thinking (*noein*) may ever come about.[8]

This passage introduces two large questions that jointly set Aristotle's research agenda in *An.* III 4–8. Searching for the distinguishing mark (*differentia*) of *nous* is equivalent to looking for how *nous* differs from other cognitive powers of the soul (and, first of all, from *aisthêsis*). Aristotle is centrally concerned with this question in *An.* III 4. It is safe to say that Aristotle has successfully answered this first question by the end of *An.* III 4. So the *pôs pote* construction in the above passage introduces another question. This second question, however, can be taken in two different ways. It can be taken *either* as a request for an explanation of how an episode of thinking comes about *or* as a call for an account of how thinking is possible in the first place. An answer to the question of how thinking—with its distinctive features of objectivity, universality, and necessity—is possible in the first place is given in *An.* III 5.[9] So at this point we are left with the second question if it is understood in the first way. In other words, we want to know how it is possible for an episode of thinking to take place. I submit that Aristotle is centrally concerned with this version of the second question in *An.* III 7. He provides us with the conceptual ingredients for an answer to the question of how an episode of human thinking is triggered. When we approach this stretch of text in this way, we immediately see that *An. III 7 is part of a larger textual, and indeed argumentative, unit which begins in An. III 4 and is not over until the end of An. III 8.*

But a full explanation of how an episode of human thinking comes about is not possible if one relies solely on the conceptual resources introduced in *An.* III 4–5 and *An.* III 6. So Aristotle is forced to take into account the role of *phantasia* in human thinking and, ultimately, to situate what he calls "the thinking capacity" (*to noêtikon*)[10] in a larger cognitive context which is not available within the narrow boundaries of *An.* III 4–5 and *An.* III 6. This explains why Aristotle is not content

[7] Is it *the soul* or rather *the agent* which pursues or avoids something? Aristotle's full answer to this question is *the agent* in virtue of having a *soul*.

[8] *An.* III 4, 429a10–13.

[9] See Chapter 2 (Section 6).

[10] Aristotle never uses this expression in *An.* III 4–5 and *An.* III 6, where he consistently speaks of *nous* and *noein*. This expression is first found in *An.* II 4, 415a17. It resurfaces in *An.* III 7, 431b2.

to build his argument on the results achieved in *An.* III 6, or to apply the principles he has discovered in *An.* III 4–5. In *An.* III 7, Aristotle goes well beyond anything established either in *An.* III 4–5 or in *An.* III 6. In fact, he goes all the way back to some of the results reached in the course of his discussion of perception and *phantasia*. At one point (*An.* III 7, 431a20–21), he even makes an explicit reference to the results reached in the discussion of how the perceptual mean, in addition to discriminating within one sense modality, discriminates across different sense modalities.[11]

In light of the above strategy, *An.* III 7 can be described as *an exercise in cognitive psychology*. By "cognitive psychology" I mean *a self-conscious attempt to apply salient principles discovered in the course of the study of embodied cognition*. These principles are now applied to the study of the [*cognitive*] *soul*. I inserted square brackets to alert the reader that this expression is an amplification of the original Greek. Aristotle speaks of soul (*psuchê*), but he must have in mind an integrated system of cognitive powers that are operationally fused together. These powers are always present in a certain kind of living body in virtue of the fact that this body possesses a certain kind of soul. More directly, the cognitive soul in question can only be a human soul, and the body in question can only be a human body.[12] On the interpretation advocated in this book, *An.* III 7 is emphatically not on a par with *An.* III 4–5 or *An.* III 6. It is something new and quite different. This last point can be restated as follows: notwithstanding the strand of unity, there are important elements of discontinuity separating *An.* III 7 from the preceding chapters. *An.* III 7 is no longer concerned with *nous* as the principle (*archê*) of human thinking (*noein*); rather, it is about the way an integrated system of cognitive powers that crucially includes the capacity for thinking (*to noêtikon*) is at work in a human body. The reference to the human body is ineliminable at this point since the soul is the first actuality of a natural body which has potentially life (*An.* II 1, 412a27–28).[13] Even when the focus is on the soul rather than the body, as is certainly the case in *An.* III 7, the treatment of the soul must make an indirect reference to the body, since the functioning of the soul crucially depends on its being present in a certain kind of body.

Adopting the interpretative approach outlined above makes it easier for us to explain why Aristotle returns to the topic of perception in *An.* III 7. Perception understood as a distinct mode of cognition was left behind at the end of *An.* III 2. Aristotle returns to it by considering the capacity for perception as a part (or

[11] The cross-reference is to *An.* III 2, 426b8–29.

[12] For a fuller attempt to define the cognitive soul, I refer the reader the Glossary (*s.v.* COGNITIVE SOUL).

[13] Aristotle goes on to say that the relevant body is organic (*An.* II 1, 412b1). By our lights, this means that the body is a tool (or instrument, *organon*) that the soul uses to discharge its power. However, this body must also be organized in a certain way for the soul to use it. This means that the body must be equipped with *organs* to work as a suitable instrument. For instance, nothing can see unless it is equipped with an appropriate sense-organ (an eye).

aspect) of a larger cognitive system. In this context, Aristotle expands on what he previously said by dealing with the question of how the activation of perception leads to the pursuit or avoidance of something across different sense modalities.

By contrast, if Aristotle's main focus remained squarely on *nous* understood as the principle of our mental phenomena, it would be difficult to explain why in *An.* III 7 he devotes so much attention to the basic model of perception and its relation to the explanation of how rational behavior depends on desire. And yet, this is how the text has been read by many, if not most, interpreters since antiquity. It is worth elaborating, briefly, on this alternative interpretation to fully appreciate what is offered in this chapter. For Themistius, Aristotle is still fully immersed in his discussion of *nous* in *An.* III 7. On his reading, the chapter marks a shift in focus, but this shift is quite different from the one I outlined above. Aristotle would no longer be concerned with theoretical *nous*: at this point, he would turn to *practical nous.* In this context, Aristotle would return to the topic of perception, and indeed would expand on it with his account of perceptual desire, because he would be operating under the working hypothesis (first introduced in *An.* III 4) that *nous* is analogous to perception.[14] A similar interpretation can be found in Ps-Simplicius and Philoponus. Both commentators think that Aristotle has exhaustively concerned himself with *nous* as the principle of theoretical thinking in *An.* III 4–6. Aristotle would now be turning his attention to *nous* as the principle of practical thinking. For both, this kind of *nous,* which crucially requires the use of *dianoia* and *phantasia,* would be the primary object of study in *An.* III 7.[15] Among contemporary interpreters of *An.* III 7, Catherine Rowett (publishing as Catherine Osborne) has also argued for the unity of the chapter along these lines. By her lights, in this chapter Aristotle defends an account of intellectual judgment by building on the parallel account of perception.[16]

Contrary to this well-entrenched exegetical tradition which makes *nous,* and in particular practical *nous,* Aristotle's research focus in *An.* III 7, I argue that *An.* III 7 is primarily concerned with the explanation of how a cognitive system, which is by definition embodied and includes the capacity for thinking as one of its constitutive elements, can engage in episodes of thinking. This is a new kind of project. While Aristotle was *before* concerned with *a definitory question,* trying to answer a *ti esti* question with respect to *nous* understood as the principle of human thought, he is *now* mostly dealing with *an explanatory question.*[17] A key question that must

[14] Themistius, *In An.* 112.25–26 and 112.33–34.

[15] Ps-Simplicius, *In An.* 263.30–264.20. Cf. Philoponus, *In An.* 558.11–31. Ps-Simplicius divides the text in a slightly different way. By his lights, the argument for *nous* as the principle of practical thinking begins in earnest only at *An.* III 7, 431a4. He thinks that the principle that establishes the priority of actuality over potentiality completes the argument for *nous* as the principle of theoretical thinking. This *divisio textus* is transmitted to the medieval commentary tradition (e.g., Thomas Aquinas).

[16] Osborne 1998: 433–466.

[17] On *An.* III 4–5 as centrally concerned with the definition of the human capacity for thinking, see Chapter 2 (Section 1).

be addressed at the outset of this project is how the relevant cognitive system is to be studied. More directly, we need to decide whether we should take a top-down or a bottom-up approach to the explanation of the cognitive soul. Apparently, Aristotle favors *a bottom-up approach*. This choice is hardly surprising if we reflect on the argumentative strategy adopted in the rest of *De anima*. This strategy goes all the way back to the analogy between souls and rectilinear plane figures ordered in a series beginning with the triangle advanced in *An*. II 3.[18] This analogy plays a pivotal role in the study of the soul understood as the principle of life. We study the different powers of the soul serially, starting from the most common, non-cognitive power (i.e., the nutritive power), continuing with the cognitive, non-rational power of perception, and ending with a discussion of the cognitive, rational power that humans alone possess among things here on earth.

This bottom-up approach is implicitly applied throughout *An*. III 7. Aristotle begins his study of how the cognitive soul operates by recalling his basic account of how perception is activated by the object of perception; he then continues with a discussion of how the non-rational pursuit or avoidance of something arises in such a system; finally, he turns his attention to the higher cognitive achievements of this soul. While the first two steps of this argumentative strategy have a more general (*zoological*) significance, the third step narrows down the discussion to the case of the *human* soul. It is only at this stage of the argument that Aristotle turns to the *rational* soul (*dianoetikê psuchê*).[19] Such a soul can only be a human soul understood as an integrated system of cognitive powers that crucially includes not only the capacity for perception but also the capacity for thinking. As soon as we realize that Aristotle concentrates his attention on how a cognitive system of this kind works, we see why the chapter contains important insights on how Aristotle conceives of the relation between perception, *phantasia*, and thought.

Adopting the bottom-up approach outlined above to the study of the cognitive soul yields some remarkable results. To begin with, Aristotle can complete his positive account of the non-rational cognitive powers of the soul. In *An*. III 7, Aristotle supplies us with his definition of non-rational desire. This definition provides a basic account of non-rational desire which is meant to apply to all forms of non-rational desire. As such, it applies to desire as is found in both human and non-human animals. This definition is arguably the most important result reached in the first part of our chapter (*An*. III 7, 431a8–14).[20] The importance of this result can hardly be overstated. Without such a definition, the treatment of the soul cannot be said to be complete. At the very least, we can say that *An*. III 7 fills a lacuna left in the previous argument.

[18] *An*. II 3, 414b20–415a13.

[19] *An*. III 7, 431a14. This is the soul that can engage in *discursive* thinking. This thinking takes the form of *propositional* thinking.

[20] For an in-depth discussion of this important passage and its philosophical implications well beyond Aristotle's *De anima*, see Corcilius 2011a: 117–169.

But there is another aspect of the argumentative strategy adopted in *An.* III 7 that I would like to underscore right from the start before engaging in an in-depth analysis of this chapter. When Aristotle turns to the higher achievements of the cognitive soul, he places special emphasis on the thinking that results in action (*praxis*). We are not told why we should focus on practical thinking at this stage of the argument. An educated guess is that *Aristotle is presupposing the practical embeddedness of human thinking*. In other words, Aristotle is tacitly assuming that the thinking that is practically oriented is *ontogenetically* prior to any other form of thinking. This does not mean, I hasten to add, that practical thinking is also *conceptually* prior to non-practical thinking. Quite the opposite: Aristotle defines *nous* in *An.* III 4–5 by focusing on theoretical rather than practical thinking. And yet, *practical thinking seems to come before theoretical thinking in the development of an individual human being.*

The thinking we encounter in a practical context has propositional structure, requires *phantasmata*, and is driven by a desire for some good. When Aristotle goes beyond this initial case and speaks of "thinking without action" (*An.* III 7, 431b10), he carries over both the first and the second feature of thinking.[21] The third feature is modified as follows: the relevant desire is no longer desire for the good of the agent but rather desire for the truth. In the end, however, all embodied (human) thinking, whether or not it results in action, turns out to be driven by desire. This conclusion is sufficiently important to deserve an explicit mention in the subtitle chosen for this chapter.

An. III 7 remains an extremely difficult, dense, and at times frustratingly elliptical stretch of text. However, I hope to show that, far from being a hopelessly disorganized and scrappy collection of ideas, the chapter as a whole

(1) is written around a single topic, *the cognitive soul*;
(2) has a main focus, the explanation of how a particular kind of cognitive soul—namely, *the rational soul*—engages in episodes of thinking;
(3) adopts a distinctive argumentative strategy, *the bottom-up approach*, which presupposes not only the *embodiment of human thinking* but also its *embeddedness in a practical context.*

A better appreciation of how *An.* III 7 fits within Aristotle's overall account of the soul prompts two final considerations. The first is this. In his treatment of *nous*, Aristotle is not immediately concerned with explaining what we nowadays call mental phenomena; instead, his first and foremost theoretical preoccupation in

[21] Let me stress, again, that *thinking without action need not be identical with theoretical thinking.* Based on what we are told in *An.* III 4–5, theoretical thinking is a special form of non-practical thinking. Among other things, theoretical thinking consists in grasping the essences. It does not take long for the reader to see that not all human thinking that does not involve action requires grasping essences as a precondition.

dealing with *nous* is to provide the elements for a definition of *nous* understood as the principle that makes those mental phenomena possible in the first place.[22] Aristotle reaches this result by isolating *nous* understood as the principle of human thinking not only from the enabling conditions of thinking but also from *phantasia* and the mental representations employed to convey the contents of human thought. Aristotle calls these mental representations *phantasmata.*[23] What we obtain, in the difficult (and still poorly understood) stretch of text known as *An.* III 3, is a *purification* of the human capacity for thinking.[24] As a result, while *An.* III 3 is an indispensable step in the overall argument of Aristotle's *De anima*, it is not itself part of Aristotle's study of the human capacity for thinking. This is why this chapter remains outside the scope of our book.[25] Our book is concerned with the essence of the human capacity for thinking, and this capacity becomes the object of study only at the outset of *An.* III 4. A direct and immediate consequence of the purification this capacity has undergone is that we are not one but two steps removed from what we would call a theory of the human mind. But now, to the extent that *An.* III 7 is concerned with the *cognitive soul* understood as an integrated set of cognitive powers that can engage in higher cognitive achievements, such as making a judgment, calculating, and indeed deliberating, it is safe to say that Aristotle is no longer concerned with isolating the distinguishing mark of *nous*: namely, the feature that separates the human capacity for thinking from the other cognitive powers of the soul. *In An. III 7 Aristotle has begun his descent from the study of nous understood as the principle of human thought to the study of the mental phenomena.* And he will continue with it through *An.* III 8. Evidence of this is that Aristotle is able, and indeed willing, to make use of some of the results he has achieved in the study of perception and *phantasia.* In *An.* III 7 Aristotle is operating at the same explanatory level as he is operating at in *An.* III 3. While it remains true that dealing with mental phenomena as such is programmatically not a part of the project attempted either in *An.* III 3 or in *An.* III 7, it is safe to say that Aristotle is no longer two steps removed from the study of the mental phenomena in *An.* III 7 (as he is in *An.* III 4–5 and even in *An.* III 6) but only one.[26]

[22] I refer the reader to Chapter 1 (Section 2).

[23] See Chapter 1 (Section 7), Chapter 5 (Section 2), as well as the Glossary (*s.v.* PHANTASMA).

[24] See Chapter 1 (Section 7) for the reasons to adopt this language.

[25] I refer the reader to Chapter 1 (Section 7) for how we (the authors of this book) understand the argument offered in *An.* III 3.

[26] At this point, one may legitimately wonder where in his research agenda Aristotle approaches directly the phenomena that fall under the heading of the mental. We submit that Aristotle deals with at least some of these phenomena in the context of what he describes as being "common to the body and the soul." Quite tellingly, this expression is used in *De anima* to refer to *another kind* of investigation (*An.* III 10, 433b20). This is most likely a reference to the *De motu animalium*, which is regarded as a contribution to the project attempted in the *Parva naturalia.* The details do not matter here. For more on how to read this reference, see Primavesi and Corcilius 2018: clxx–clxxvi. What is immediately relevant is that the short essays collectively known as *Parva naturalia* (augmented by *De motu animalium*) are concerned with *psychophysical phenomena.*

This final remark helps me turn to my second consideration. Along with *An.* III 6, *An.* III 7 provides the much-needed expansion of the core case of thinking advanced in *An.* III 4–5. By the end of *An.* III 7, Aristotle is confident that he has given us a full theory of human thought understood as a template for the explanation of mental phenomena. While an explanation of mental phenomena is beyond the scope of Aristotle's *De anima*, providing a theory for how to explain embodied cognition is part and parcel of the project attempted in the treatise. Among other things, this means that a perceptive philosopher who is looking for continuity between the ancient study of the soul and the modern study of the mind will find elements of continuity between Aristotle's theory of the soul and the contemporary philosophical reflection on the nature and working of the mind, even though the theoretical framework adopted by Aristotle remains quite different from ours.

2. The priority of actual thinking

Aristotle opens his investigation by stating that actual knowledge (*epistêmê*) is the same as its object (*An.* III 7, 431a1–2). This sentence is ambiguous in more than one way. To begin with, it is not clear how much we should read into the word *epistêmê*. One might be tempted to think that the *epistêmê* in question is equivalent to *scientific* knowledge. This knowledge crucially depends on grasping essences understood as those items that are taken to be primary in the explanation of the relevant scientific facts.[27] This reading does not seem to be required. It is better, indeed safer, to think that when Aristotle speaks of *epistêmê*, he has in mind knowledge in general without presupposing the theory of scientific knowledge outlined in the *Posterior Analytics*. But actual knowledge is also ambiguous in another way. It is not clear whether actual knowledge refers to the disposition to engage in thinking, which is a first actuality, or to the activity of thinking, which is a second actuality. Since one of the results Aristotle hopes to establish in the first part of *An.* III 7 is that activity (*energeia*) is different from change (*kinêsis*) in the sense that all *kinêsis* is *energeia* but not all *energeia* is *kinêsis*, Aristotle must be referring to the activity of thinking rather than to the disposition that gives rises to episodes of thinking. In other words, he must be referring to thinking as second actuality.[28]

Aristotle argues that the activity of thinking, taken in abstraction from all the individual thinkers, is always prior to the power or capacity (*dunamis*) of thinking.

[27] An epistemological interpretation of the Aristotelian notion of essence based on the practice of Aristotle's scientific explanation was suggested in Chapter 1. On this suggestion, the essence of *X* is a necessary and universal feature (or a combination of necessary and universal features) of *X* taken to be primary in the explanation of scientific facts about *X*. The expression "explanatory essentialism" was adopted in that context. For a brief introduction to this expression and its significance in the context of Aristotle's scientific enterprise, see Glossary (*s.v.* EXPLANATORY ESSENTIALISM).

[28] For more on the origins of this language and the nature of the conceptual distinction between *energeia* and *kinêsis*, see Menn 1994: 73–114.

This claim is not new; on the contrary, we have already encountered it at *An.* III 5, 430a20–21. However, this claim is now supported by a metaphysical principle that does not appear to allow for exceptions: every instance of coming to be (becoming) *F* presupposes the existence of something that is *F* in actuality (*An.* III 7, 431a3–4). This metaphysical principle describes, at the most general and abstract level, how an agent that is actually *F* and a patient that is potentially *F* come together so as to give rise to an instance of coming to be *F* (or becoming *F*). The wording of the principle is carefully crafted to apply to cases where the transition from potentiality to actuality is a straightforward case of change (*kinêsis*), as well as to cases where that transition is an activity (*energeia*). In both cases, we are dealing with instances of coming to be or becoming (*gignesthai*).[29]

Aristotle does not stop to explain, let alone to defend, the priority of actuality over potentiality. He is content to invoke a general principle whose application goes beyond the narrow boundaries of the study of the cognitive soul. At least for Aristotle, the task of elucidating this principle pertains to another philosophical project: namely, first philosophy.[30] In his recent essay on *An.* III 7, Klaus Corcilius has convincingly argued that this principle is applied to a number of cognitive activities starting from the case of thinking. In other words, this principle is the common element that unifies the different parts of the chapter.[31] I will look at how Aristotle applies this principle beyond the case of thinking momentarily. For the time being, I would like to stress that the application of this principle to the case of thinking generates the following important result: *while it is true that thinking is an emergent phenomenon at the level of the individual mind, thinking in general must be a primitive reality.*[32] Put differently, and more boldly: there must be at least one active *nous* engaged in actual thinking as a precondition for the possibility of our individual thinking. This may strike most of us as a surprising outcome; and yet, this is a widely shared view in antiquity. It is endorsed not only by Plato and Aristotle but also by some of the most prominent philosophers working within the Platonic and Aristotelian traditions (most notably, Alexander of Aphrodisias, Plotinus, and Averroes).

The fact that this view is widely shared in antiquity (and beyond) does not make it true. Still, it is quite telling that this view is the starting point for the *tour de force* attempted in *An.* III 7. This *tour the force* brings us back full circle to the activity

[29] This language is reminiscent of how Aristotle refers to change in *Phys.* I, which is the most general introduction to the study of nature. It appears that, in Aristotle's mind, *genesis* covers both *energeia* and *kinêsis*.

[30] The priority of actuality (*energeia*) over potentiality (*dunamis*) is defended in the whole of *Metaph.* IX 8.

[31] Corcilius 2020a: 185–219.

[32] By saying that thinking is an emergent phenomenon at the level of the individual, I do not mean to suggest that thinking is a supervenient phenomenon. At this point, it should be abundantly clear that Aristotle adopts a non-reductive approach to the explanation of thought and thinking even at the level of the individual mind.

of thinking at the end of the chapter (*An.* III 7, 431b17).[33] In other words, Aristotle starts out by stating the priority of actual thinking over potential thinking and returns to actual thinking at the end of a long and tortuous argument that takes its lead from a discussion of the basic model of perception. This argumentative strategy suggests the following observation. While the opening lines of the chapter have been regarded as a repetition that can be omitted (Themistius in his paraphrase of Aristotle's *De anima*), or as a fragment that is out of place (Alexander of Aphrodisias in his lost commentary on Aristotle's *De anima*),[34] they amount to a theoretical statement committing Aristotle to the *non-derivative nature of thinking.* For Aristotle, thinking is a basic, and indeed necessary, ingredient of the world.[35] Aristotle is not simply repeating what he has already stated in *An.* III 5. Far from being an expendable repetition, or even worse an intrusive gloss, this opening statement shapes, and indeed controls, the subsequent discussion. Placed at the outset of the attempt to offer an account of how episodes of thinking occur in a complex cognitive system such as a rational soul, the priority of actual thinking over potential thinking signals that the bottom-up approach Aristotle takes in *An.* III 7 is not just a heuristic device but rather a principled approach yielding explanatory fruits.

3. Getting off the ground

What immediately follows in the text is the application of the principle stating the priority of actuality over potentiality to the basic model of perception. Ross places the entire discussion of the basic model of perception within em dashes (*An.* III 7, 431a4–7). Following Torstrik, he takes this discussion to be a fragment which does not follow from the opening statement in which Aristotle announces the priority of actual thinking over potential thinking. Before being conceptual, the challenge (graphically presented by printing the text within em dashes) is grammatical. We need to spell out how Aristotle negotiates the transition from the clause stating the priority of actuality over potentiality at the level of thinking to the application of the same principle at the level of perceiving. An attempt to meet this challenge is offered by Klaus Corcilius, who has suggested reading the *men solitarium* at *An.* III 7, 431a4, as an apodotic *men*: that is, as a *men* signaling the consequence (namely, the apodosis) of what is said in the previous part of the syntactical construction.[36]

[33] Aristotle speaks of *nous* rather than *epistêmê* in actuality: however, I do not think that this linguistic variation is significant.

[34] The information on Alexander is preserved by Philoponus (Philoponus, *In An.* 558.4–8).

[35] Recall that Aristotle is committed to a strong version of eternalism. By his lights, the world is of necessity (*ex anankês*) eternal. This means that thinking is not only a basic but also a necessary feature of the world. For more on the eternalist position defended by Aristotle, see Falcon 2021: 7–22.

[36] Corcilius 2020a: 197–198.

If *men* at *An.* III 7, 431a4, is taken in this peculiar way, then Aristotle is *contrasting* thinking and perceiving. According to Corcilius, this contrast gets the *whole* argument advanced in *An.* III 7 off the ground. But how exactly does Aristotle intend this contrast to work in his overall argument?

For Corcilius, Aristotle takes the priority of actuality over potentiality for granted in the case of actual knowledge (*epistêmê*); *by contrast*, Aristotle does not think that this priority is clear in the case of perception, so he turns to the basic model of perception to show that this principle holds in this case as well as in more complex forms of embodied cognition that depend on perception. The adoption of this strategy brings Aristotle all the way back to the case of thinking at the end of *An.* III 7. On this reading, the chapter is an instance of ring composition in which the opening statement generates a discussion that ultimately leads us back full circle to our original starting point. While embodied cognition is the main theme of the chapter, the beginning and the end of the chapter are about a form of cognition that is not, or at least not essentially, embodied. In this case, Aristotle is entitled to assume the identity between *F* and the thought of *F*, since this is an identity that Aristotle has already established for theoretical knowledge:

> In the case of objects without matter, that which thinks and that which is thought are identical, because theoretical knowledge is identical with what is known in this way.[37]

So much for how Corcilius reads the contrast between thinking and perceiving. I read this contrast in a slightly different way. Except for the very end of the chapter, where Aristotle asks (but does not answer) a question that pertains to the cognition of separate substances (i.e., disembodied intellects), the chapter appears to be concerned with embodied cognition of enmattered objects. Within embodied cognition, thinking plays a special role, since the chapter is ultimately meant to explain how episodes of thinking occur in a cognitive soul that is an integrated system of perception, *phantasia*, and thought—in short, how episodes of *human* thinking come about. However, the priority of actuality over potentiality is not immediately evident in the case of human thinking; *by contrast*, it can be established for the basic model of perception. Hence, Aristotle turns his attention to this case to show that the principle holds not only for perception but also for cognitive achievements of ascending complexity that crucially involve the exercise of perception. This argumentative strategy is best described as bottom-up; it takes us all the way to the case of thinking, which was also the starting point of the argument. Therefore, it is only at the very end of the chapter that Aristotle can vindicate his opening claim.

[37] *An.* III 4, 430a3–5.

When applied to embodied cognition, the priority of actuality over potentiality states that every process-related form of cognition of *F* requires the agency of something that is *F* in actuality so that it can function as the triggering cause of the entire process. Why is this principle not immediately evident in the case of thinking? We are not told why, but a suggestion is easily at hand: once acquired, knowledge does not need to be triggered by an external cause. Rather, it can be activated by the knowers on their own initiative. The autonomy of *nous*, which does not need to be activated by anything external, is a familiar enough phenomenon. Aristotle has already registered this phenomenon in connection with the acquisition of knowledge:

> When it [i.e., *nous*] has become each single [object of knowledge] in the manner in which we say that someone actually possesses knowledge—*that occurs when one is able to be active through oneself*—even then it is still potential in some way; not, however, as it was before learning or discovering.[38]

The autonomy of *nous* is introduced early on in *De anima* in connection with the discussion of perception. There, it is registered as a basic difference setting the activities of thinking and perceiving apart.

> Perceiving in actuality (*to aisthanesthai to kat'energeian*) is spoken of in a similar way to contemplating (*theôrein*). But there is a difference because the things that are capable of producing the activity of perceiving are external (the visible, the audible, and the remaining objects of perception). The reason is that actual perception (*ê kat'energeian aisthêsis*) is of the particulars, whereas knowledge (*epistêmê*) is of the universals, and these are in a way (*pôs*) in the soul itself. *This is why thinking* (*noêsai*) *is in one's control whenever one wishes, whereas perceiving* (*aisthanesthai*) *is not, since an object of perception must be present.*[39]

In light of the autonomy claim, which states that thinking is in our control in the sense that we can switch from potential to actual thinking at will, Aristotle may be thinking that the best way to establish the priority of actuality over potentiality in the case of embodied cognition is by reflecting on how the perceptual capacity is activated by an external object of perception in the basic model of perception.[40] For one thing, perception is a more familiar case to us. For another, we already have a whole theory in place that can help us see how something that is *F* in actuality (the

[38] *An.* III 4, 429b5–10.

[39] *An.* II 5, 417b18–26.

[40] A full discussion of the autonomy claim goes beyond the scope of this chapter. The reader will find an insightful discussion of this claim in connection with the passage from the end of *An.* II 5 in Corcilius 2009: 1–15.

object of perception) brings something else that is potentially *F* (the perceptual capacity present in the perceiver) into actuality.[41] Hence, Aristotle may feel entitled to turn to perception in order to show how the priority of actuality over potentiality holds in this case.

Let us recall the relevant passage where the actuality principle is established for perception:

> But at least [in the case of the perceptual capacity] it is clear that the object of perception brings the perceptual capacity from being in potentiality to being in actuality, since [the object of perception] is not affected or altered.[42]

The words in square brackets amplify the translation. They also disambiguate the Greek text. We can supply either the object of perception (*to aisthêton*) or the perceptual capacity (*to aisthêtikon*) as the grammatical subject of the final clause (the *gar*-clause). Both supplements are acceptable from a doctrinal point of view, since it is true for Aristotle that neither the object of perception nor the perceptual capacity is affected or undergoes any qualitative change during an act of perception. While Aristotle admits that there is some qualitative change in the sense-organ (*to aisthêterion*), he does not think that the perceptual capacity itself (*to aisthêtikon*) is affected. Given this grammatical and doctrinal context, the vast majority of the interpreters of Aristotle's *De anima* read the Greek text as saying that the *perceptual capacity* is not altered or affected during the act of perception.[43] And yet, this reading is far from being compelling when the larger argumentative context is taken into account. In fact, this reading obfuscates, if not even spoils, the overall train of thought. Recall that Aristotle is turning to perception precisely because he hopes to establish the priority of actuality over potentiality for perception.[44] Applied to perception, this principle states that the presence of the object of perception in actuality is a necessary condition for the activation of the perceptual capacity. If the object of perception is the subject of the final sentence, then Aristotle is telling us that the object of perception in actuality, which is the triggering cause of perception, is not itself affected and does not undergo any qualitative change during an act of perception. In other words, the object of perception in actuality is the *unmoved mover* that explains how a causal chain of changes that begins from the object of perception and ends in a sensory affection takes place.

[41] There is no question that Aristotle is relying on his account of perception in *An.* III 7. In addition to the distinction between *energeia* and *kinêsis*, he refers twice to the perceptual mean (*mesotês*). Aristotle does not stop to explain what he means by these technical concepts. Evidently, he is counting on his reader to be able to follow him when he applies them in *An.* III 7.

[42] *An.* III 7, 431a4–5.

[43] Corcilius 2020a: 191–195 and Menn 1994: 110n49 are notable exceptions to the rule.

[44] Here I am adopting the reading defended in Corcilius 2020a: 191–195.

4. Aristotle's bottom-up approach in *An.* III 7

Once Aristotle has shown how the priority of actuality over potentiality holds for perception, he introduces the following analogy: "perceiving is similar, then, to mere saying and thinking" (*An.* III 7, 431a8). In Section 1 of this chapter, I argued that this move is the most obvious strand of continuity between *An.* III 6 and *An.* III 7. Recall that, toward the end of *An.* III 6, Aristotle has already equated propositional thinking to a certain kind of saying: namely, the saying that takes the form of saying something of something else (*An.* III 6, 430b26–27: *ti kata tinos*).[45] The propositional structure involved in this type of thinking (and saying) entails that this thinking (and saying) is always either true or false. Aristotle goes out of his way to stress that this is not the only kind of thinking, since grasping essences is a more basic type of thinking. While an essence can be conveyed in propositional form to the extent that it can be expressed in a definition that says what the thing really is, our thinking of essences does not take propositional form, at least for Aristotle; rather, it is very like seeing an exclusive object of perception (*An.* III 6, 430b27–29). We encounter here, for the first time, the implicit idea that seeing white is equivalent to bare saying. This does not mean that "bare saying" must be equated with the activity of grasping the essences as outlined at the end of *An.* III 6. By "bare saying" Aristotle may mean, more modestly, the activity of entertaining *simple* (as opposed to *combined*) thoughts. These simple thoughts are among the *adiaireta* introduced at the outset of *An.* III 6 (430a26–28).[46]

If we keep in mind this larger context, we should no longer be surprised to discover that Aristotle builds his account of how the cognitive soul pursues or avoids something on the analogy between perceiving and thinking, on the one hand, and saying, on the other:

> Perceiving is similar, then, to mere saying and thinking; however, whenever [perception] is pleasant or painful, [the soul][47] pursues or avoids as if affirming or negating.[48]

The following claims can be extracted from this passage:

(1) Perceiving an exclusive object = bare saying.
(2) Perceiving something pleasant = saying something of something else.

[45] See Chapter 3 (Section 3) for a full discussion of the context in which this claim is introduced.
[46] More on this front in Chapter 3 (Section 3).
[47] The subject is not explicitly stated. However, the participles (*kataphasa ê apophasa*) require a feminine subject. The most natural supplement is the soul (*psuchê*). What Aristotle really means, of course, is that the *animal* by virtue of having a soul pursues or avoids something *as if it were* affirming or negating something of something else.
[48] *An.* III 7, 431a8–10.

(3) Perceiving something painful = saying something of something else.
(4) Pursuing something pleasant = affirming something of something else.
(5) Avoiding something painful = negating something of something else.

Let me start my analysis of these claims by clarifying that I take perceiving something pleasant or painful to be equivalent to perceiving something to be pleasant or to be painful. This equivalence allows us to rephrase (2) and (3) by adopting the *ti kata tinos* structure. But this does not mean that Aristotle is equating all perceiving to perceiving that something is the case. In fact, the notation "=" is not meant to express an identity claim. On the contrary, Aristotle is very careful to avoid giving the impression that he is putting forward an identity claim. He states that whenever the perception of the object is pleasant or painful, the cognitive soul pursues or avoids it *as if it were* affirming or negating (*An*. III 7, 431a9–10). Considering this wording, we should stop short of committing Aristotle to the view that the pursuit of the pleasant or the avoidance of the painful presupposes or involves the ability to judge that something is good or bad.[49]

This first clarification leads to a second. I speak of *cognitive soul* (rather than *rational soul*) because Aristotle is not yet concerned with the rational pursuit or avoidance of something. At this stage of his argument, Aristotle is still dealing with perception and how the discrimination of pleasant and painful things prompts the cognitive soul to pursue and avoid them. Since the cognitive soul in question can be the soul of a non-rational animal, what Aristotle says in this stretch of text has a more general (*zoological*) significance. It can be used to explain non-rational (*animal*) behavior.

With these two clarifications in place, we can now look at the information conveyed in (1)–(5). While there is a clear syntactic difference between (1), on the one hand, and (2)–(5), on the other, there is no clear syntactic difference among (2), (3), (4), and (5). Affirming or negating amounts to saying something of something else. In all four cases, we are presented with a *ti kata tinos* structure: namely, with the predicative structure already introduced in *An*. III 6. But if there is no clear syntactic difference among (2), (3), (4), and (5), we cannot say that for Aristotle pursuing the pleasant or avoiding the painful is a clearly demarcated step from perceiving something pleasant or perceiving something painful. More directly, and more precisely, we cannot say that the soul *first* perceives something pleasant or something painful and *then* pursues or avoids it. By Aristotle's lights, perceiving something pleasant or painful is *ipso facto* pursuing or avoiding it. It is quite telling that Aristotle goes on to say that the capacity for pursuit and the capacity for avoidance are not different from one another or from the perceptual capacity; rather, it is only their *being* that is different (*An*. III 7, 431a13–14). We can restate this point

[49] For a full discussion of this aspect of Aristotle's account of the formation of non-rational desires, see Corcilius 2011a: 122–127 (with reference to alternative lines of interpretation).

by saying that, at least for Aristotle, there are not three distinct capacities in the cognitive soul but only one applied in three different ways. In other words, there is only one capacity, but this capacity is either taken by itself (as in perception) or taken in relation to how the cognitive soul (or, rather, the animal in which the cognitive soul is realized) reacts to that which is good (pleasant) or bad (painful) for it.

Aristotle tells us that the activation of the perceptual mean (*aisthêtikê mesotês*) with respect to the good (pleasant) or the bad (painful) as such is a necessary and sufficient condition for the explanation of why the cognitive soul (or the animal in which the cognitive soul is realized) pursues or avoids something. The addition of the qualification "as such" is important. An episode of perception always has a perceptual content. But it is not because of that perceptual content that the cognitive soul (the animal) pursues or avoids something, but rather because the cognitive soul (the animal) perceives the content of perception to be good (pleasant) or bad (painful).

Here we have reached a definition of non-rational desire (*orexis*) as an immediate consequence of feelings of pleasure and pain.[50] Among other things, this passage as a whole sheds some light on why Aristotle can be so confident (in *An.* II 2) that where there is perception there are also feelings of pain and pleasure, and in turn there is also non-rational desire (*epithumia*) *of necessity* (*ex anankês*) (*An.* II 2, 413b23–24).[51] Contrary to what some interpreters have argued, Aristotle is not making a conceptual point; rather, he is making an observation as to how, in general, embodied cognition in a hylomorphic compound of soul and body works here on earth. In other words, his reference to necessity in *An.* II 2, 413b24, is a reference to *physical* rather than *conceptual necessity*.[52]

But how does Aristotle explain pursuit and avoidance in a more complex cognitive system such as a rational (human) soul? Aristotle begins answering this large question in the following stretch of text:

> *Phantasmata* belong to the rational soul like percepts (*aisthêmata*), and whenever [the objects represented by the *phantasmata*][53] are good or bad, [the soul] affirms or negates, and pursues or avoids. That is why the soul never thinks without a *phantasma*.[54]

[50] This pivotal passage has been discussed extensively by Klaus Corcilius, who has considered it central for a reconstruction of Aristotle's conception of non-rational desire. See Corcilius 2008a: 79–82, 103–108; Corcilius 2011a: 117–143.

[51] For Aristotle there are three forms of desire: rational wish (*boulêsis*), spirited desire (*thumos*), and appetitive desire (*epithumia*). While the first is a rational desire, the second and the third are distinct and irreducible forms of non-rational desire. The non-rational desire defined in *An.* III 7, 431a10–14, is the non-rational form of desire that is called *epithumia*.

[52] *Pace* Hamlyn 1993^2: 89–90, who thinks that Aristotle is hopelessly confused here. But it is not difficult to see that Aristotle is presupposing the results he has achieved in his study of living beings.

[53] One might be tempted to supply "*phantasmata*." Upon reflection, however, Aristotle cannot mean *phantasmata*; he must mean *the objects represented by the phantasmata*. I owe this point to Robert Roreitner.

[54] *An.* III 7, 431a14–17.

A rational soul is a special kind of cognitive soul. More precisely, the rational soul is an integrated system of cognitive powers that can engage in discursive thinking. The Greek word for this kind of thinking is *dianoia*. Aristotle does not stop to tell us what kind of thinking he has in mind when he speaks of discursive thinking. However, we can gather some clues from the way he explains the actual pursuit or avoidance of something. Aristotle tells us that the rational soul affirms or denies that something is either good or bad. At the very least, we can infer from the language adopted in this passage that this soul is able to engage in *propositional thinking* so as to *judge* that something is good or bad.[55] According to *An.* III 6, this sort of thinking is always true or false. Among other things, this means that the rational soul can also make *mis*judgments. In other words, the rational soul can judge something to be good while it is in fact bad (or vice versa). A judgment (or a misjudgment) of this sort is sufficient to explain why the rational soul pursues or avoids something. There is no textual evidence that Aristotle sees any explanatory (causal) gap between a judgment and the actual pursuit or avoidance of something. Quite the opposite: whenever the rational soul affirms that something is good (or denies that it is so), then the rational soul *ipso facto* pursues or avoids it.

This conclusion is consistent with the account offered in *De motu animalium.* I have in mind the well-known passage where Aristotle introduces the so-called practical syllogism (*Mot. An.* 7, 701a7–25). For Aristotle, the conclusion of such a syllogism is an action (*praxis*) rather than a propositional thought specifying an action (*praxis*). In other words, there is no logical (let alone causal) space between the conclusion of the syllogism and the beginning of the action.[56] Furthermore, in *De motu animalium*, Aristotle emphasizes, pointedly and repeatedly, that the relevant action follows *immediately* or *right away* (*eutheôs, euthus*) from the premises (provided that there is no external hindrance).[57] This emphasis suggests that, in his view, the two premises are jointly sufficient for action.

What Aristotle tells us in *An.* III 7 may serve as a corrective to a too narrow reading of the practical syllogism.[58] In this stretch of text, Aristotle is not content to say that the soul pursues what it judges to be good and avoids what it judges to be bad. He adds that the soul never thinks without a *phantasma* (*An.* III 7, 431a16–17. Cf. *Mem.*1, 449b32–450a1, where Aristotle offers a fresh argument for this claim; more on this below). This claim suggests that judgments resulting in action entail

[55] Since Aristotle is careful not to ascribe the capacity for making judgments to the non-rational soul, but he singles out this capacity for the rational soul, it is safe for us to infer that the capacity to make judgments is the distinguishing mark of this second kind of soul. All its judgments take the form of a *ti kata tinos* thinking.

[56] *Mot. An.* 7, 701a11–13, 20, 22–23. See the commentary by Klaus Corcilius in Primavesi and Corcilius 2018: 128–133. For an in-depth discussion of the so-called practical syllogism and the causal relation that Aristotle establishes between thought and action in his explanation of action, I refer the reader to Crubellier 2004: 9–15; Corcilius 2008b: 163–184; Morel 2008: 185–196.

[57] *Mot. An.* 7, 701a14, 15, 22.

[58] I have especially in mind the reading defended in Cooper 2020: 345–386.

the use of *phantasmata*, and that thought is only *indirectly* responsible for action via the use of *phantasmata*. This is also the considered view defended in *De motu animalium*, where Aristotle argues that whenever one thinks one should walk, one walks right away (provided that there is no external hindrance).[59] Quite tellingly, Aristotle goes on to provide a causal chain in which *phantasia* prepares desire, desire prepares the affections, and the affections bring the instrumental parts of the body into a suitable condition.[60] In this case, it is the thought-accompanying *phantasia* that brings about the episode of desire, not thought itself.[61] I note, in passing, that the view that thought is only indirectly responsible for action (via *phantasia*) is consistent with what we are told in a difficult, too often neglected, or easily misunderstood, passage in *Part. An.* I 1, where Aristotle argues that *nous* is not an origin of motion.[62]

To understand the role that Aristotle assigns to *phantasmata* in his account of action we need to appreciate what is implied by the claim that a *phantasma* belongs to the cognitive soul like a percept (*aisthêma*) (*An.* III 7, 431a15).[63] For Aristotle, the percept is the primary effect of an act of perception. By contrast, the *phantasma* is only a side-effect of an act of perception.[64] Yet, it is a causally efficacious side-effect. More to the point, it is a causally efficacious side-effect that not only persists in the soul but also inherits its content from the percept via its causal effect on the perceiver.[65] As a result, a *phantasma* can take the casual role of the percept in a causal chain resulting in the pursuit or avoidance of something—in brief, resulting in an action.[66]

At least at the level of the causal process, the explanation of rational behavior offered in *An.* III 7 is structurally like the explanation of non-rational behavior. In both cases, Aristotle posits the existence of a triggering cause that activates the cognitive soul. However, his account suggests that in the case of the rational soul there is no need to posit an external triggering cause equivalent to the object of perception. An *internal* triggering cause—that is, a *phantasma*—is sufficient to explain why the rational soul pursues or avoids something. This is equivalent to saying that

[59] *Mot. An.* 8, 702a15–17.

[60] *Mot. An.* 8, 702a17–21.

[61] For helpful remarks on this passage, see Rapp 2020b: 49–50.

[62] *Part. An.* I 1, 641a32–b10. For a full discussion of the philosophical, and indeed architectonic, implications of this passage, I refer the reader to Chapter 6 (Section 5).

[63] For a definition of percept, see the Glossary (*s.v.* Aisthêma). The reader should note that we, the authors of this book, refrain from translating *phantasma*. We explain the reason for this choice in the Glossary (*s.v.* Phantasma).

[64] For the idea that the *phantasma* is a leftover of an episode of perception, see *Insomn.* 3, 461a21–22. For an introduction to the topic of *phantasia*, I refer the reader to Frede 1992: 279–295, who argues that *phantasmata* are produced while perception is still in operation (284).

[65] *An.* III 3, 429a4–5. For a recent discussion of this claim, I refer the reader to Dorothea Frede (in Frede 2020: 64–70).

[66] I only add that the fact that the *phantasma* is like a percept does not mean that the *phantasma* must be a pictorial or visual representation of the percept. For more on this important point, see Wedin 1988: 90–99.

a *phantasma* can functionally replace a percept in the explanation of how the pursuit or avoidance of something is triggered in the case of the rational soul. Hence, the rational soul never thinks without a *phantasma* (*An.* III 7, 431a17).

The claim that the rational soul never thinks without a *phantasma* has attracted considerable attention, since it appears to establish a general point about human thinking: we *never* think without a *phantasma*. However, this conclusion is often recalled in isolation from its surrounding context as if it were a dislocated fragment.[67] To correct this lamentable practice, I would like to recall how the overall argument has been unfolding so far. The starting point of the argument is the metaphysical principle that every instance of coming to be (or becoming) *F* presupposes the existence of something that is already *F* (*An.* III 7, 431a3–4). This principle is invoked to establish the priority of actual thinking over potential thinking. However, the special power of thought to activate itself is an obstacle, if not even a potential counterexample, to the priority of actual thinking. This prompts Aristotle to return to the basic model of perception in order to show that, *at least in the case of perception*, the actuality principle holds. This leads us to a discussion of how pursuit or avoidance occurs in the presence of an object of perception. When Aristotle turns to the rational soul, he tells us that a *phantasma* typically replaces the object of perception as the ultimate relevant triggering cause.[68] Hence, saying that the rational soul never thinks without a *phantasma* is equivalent to claiming that every episode of human thinking requires a *phantasma* as its triggering cause.[69] An important corollary of this reading is this: the claim that the rational soul never thinks without a *phantasma* applies, directly and immediately, to *practical thinking*; it remains to be seen how this result can be extended to thinking that does not result in action. More on this front in due course.[70]

Saying that the rational soul never thinks without a *phantasma* commits Aristotle to the view that *phantasmata* are necessary for (at least practical) thinking. However, saying that this soul never thinks without a *phantasma* does not commit Aristotle to the stronger claim that thoughts (*noêmata*) are identical with *phantasmata*. It is quite telling that when Aristotle goes beyond his basic account—I refer the reader to the next section for a fuller discussion of the larger context in which the claim occurs—he restates this point by saying that the capacity for thinking (*to noêtikon*) thinks the [perceptible] forms *in* the *phantasmata*

[67] This practice is surely encouraged by the widespread perception that *An.* III 7 is a collection of disconnected, or only loosely connected, thoughts.

[68] Although at this point the focus of the argument has shifted to the *rational* soul, one may wonder whether this claim can be extended to the cognitive soul in general. Put differently, one may wonder whether the non-rational behavior of a non-human animal can be triggered by a *phantasma* understood as a casually efficacious residue or by-product of an act of perception. My answer to this question is affirmative: the *phantasma* can replace the *aisthêma* also in the case of a non-human (non-rational) agent.

[69] Cf. Corcilius 2020a: 204.

[70] Aristotle will show that all embodied (human) thinking requires *phantasia*. See Section 7 in this chapter.

(*An.* III 7, 431b2).[71] By rewording his position in these terms, Aristotle makes it clear that he does *not* identify thoughts with *phantasmata*. His considered view is that the content of a thought is not identical with a *phantasma*, but it is always thought along with a *phantasma*.[72]

Clarifying the relation between thought and *phantasia* has been on Aristotle's agenda since the very beginning of *De anima*. Already in *An.* I 1 Aristotle wondered whether thinking is identical with *phantasia* or whether it cannot take place without *phantasia* (*An.* I 1, 403a8–10). What is ultimately at stake is the ontological separability of embodied (human) thinking. More directly, if embodied (human) thinking is identical with *phantasia*, or even if it cannot take place without *phantasia*, then embodied (human) thinking cannot exist without a (human) body.[73] *An.* III 7 allows us to make a significant step toward answering this question. It appears that the sort of thinking that is instantiated in a rational soul when the latter is engaged in the pursuit or avoidance of something is ontologically inseparable from the body.

5. Beyond the basic account of perception

Up to this point, Aristotle has offered us a basic and highly abstract account of how the cognitive soul pursues or avoids something. It is a *basic* account because Aristotle has not explained how the cognitive soul responds to the perceptual stimuli across different sense modalities. It is also a *highly abstract* account because Aristotle has not offered a physiological account of how this response is activated in the living organism (the animal). As Aristotle moves on (and indeed forward) with his argument, he makes reference to the existence of a suitable perceptual medium (e.g., air) acting in a certain way on a suitable sense-organ (e.g., the eye-jelly) (*An.* III 7, 431a17). He also notes that the eye-jelly must act in a certain way on something else (*An.* III 7, 431a18). At this stage of his argument, Aristotle envisions a more complex causal story originating from the object of perception understood as the *unmoved* mover and involving at least three (non-expendable) *moved* movers. They are the perceptual medium, the primary sense-organ, and a third unspecified moved mover. Philoponus identifies this third (non-expendable) moved

[71] For the significance of this claim in connection with *An.* III 8, see Chapter 5 (Section 3).

[72] It is emphatically not part of Aristotle's theory that intellectual cognition *in general* involves *phantasia*. On the contrary, Aristotle posits the existence of a finite number of disembodied intellects that are always engaged in thinking without being capable of *phantasia*. Recall, however, that *An.* III 7 is crucially concerned with *embodied* cognition. This is a direct consequence of the bottom-up approach adopted in the chapter. For more on this point, I refer the reader to Section 1 of this chapter as well as to the concluding section, Section 7.

[73] For more on the *nous* and *phantasia*, see Chapter 1 (Section 7). On the (in)separability of *nous* from body, I refer the reader to Chapter 6 (Section 7).

mover with innate (or connate) *pneuma*.[74] But this is emphatically not the only way we can try to fill in the gaps left in Aristotle's account.[75]

Rather than elaborating further on the nature and role of the third moved mover, Aristotle goes on to say that an analogous chain of movers must be in place in the case hearing: in other words, just as in the case of sight, so also in the case of hearing (*An.* III 7, 431a18–19).[76] With these few strokes, Aristotle goes beyond the basic model of perception in two different but related ways. First, he considers two different sense modalities at once. Second, he gestures at the existence of a fuller causal account that explains how the perceptual stimuli coming from the immediate surrounding are transmitted within the animal from the peripheral sense-organs to the center of the perceptual system. Quite tellingly, Aristotle adds that there must be a common endpoint to these two distinct but analogous causal chains. This endpoint is described as a single thing and a single mean (*An.* III 7, 431a17–19). This mean (*mesotês*) must be the same as the one mentioned at *An.* III 7, 431a11. Aristotle's immediate concern is to disabuse his reader of the idea that there are (as many as) five peripheral perceptual means in addition to a centralized mean that jointly explain how the animal responds to the external stimuli. His view is that there is a single perceptual mean located at the center of the perceptual system by which the animal is susceptible to the perceptual stimuli coming from the immediate environment. While one in number, this *perceptual* mean is activated in (up to) five different ways.

Although his language is elusive, Aristotle has clearly indicated that a more robust physiological account explaining how the animal pursues or avoids something is in principle available to us. And yet he has also stopped short of giving such an account. It is easy to imagine a disappointed ancient or modern reader wanting to know more about how this perceptual system actually works: for instance, how the information is transmitted from the periphery to the center, and what role this third moved mover (most likely the *pneuma*) plays. None of this is offered to us in *An.* III 7. To understand Aristotle's overall strategy we must bear in mind that his *De anima* is programmatically concerned with the soul as the first actuality of a natural body that has potentially life. While the soul so understood is always present in a body, the natural, organic body as such is not an object of study in Aristotle's *De anima*.[77] Therefore, the very few (but always precise) references

[74] Philoponus, *In An.* 560.10. Cf. Philoponus, *De Int.* 99.2 ("*spiritus visivus*").

[75] A full discussion of the physiology of perception, including a thoughtful discussion of possible candidates for the role of third moved mover (blood, pneuma, or the blood vessels themselves) is offered in Roreitner 2020: 288–309.

[76] For this reading of 431a17–19, see also Osborne 1998: 438 (*contra* Ross, who adds suspension points in his editions of *De anima*, both the *editio maior* and the *editio minor*, to signal a lacuna).

[77] It is worth recalling the opening lines of *De sensu* where, with reference to the investigation into the soul, Aristotle states quite clearly that he has made determinations about the soul *by itself and its capacities taken as parts of the soul* rather than about the compound of form and matter that are the ensouled living beings, either animals or plants (*Sens.* 1, 436a1–2).

to the natural, organic body made in *An.* III 7 must be taken for what they are: a reminder that a rich physiological account of how ensouled body works can be supplied, although not in the course of the study of the soul. At least for Aristotle, offering such an account is the task of the study of what is common to the soul and the body, which is the standard way in which Aristotle refers to the project attempted in his *Parva naturalia* augmented by *De motu animalium*.[78]

But there is at least one more aspect of the overall strategy adopted in this stretch of text which deserves a few words of elaboration. In *An.* III 7, Aristotle not only offers a discussion of cognitive achievements of ascending complexity but also takes a bottom-up approach to the study of embodied cognition. Considering this overall strategy, it is not surprising to see that he returns to perception in order to provide a more complex account of how the cognitive soul responds to the stimuli coming from the surrounding environment. But while this account is surely at work as Aristotle turns to higher cognitive achievements—I mean those that crucially involve a rational soul and the capacity for thinking—it is not necessary as a model for how the rational soul responds to the stimuli from the immediate environment. The view that the account of how the perceptual mean discriminates across sense modalities provides us with a model for understanding how the rational soul works is the standard reading of *An.* III 7, 431a17–b1. On this reading, most recently defended by Catherine Rowett, the extended discussion of how the single mean discriminates across different sense modalities serves to elucidate how the rational soul pursues or avoids something.[79] However, this reading is far from being compelling if one takes, as both Rowett and I do, the *hôsper* in line 17 as part of a sentence that establishes the existence of two analogous causal stories (one for sight and another for hearing) for how the perceptual input reaches the single perceptual mean located at the center of the perceptual system. Once we read *hôsper* in this way, there is no textual evidence that Aristotle is looking back to the rational soul.[80] On the contrary, everything suggests that Aristotle is making a fresh point in order to introduce a new, more complex account of perception.

[78] For the expression "common to the body and the soul," see *Sens.* 1, 436a6–12, combined with *An.* III, 10, 433b19–21. The significance of this expression in the context of Aristotle's explanatory project is explored in Morel 2006: 121–139, Johansen 2006: 140–164, and Rapp 2020a: 273–302 (especially 288–291). For an attempt to provide the full physiological story of how perceptual stimuli are transmitted from the perceptual periphery to the center, I refer the reader to Corcilius and Gregoric 2013: 52–97.

[79] Osborne 1998: 438. Her reading is an updated version of the standard line of interpretation that makes the argument offered in *An.* III 7 dependent upon a tacit parallelism between perception and thought. The assumption that Aristotle is comparing sense-perceiving and thinking is shared by Finamore 1989: 27–41.

[80] On the standard line of interpretation (already defended in Simplicius, *In An.* 268.29–230.18) the *hôsper* would point backward to the rational soul. It would establish a parallelism between the perceptual mean and the rational soul. Moreover, Aristotle would now return to perception as something more familiar and better known to us. His discussion of how the perceptual mean discriminates would serve as a model for how the rational soul makes intellectual judgments.

Admittedly, this new, more complex account feels like an expendable addition.[81] It is quite telling that the reader can jump from the claim that the rational soul never engages in thinking without a *phantasma* (*An.* III 7, 431a16–17) to the claim that this soul has the capacity to think the [perceptible] forms in a *phantasma* (*An.* III, 431b2–3) without apparent loss of information.[82] Still, we may want to resist the conclusion that the stretch of text beginning at 431a17 and ending at 431b1 is a later interpolation that interrupts the main argument.[83] At the same time, however, we must concede that this stretch of text is not well integrated with what immediately precedes and follows in the argument.[84] While it is true that the reference to the existence of a single perceptual mean located at the center of the perceptual system provides an important element of continuity with the basic account of perception offered in the first part of *An.* III 7, this element alone is not sufficient to conclude that the text as a whole was originally written as part of the argument.[85]

If the interpretation offered so far is on the right track, Aristotle is now envisioning a more complex causal story dealing with the perception of something across different sense modalities. But how can the perceptual mean discriminate the perceptual input coming from different sensory modalities at once? This is a question that Aristotle has already answered in *An.* III 2. There, he has employed the image of a point *C* that divides the line *AB* into two segments: namely, *AC* and *CB*. One and the same point *C* is at once the end of *AC* and the beginning of *CB*. As such it is at once one and two.[86] The perceptual mean is analogous to such a point in the sense that it is an indivisible and unextended entity that can be activated with respect to two (or more) different sense modalities at once. For instance, it can discriminate simultaneously sweet and hot. This idea is restated in *An.* III 7, where we are told that the perceptual mean is a boundary (*horos*). Think, again, of how *C* divides *AB*. In this case, *C* serves as the boundary between *AC* and *CB*. In *An.* III 7 Aristotle goes beyond what he has already said in *An.* III 2, since his most pressing concern is to establish that the relation that holds between the hot and the sweet in the perceptual mean is the same as the relation that holds between the perceptual properties in the object of perception. Here is the relevant text:

> There is some one thing, and it is so as a boundary; and these [things] too, being one by analogy and in number, are in relation to each other as those [other things] are to one another.[87]

[81] This is already noted by Klaus Corcilius (in Corcilius 2020a: 204–207).

[82] Unsurprisingly, Themistius omits this stretch of text in his paraphrases of *De anima*. At the very least, Themistius felt that this was an expendable addition to the main argument.

[83] *Contra* Shields 2016: 339 ("possibly a scholiast's interpolation"). I do not see how it could be any easier to explain why someone would make such an extravagant interpolation.

[84] Trendelenburg 1877: 426 ("*negligenter addita*").

[85] The cross-references to *An.* III 2 in 431a20–21 do not help us establish that the text belongs here. At most, it can be used to establish that this stretch of text is not a later interpolation.

[86] *An.* III 2, 427a9–14.

[87] *An.* III 7, 431a21–23.

The things that are one by analogy and one in number are the things discriminated by the perceptual mean when it discriminates the hot and the sweet. They are one by analogy because the hot is to the cold as the sweet is to the bitter. The claim is that the perceptual mean is hot and sweet at once because there is a single object of perception that is both hot and sweet. Moreover, the relation that holds between the hot and the sweet in the *subject* of perception ("these [things]") can be traced back to the perceptual properties present in actuality in the *object* of perception ("those [other things]"). This conclusion is an application of the principle that establishes the priority of actuality over potentiality. We have already seen that this principle is the glue that holds together the different sections of *An.* III 7 and allows us to read a single argument unfolding in the chapter. Aristotle has shown that this principle is at work in the basic model of perception when he has shown that an episode of perception of *F* requires the agency of something that is *F* in actuality. He now shows us that the perception of *F* & *G* (where *F* & *G* are modally specific perceptual qualities) requires the agency of something that is *F* & *G* in actuality.

In the final stretch of text, Aristotle illustrates how it is possible for one and the same indivisible and unextended perceptual mean to discriminate across different sense modalities. Discriminating within a sense modality is equated to the capacity to discriminate different values within one and the same scale. There is a maximum and a minimum value in the scale, with all the other values being intermediate. For instance, all the colors are intermediate in a scale that has white and black as the two extreme colors. For the perceptual mean to discriminate a color is to take on a certain value in this scale. A similar point can be made with respect to hot and cold as the extreme values on the scale of temperature.[88] The perceptual mean discriminates not only within a given scale but also across different scales, provided that the extreme values on the scale are treated as standing in an analogous proportion. Aristotle illustrates this point with the help of the following proportion:

$$A\,(\text{white}) : B\,(\text{black}) :: C : D$$

The values of *C* and *D* are not specified in the text. We only need to posit that *C* and *D* are extreme terms on a homogeneous scale that is different from, but analogous to, the scale of colors. If so, *C* and *D* play a role that is functionally analogous to the one that white (*A*) and black (*B*) play in the scale of colors. Aristotle tells us that the proportion holds also *in alternando*. In other words, the extremities can be arranged as follows:

$$A\,(\text{white}) : C :: B\,(\text{black}) : D$$

[88] I note, in passing, that hot and cold are not absolute values but are always relative to the perceptual capacity. In this context, it is worth recalling Aristotle's observation that the excesses of the object of perception (e.g., what is too hot or what is too cold) destroy the respective sense-organs (*An.* II 12, 424a28–32).

But this means that one and the same perceptual mean can discriminate not only black and white but also white and *C* (regardless of the value assigned to *C*).

In a final, elliptical sentence Aristotle adds that the same result can be achieved if the starting point are two heterogeneous terms such as white and sweet. In this case, we should posit the following proportion:

white : sweet :: black : bitter

in order to obtain, by conversion,

white : black :: sweet : bitter.[89]

6. Human thinking explained

In *An.* III 7, 431a17–b2, Aristotle goes beyond the basic account of perception by explaining how the cognitive soul is susceptible to perceptual stimuli across different sense modalities. When this explanation is finally in place, Aristotle returns to the rational soul (*dianoêtikê psuchê*) understood as an embodied cognitive system in which perception, *phantasia*, and the capacity for thinking (*to noêtikon*) work together. The transition to the rational soul happens in *An.* III 7, 431b2, where Aristotle credits the capacity for thinking with the power to think the [perceptible] forms in *phantasmata*. Whenever this capacity is exercised, we are confronted with an episode of human thinking. The content of human thinking is not identical with the *phantasmata*, but it crucially depends on their presence.

Aristotle has already established that as perceptual residues *phantasmata* have the power to activate the rational soul and prompt it to pursue or avoid something. As such, *phantasmata* can function as casual substitutes for perception in the case of action. Consequently, the rational soul can pursue or avoid something in the presence as well as in the absence of perception. In the absence of perception, the rational soul can pursue or avoid something by attending to a *phantasma*.[90] This point is now illustrated with the help of a more complex example. This is an example that requires the cognitive soul, which in this case is a rational soul, to be susceptible across different sense modalities:

> For instance, perceiving a beacon, that it is fire, seeing with the common [sense] the fire to be moving, one recognizes that it is an alarm signal. And, at times, on the basis of *phantasmata* or thoughts in the soul, just as if seeing, [one] calculates and deliberates about future things with reference to present things; and whenever

[89] I owe the reading of the final sentence to Bodéüs 1993: 237n2.
[90] None of this is really new. See *An.* III 7, 431a14–16.

> [one] says that the pleasant or painful is there [in the future], here [in the present] one avoids or pursues—and, generally speaking, this is the case in action.[91]

The example of the alarm signal has been intensely discussed in the secondary literature.[92] The most important interpretative decisions made in the above translation are the following two. To begin with, the content of perception is expressed in propositional terms: in other words, one perceives *that* a beacon is fire. Since Aristotle is concerned with a cognitive system that has the capacity for thinking in addition to the capacity for perception, I do not find it problematic to ascribe to such a system the capacity to perceive that something is the case.[93] Moreover, I supplement the Greek word *koinêi* with the noun *aisthêsei* so as to read "common sense." The common sense is that which allows the perceiver to see the beacon-fire to be moving in a certain way.[94] This beacon-fire is moving in a certain way so as to signal the presence of an approaching enemy.[95] The meaning attached to the motions of the beacon-fire is the result of a previous agreement. As such, the moving beacon-fire is a *conventional signal* that only a rational soul can grasp. We can restate this point by saying that grasping an alarm signal involves perception, but it is not itself a perceptual act. It does not take long to see that grasping an alarm signal amounts to grasping the *symbolic meaning* associated with the movements of the beacon-fire.[96]

Aristotle introduces the example of the alarm signal to illustrate how the *rational soul* is moved to action "outside perception" (*An.* III 7, 431b3). As Aristotle introduces the example of the beacon-fire, he is already engaged in the attempt to explain how the soul is activated by attending to the relevant *phantasmata* (*An.* III 7, 431b4–5).[97] In our example, the relevant *phantasma* is that of the beacon-fire, which represents an approaching enemy. This *phantasma* is equivalent to a mental representation the content of which is an approaching enemy. It replaces the external object as the triggering cause of action. To be as clear as possible: one does not act because one sees an enemy to be approaching; as a matter of fact, one only sees a beacon-fire to be moving; however, by seeing a moving beacon-fire *and*

[91] *An.* III 7, 431b2–10.

[92] For an extensive discussion of this passage with a review of alternative interpretations, I refer the reader to Gregoric 2007: 112–123.

[93] The alternative would be to take the *hoti* clause to introduce the explanation of why the beacon is perceived. In other words, the beacon is perceived *because* it is fire (Gregoric 2007: 117–118).

[94] For this reading, see Simplicius, *In An.* 274.5–17.

[95] For a moving beacon-fire as a conventional alarm signal, see Thucydides, *Hist.* II 94; *Hist.* III 22; *Hist.* III 80; *Hist.* VIII 102.

[96] The view that grasping the alarm sign is nothing more than a perceptual act is defended in Gregoric 2007: 121. On this alternative reading, the perceiver sees the alarm signal by means of the common sense. The idea that motivates this reading is that the possession of a rational soul expands the scope of the things in the world that we can perceive. On this reading, we literally see the alarm signal rather than seeing a moving beacon-fire and then inferring from its moving that it is an alarm signal indicating that an enemy is approaching.

[97] *Contra* Gregoric 2007: 121, who thinks that the soul is moved to act by seeing the alarm signal. See previous footnote.

thinking that there is an approaching enemy, one responds to what one sees by engaging in action. In this case, the *phantasma* of the approaching enemy functions as the representational and causal substitute for the external object of perception (the approaching enemy).

The response may range from preparing for combat, to fleeing, to sending an embassy to the enemy to indicate willingness to accept reasonable conditions of peace—or whatever else is appropriate and relevant in the situation. In the stretch of text that begins at *An.* III 7, 431b6, Aristotle provides us with an outline of how the agent works out what to do. The agent calculates and deliberates (*logizetai kai bouleuetai*) and does so by using *phantasmata* or thoughts (*noêmata*) as if seeing them. Aristotle mentions both *phantasmata* and thoughts since he has committed himself to the view that thoughts are only indirectly efficacious via *phantasmata*. His view, however, is that there is always a thought behind a *phantasma* (recall that, for Aristotle, we think the [perceptible] forms in the *phantasmata*).[98] In other words, the "or" (Greek: *ê*) is best understood as introducing a clarification, or as making the point more precisely: *phantasmata or rather* thoughts (this is a limitative *ê*). Calculation and deliberation are the distinctive marks of practical thinking. In his ethical theory, Aristotle tells us that deliberating is the same as calculating and he describes the part of the soul that can engage in both activities as the calculating part of the soul (*to logistikon*).[99] Calculation and deliberation require the ability of the agent to think about possible future outcomes as well as the ability to relate them to the present situation. It does not take long to see that *phantasia* plays an *ineliminable* role in accomplishing this cognitive feat. The future outcome is not something that is directly available to perception; rather, it is something to which the agent can relate via a suitable *phantasma* (or a combination of *phantasmata*). The *phantasma* of something that is pleasant or painful in the future is that which motivates the agent to pursue or avoid something in the present (*An.* III 7, 431b8–10). What Aristotle says is evidence that he thinks of *phantasia* as involving pain and pleasure. It is because the prospective good or bad is presented as pleasant or painful that the agent is motivated to act in a certain way. The agent would not be moved to action if the agent could not envisage a certain outcome as pleasant or painful.[100]

At the end of this section, Aristotle makes it very clear that he has given us a model for action *in general* ("and generally speaking this is the case in action").[101]

[98] *An.* III 7, 431b2.

[99] *EN* VI 2, 1139a11–15.

[100] This pleasure- (or pain-) involving aspect of *phantasia* seems to be entailed by the causal role that a *phantasma* is meant to play in the explanation of action. Recall that the cognitive soul is activated by what is perceived as good or bad (*An.* III 7, 431a10–11). Likewise, the rational soul is activated by what is envisaged as good or bad (as desirable or undesirable).

[101] *An.* III 7, 431b10. Ross changes the proposition *en* into the numeral *hen*, which he renders as follows: "and, generally speaking, [the agent] will do one thing and another" (Ross 1961: 307). But as a rule, we do not want to change the transmitted text except when it does not really make sense. In fact,

Let us stop, briefly, to appreciate what Aristotle has been able to accomplish in this stretch of text. In a few big strokes, Aristotle has provided us with *an outline* of what is distinctive of human practical thinking: namely, calculation, deliberation, and *phantasia*. By dealing with cognitive situations of ascending complexity, he has first shown how the soul is activated by an external object of perception across different sense modalities, and then he has shown how a *phantasma* can take the role of the external object in virtue of the fact that the content of the *phantasma* derives from an episode of perception.[102] By so doing, Aristotle has explained how *phantasia* enters into the explanation of an episode of practical thinking. By his lights, *phantasia* is responsible for presenting the rational soul with the *phantasma* of something pleasant or painful. The prospective pleasure or pain is enough to motivate the rational soul to engage in an episode of (goal-directed) action. It is also worth stressing that this account of how practical thinking comes about remains highly sketchy and is ultimately incomplete in more than one way. For instance, there is no reference to the kind of *phantasia* that is involved in calculation and deliberation—the activities that are regarded as constitutive of practical thinking. Aristotle will return to this topic when dealing with animal locomotion. In that context, he distinguishes between perceptual *phantasia* and calculative (or deliberative) *phantasia* (*An.* III 10, 433b29–30 combined with 434a5–7).[103]

As soon as a general (i.e., abstract) model for the explanation of thinking that results in action is in place, Aristotle turns to *non-practical* thinking:

> And what does not involve action, namely the true and the false, is in the same genus as the good and the bad, except that they differ as to whether they are without qualification and relative to someone.[104]

Thinking that results in action is practical thinking. In this passage, we are told that this thinking is always relative to an agent in the sense that what turns out to be good or bad to the rationally calculating soul is the starting point of action (where action is understood as the pursuit of what is good for the agent or, alternatively, the avoidance of what is bad for the agent). By contrast, thinking that does not involve action (non-practical thinking) is concerned with truth and falsehood without qualification. Such a thinking is not relative to any thinker. An educated guess is that the non-practical thinking Aristotle has in mind here is the one first introduced in *An.* III 6. Recall that *An.* III 6 has given us the conceptual elements to

the transmitted text makes perfectly good sense as soon as we realize that these few words are meant to signal to the reader that she is given a model for how to think about action (*praxis*) in general.

[102] Recall that *phantasia* is a motion arising from actual perception (*An.* III 3, 459a10–18).

[103] For more on these two kinds of *phantasia*, I refer the reader to Chapter 1 (Section 7).

[104] *An.* III 7, 431b10–12.

go beyond the basic model of thinking outlined in *An.* III 4–5 (grasping essences). In *An.* III 6 Aristotle has introduced the idea that thoughts combine so as to produce compositional thinking: namely, thinking that combines thoughts and as such can be true or false (*An.* III 430a26–b6).[105] There is, however, a caveat: while in *An.* III 7 Aristotle is centrally concerned with embodied cognition, there is no clear evidence that *An.* III 6 shares this focus. Notwithstanding this shift in focus, *An.* III 6 and *An.* III 7 jointly contribute to providing the key elements for an account of human thinking.

Practically oriented thinking is discussed *before* non-practically oriented thinking in *An.* III 7. Aristotle marks the transition from the former to the latter with the claim that both kinds of thinking fall under one and the same genus: namely, embodied (human) thinking (431b11). This is an arresting claim considering what Aristotle says elsewhere. I have especially in mind *NE* VI 1–2 (= *EE* V 2), where Aristotle tells us that practical thinking and theoretical thinking can be traced back to different capacities of the soul.[106] The tensions that are felt when these two texts are juxtaposed may be resolved if we bear in mind that Aristotle approaches theoretical and practical thinking from different points of view. In *An.* III 7 Aristotle is concerned with the question of how an episode of thinking comes about. Aristotle is confident that he can offer a single account of how thinking is triggered. As a result, *from the causal point of view*, episodes of theoretical thinking and episodes of practical thinking pertain to the same genus. This is emphatically not a trivial result; on the contrary, it takes a whole argument leading up to this conclusion. More to the point: this is arguably one of the most important results reached in *An.* III 7. In fact, it is a conclusion for which the ground was prepared already in *An.* III 6, where Aristotle establishes that all thinking has a propositional structure. But this does not mean that the nature of theoretical thinking and practical thinking are the same. It remains true that, at least for Aristotle, there are two different kinds of thinking: namely, practical and theoretical thinking. As such, they can be traced back to different capacities of the (rational) soul. In *NE* VI 2 (= *EE* V 2), Aristotle refers to them as *to logistikon* and *to epistêmonikon*.[107] There, he refers to them as parts of the soul, but this is a non-technical use of the term "part."

But why has Aristotle opted to discuss practically oriented thinking *before* non-practically oriented thinking? Aristotle does not stop to elaborate on the reasons for his overall argumentative strategy. He remains silent not only on the adoption of the bottom-up approach to embodied cognition but also on the order of discussion adopted in the chapter. Still, it is not difficult to defend his overall approach to embodied (human) thinking on the ground that, both *historically* and *ontogenetically*, practical thinking precedes non-practical thinking. Aristotle himself is

105 See Chapter 3 for more on the nature of synthetic propositional thinking.
106 Aristotle calls them *to epistêmonikon* and *to logistikon* (*NE* VI 1, 1139a11–14).
107 *NE* VI 2 (= *EE* V 2), 1139a11–12.

committed to this view in the *Metaphysics* when he notes that people turned to wisdom only when the necessities of life, as well as the things that contribute to ease and recreation, were finally available.[108] But what are the features of thinking discovered in the study of practical thinking that can be safely ascribed to both practical and non-practical thinking? They appear to be at least two: the ability to engage in complex forms of thinking via the use of *phantasmata*, and the desire-driven nature of all human thinking. Both features can be traced back to the claim that any episode of human thinking is triggered by a *phantasma* playing the role of causal substitute for the external object.[109]

When this general outline of the nature of non-practical thinking is in place, Aristotle turns to a particular case of non-practical thinking: mathematical thinking. What interests Aristotle is the abstract nature of mathematical thinking. His primary concern is to explain how abstract thinking is possible in the first place. Here too we must posit the existence of a *phantasma* as the starting point of any episode of thinking. In Aristotle's example, this *phantasma* is that of a hylomorphic compound such as the snub. Recall that the snub is invoked as the model for how we should think of the hylomorphic compound in *An.* III 4. There, we are told that the snub is "a this in that."[110] More concretely, snubness is concavity realized in human flesh and human bone (a human nose). Thinking of concavity entails the ability of the rational soul to think of the form (i.e., concavity) separately from its relevant matter (human flesh and human bone). Of course, this does not mean that mathematicians start each time from imagining the snub when they think about concavity. It only means that concavity is available as a mathematical object through a process of abstraction. Unlike Plato, Aristotle does not believe that there exist separate mathematical objects. Rather, his view is that "[one] thinks of the mathematical objects, which are not separate [entities], *as if* separate" (*An.* III 7, 431b15–16).

It may be worth pausing here to recall that Aristotle elaborates further on the use of *phantasmata* in mathematical thinking in *Mem.* 1. There too Aristotle states that it is not possible to engage in thinking without *phantasmata* (*Mem.* 1, 449b31–450b1). In the ensuing *gar*-clause, however, Aristotle offers a set of fresh considerations in support of the claim that thinking requires *phantasmata* but cannot be reduced to them. These considerations are made by reflecting on the case of mathematical thinking. When we prove a geometrical theorem about a triangle—say, the theorem that the sum of the internal angles of any triangles is equal to two right angles (180 degrees)—we always draw the image of a triangle either on a blackboard or in the sand. This image always has a particular size

[108] *Metaph.* I 2, 982b11–28.

[109] For a discussion of these two features of human thinking, I refer the reader to Corcilius 2020a: 212–214.

[110] *An.* III 4, 429b14. Cf. *Metaph.* VII 5, 1030b18.

even if the geometrical proof does not depend on the triangle having any specific size; rather, it depends on the fact that the triangle is a closed plane figure bounded by three rectilinear sides. Likewise, the operation of thinking is always accompanied by *phantasmata*, but these *phantasmata* are only incidental on thinking.

Mathematical thinking, as an instance of *abstract* thinking, is the final topic on the agenda of *An.* III 7. It is quite telling that Aristotle ends his account of thinking with the following claim: "generally speaking, *nous* in actuality is the same as the objects it thinks" (*An.* III 7, 431b17). This final remark brings us back full circle to what we were told at the outset of *An.* III 7, when we were told that "actual knowledge (*epistêmê*) is the same as its object" (*An.* III 7, 431a1–2). In both cases, Aristotle is referring to the activity of thinking. In thinking *F* (where *F* is any suitable object of thought such as concavity), *nous* becomes *F*. In this scenario, the actual thought of *F* is identical with the object of thought *F*.

7. Embodied cognition as the focus of *An.* III 7

Mathematical thinking is the last form of embodied cognition that Aristotle takes into account in *An.* III 7. Dealing with mathematical objects which are not separate entities but can be treated *as if* they were separate entities prompts a final question pertaining to the possibility of *our* thinking of truly separate entities: that is, entities that are not enmattered and cannot be treated as separate by means of abstraction. By Aristotle's lights, there do exist such entities. In *An.* III 4, he has distinguished three kinds of objects of thought: essences of natural, material objects (i.e., essences of hylomorphic compounds), abstract mathematical essences, and essences without matter (i.e., immaterial essences).[111] At the end of *An.* III 7, he turns to the immaterial essences existing as disembodied intellects.[112] He wonders whether, and eventually how, a *nous* that is not separate from magnitude—or, if you prefer, a *nous* that is an integral part of the soul and as such is inseparable from the organic, natural body in which it is realized—can have knowledge of something that is separate from matter not by an act of thought but because it is by its own nature a disembodied intellect.

[111] I refer the reader to the discussion of these three types of essences offered in Chapter 2 (Section 3).

[112] *Pace* Alexander of Aphrodisias (*apud* Philoponus, *De Int.* 110.23–28, who refers to the lost commentary on Aristotle's *De anima* written by Alexander), there are no separate forms in Aristotle's metaphysics but only disembodied intellects. In Aristotle's original hylomorphism, forms are always, both conceptually and ontologically, related to a species-specific matter. As part of a self-conscious attempt to enlarge the scope of Aristotle's hylomorphism, Alexander extends the concept of form beyond its original scope. For a perceptive presentation of the exegetical project attempted by Alexander, and its philosophical implications for the overall interpretation of Aristotle, I refer the reader to Rashed 2007. Thanks to Alexander, the idea of separate forms (rather than disembodied intellects) resurfaces in the commentary tradition. See, e.g., Themistius, *In An.* 114.31–115.9.

It does not take long to see why this is a pressing question for Aristotle. A main lesson that we are expected to take away from *An.* III 7 is that all embodied cognition, whether it is perceptual or intellectual, requires a triggering cause. We have seen that in the case of intellectual cognition, a *phantasma* kicks in to initiate an episode of human thinking. For Aristotle, this is true for both practical and non-practical thinking. So, according to Aristotle, *phantasia* plays an ineliminable cognitive role in all human thinking. But since *phantasmata* are remnants of an act of perception, humans only have *phantasmata* of *perceptible* objects. By contrast, separate objects such as disembodied intellects are by definition *imperceptible* objects since they are separate from matter (they are matterless). How can, therefore, an episode of human thinking be initiated in the absence of a *phantasma*?

Aristotle does not answer this question. Instead, he tells us that this is a question that has to be investigated later (*An.* III 7, 431b19). Since Aristotle never returns to this topic in his *De anima*, we must infer that dealing with the cognition of separate objects goes beyond the boundaries of the investigation of the soul as envisioned in the *De anima*, or at least that this issue cannot be fruitfully pursued with the conceptual resources developed in *De anima*.[113] In all probability, this is a topic to be pursued in the context of first philosophy. Based on what we have seen so far, we can only say that from the fact that *phantasmata* are necessary for human thought it does not follow that the objects of thought (*noêta*) require *phantasmata*. Moreover, it does not take long to see that the philosophical ambition driving the investigation that is conducted in *Metaph.* XII (*Lambda*) requires an embodied *nous* (i.e., a human *nous*) to be able to engage in a search for something that is entirely separate from matter. Still, there may be significant limitations to what can be accomplished by an embodied *nous* (a human *nous*) once it is concerned with a separate substance. An educated guess is that such a *nous* can grasp the separate substances not *per se* but only *per aliud*: that is, insofar as the latter perform the role of first principles of the perceptible substances. In other words, we learn about the separate substances, and deal with them, only insofar they are causally connected to the perceptible substances.[114]

Historically, it is interesting to note that the question that brings the argument offered in *An.* III 7 to an end has been understood in two different ways in the exegetical tradition. For those like Alexander of Aphrodisias who think that human *nous* is not ontologically separate from the body, the final question takes

[113] Why not assume that Aristotle has forgotten to fulfill the promise made at the end of *An.* III 7? Since his *De anima* is one of the best and most vivid examples of how self-consciously disciplined Aristotle is as an investigator of the natural world, it is simply unacceptable to suggest that he may have forgotten about this item on his research agenda. The reader will find additional reflections on this front in Chapter 5 (Section 2). They are to be combined with what is said here.

[114] Such an idea was already suggested by Alexander of Aphrodisias in his lost commentary on Aristotle's *De anima* (*apud* Ps-Simplicius, *In An.* 279.30–32: "it is from inseparable objects that *nous* is referred to the separate objects"). For an attempt to explore this idea and its theoretical implications, I refer the reader to Roreitner 2021a: 264–266.

the following form: how can the intellect, *though* not separate from the body, understand separate objects such as the disembodied intellects? For those like the Platonic commentators who think that *nous* is ontologically separate from the body, the question becomes: how can the intellect, *while* not separate from the body, understand separate objects? These alternative readings are recalled by Philoponus, who as a Platonist philosopher (and a Christian thinker) takes the question in the second way.[115] His interpretation prevailed in the subsequent exegetical tradition.

By way of conclusion, I would like to recall the most salient aspects of the reading developed in this chapter. They are important for the argument advanced in this book. To begin with, contrary to the standard reading of *An.* III 7, I argued that in this chapter Aristotle is concerned not with *nous* but rather with the soul (*psuchê*). More precisely, I argued that Aristotle is concerned with a *cognitive soul* that has *nous* as one of its essential components.[116] Aristotle refers to this soul as the *rational soul* (*dianoetikê psuchê*).[117] Among other things, this soul can engage in discursive reasoning (*dianoia*). Such reasoning has a propositional nature and is central to both practical and non-practical thinking. The rational soul so understood is an integrated system of cognitive powers that crucially includes (but is not limited to) perception, *phantasia*, and the thinking capacity (*to noêtikon*).[118] In *An.* III 7, Aristotle gives us an outline of how this integrated cognitive system works when it is triggered by the relevant cause (either an external object of perception or an internal *phantasma* that functions as a causal substitute for the external object of perception). On the reading developed here, the most significant results reached in the chapter are two. The first is that *phantasia* plays an ineliminable role in all episodes of human thinking.[119] The second is that all episodes of human thinking are driven by desire. While episodes of practical thinking are motivated by the desire for the good of the agent, episodes of theoretical thinking are prompted by the desire for the truth.[120]

But there is at least another notable result reached in connection with the topic of desire that deserves to be mentioned as a fitting conclusion to this chapter. We have seen that in the first part of *An.* III 7 Aristotle gives us an account of the

[115] Philoponus, *De Int.* 110.23–32.

[116] For the claim that *nous* is a part or component of the soul, see *An.* III 4, 429a10, 429a22. Cf. *Part. An.* I 1, 641a31–b10. For a full discussion of this second passage, and its significance for how Aristotle thinks about his treatment of *nous*, I refer the reader to Chapter 6.

[117] *An.* III 7, 431a14.

[118] Such a cognitive system possesses other cognitive powers. Among them, I would like to single out the capacity to remember (memory). By Aristotle's lights, memory is not a basic power of the soul but depends on the possession and use of perception and *phantasia*, so his treatment is deferred to the short essay *On Memory* (*De memoria*). The discussion of memory falls squarely within the project of the *Parva naturalia*. For a discussion of Aristotle's account of memory and its place in Aristotle's larger explanatory project, I refer the reader to Falcon and Corcilius 2022: 12–30.

[119] For more on this front, see Chapter 5.

[120] This aspect of the account of thinking is brought to light in Corcilius 2020a: 212–214.

formation of desire. The desire in question must be non-rational since Aristotle is concerned with how the cognitive soul in general is activated by an external object of perception. On this account, a non-rational desire to pursue or to avoid something arises as soon as the cognitive soul is activated with respect to the perceptual mean toward the good or the bad as such. Since Aristotle does not mention *phantasia* in this connection, we can safely infer that he does not regard *phantasia* as necessary for the formation of a non-rational desire. Apparently, *phantasia* is necessary only for the formation of a rational desire.[121]

[121] I owe this point to Corcilius 2020b: 321n54.

5

An. III 8: concluding theorems about human *nous*

1. Introduction

On the face of it, the argument of *An.* III 8 is relatively easy to follow, at least if we compare it with the exceedingly difficult preceding chapters on *nous*. The chapter announces itself as a summary of what has previously been said about the soul. It is relatively short and exhibits a more or less clear structure, falling into two major parts: while the first introduces, and motivates, the claim that the cognitive soul (perception and *nous*) "is somehow all beings" (hereafter "identity thesis"), ending with the famous comparison of the cognitive soul with the hand, the second states that intelligible objects are "in" perceptible things and that for that reason perception is a necessary condition for the cognition of intellectual objects ("empiricist claim" in what follows, for ease of reference), with a short but related coda on the role of *phantasia* in intellectual cognition. But looking at the chapter in this way merely scratches the surface of the text, isolating its contents from the larger argument. In fact, *An.* III 8 does not merely summarize the previous treatment of the cognitive capacities of the soul; rather, it summarizes it in such a way as to address the major philosophical questions about the nature of cognition that were raised early on in *An.* I. The chapter draws momentous conclusions from the previous treatment of perception and *nous* by situating the cognitive soul in Aristotle's ontology of the physical world in a way that invites comparison with Plato's simile of the line. Taking all this into account, it is probably not an overstatement to say that *An.* III 8 contains Aristotle's final word on the nature of human cognition and the place of cognition in the world. As it turns out, Aristotle is a proponent of the old and venerable like-is-known-by-like theory of cognition (hereafter LKL theory), even if only a highly qualified version of that theory. He claims that the cognitive soul, when actual, is identical with its objects—but only in form and in potentiality. It also turns out that Aristotle is a great optimist about our cognitive capacities.[1] He argues that the cognitive soul can cognize all beings. The identity thesis is merely

I would like to thank Andrea Falcon, Robert Roreitner, and Michel Crubellier for their feedback on previous versions of this chapter.

[1] On Aristotle's perceptual optimism, see Gregoric 2019: 543–560. Cf. Crubellier 2020: 277, who rightly speaks in that connection of an "*optimisme épistémologique*."

Aristotle on the Essence of Human Thought. Klaus Corcilius, Andrea Falcon, and Robert Roreitner, Oxford University Press.
 DOI: 10.1093/9780198921820.003.0005

the logical consequence of these two important philosophical theses. We will have to see what these mean and whether or not Aristotle succeeds with his theory.

Apart from the formidable philosophical difficulty of the chapter's contents, we face also the interpretative challenge posed by Aristotle's statement that "it seems that there is nothing beside perceptible magnitudes."[2] This statement seems to contradict Aristotle's otherwise well-attested ontological commitment to the existence of separate substances, a commitment that is restated in *De anima* itself. This, in turn, raises the further issue of the scope of the argument offered in the chapter. In the end, the question is whether *An.* III 8 is about cognition *per se* and without qualification, so as to include the cognition of separate substances, or whether the chapter (very much like *An.* III 7) is concerned with the embodied cognition of brute animals and human animals to the exclusion of the cognition of separate substances. This is arguably *the* central interpretative question of *An.* III 8.

In connection with this question, *An.* III 8 also raises related questions about its place in the overall argument of Aristotle's *De anima* as well as in the larger context of Aristotle's science of living things. With *An.* III 8, the treatment of the intellectual capacity as the third canonical part of the soul ends. This treatment is followed by what looks—at least from a methodological point of view—like a very different discussion of the locomotive capacity in *An.* 9–11. This raises the further issue of the relation between *An.* III 8 and *An.* III 9 and the role of *An.* III 8 in the overall program of the treatise. Unfortunately, I cannot adequately address these very interesting and important issues here.

Previous commentators have been comparatively brief on the chapter. While some of them doubted its coherence, others even questioned its authenticity.[3] If we go by the number of pages devoted to the explication of *An.* III 8, the chapter is among those that have attracted less attention from commentators since antiquity.[4] The argument of the present chapter falls into two major parts: the first is concerned with *the identity thesis*, the second with the *empiricist claim.*

2. Part I: the identity claim and the hand

The chapter begins with a promise to "summarize" (*sunkephalaiôsantes*; *An.* III 8, 431b20)[5] the previous treatment of the soul, only to make the bold initial assertion

[2] *An.* III 8, 432a3–4.

[3] Most notably, Hamlyn 1993^2: 149. In his new Clarendon translation, Christopher Shields cautiously raises some doubts and uncertainties (Shields 2016: 341–347).

[4] This is the case for Philoponus, Pseudo-Simplicius, Sophonias, and Themistius and, among the modern interpreters, for Trendelenburg, Rodier, Hicks, and Polansky. Alexander of Aphrodisias, in his own *De anima*, offers a very instructive (albeit short) discussion of the claim that the soul is somehow all things that can be applied to Aristotle as well. Hegel is doubtful of the authenticity of this and the previous chapter. He writes that *An.* III 7–8 contain explications of *An.* III 4–5 and that they look like the work of a commentator (*Vorlesungen zur Geschichte der Philosophie* Bd. II: 216, Anm.).

[5] For a discussion of Aristotle's use of this expression, see Rodier 1900: 520.

that "the soul is somehow all beings" in the immediate sequel. Aristotle starts by spelling out the identity claim in more detail and continues with an argument in which the claim is explicated: "it must be investigated in which way this is the case" (*An.* III 8, 431b23–24). The simile of the hand ends the first part with a poignant image which is meant to capture the gist of the previous discussion of the cognitive soul. Let us go through the arguments in turn.

An. III 8, 431b22–23 restates the initial formulation of the identity claim in a disjunctive fashion, distributing beings over the different cognitive capacities. Aristotle says that beings (*ta onta*[6]) are either objects of perception or objects of knowledge. He also says that knowledge is somehow identical with the objects of knowledge, and perception is somehow identical with the objects of perception. Aristotle does not explain or justify this important assertion.[7] However, the whole discussion of cognition from *An.* II 5 to *An.* III 4 relies on the idea that cognition involves the assimilation of the cognitive capacities to their objects. The result of that assimilation should be some kind of identity between cognition and its objects. At this point in the argument, therefore, the identity claim should not come as a complete surprise, even if the blunt identification of the entire cognitive soul with *all* beings does bring out a consequence that has not been drawn explicitly before. It also should be clear at this point of the argument that Aristotle believes that our cognitive capacities (perception and *nous*) equip us with the means to cognize everything there is. He has advanced this claim on various occasions in connection with perception and *nous* severally, but not with respect to the cognitive soul as a whole.[8] Now, the conjunction of the two statements above suffices to yield the identity claim.

Aristotle's commitment to the identity thesis would thus be a good reason for taking the terms "knowledge" (*epistêmê*) and "capacity for knowledge" (*epistêmonikon*) employed in *An.* III 8, 431b23 and 27 as equivalent to, and interchangeable with, "thinking" and "capacity for thinking" (*nous*). But we can also arrive at this conclusion from a separate route, when we note that Aristotle has used the term *epistêmê* for the act of intellection before (*An.* III 4, 430a20; *An.*

[6] The definite article in *ta onta* suggests exhaustivity in the sense of "all beings."

[7] The πάλιν in the first sentence of the chapter can, but need not, be taken as meaning "again" (i.e., "[once] again"). This is how Hicks seems to want to take it "over again" (Hicks 1907: 543). However, since Aristotle did not make this claim previously in the argument of *De anima*, and since πάλιν also can be used to mark a transition from one step to the next step in an inquiry or exposition, this is how I translate πάλιν. I thank Michel Crubellier for reminding me of this. See also *Index Aristotelicus, s.v.* πάλιν: "πάλιν *omnino progressum in narrando, enumerando, querendo significat*" (559b13). Trendelenburg suggests reading πάλιν as picking up on previous philosophers' claims that the soul is all things which Aristotle here, according to Trendelenburg, reasserts but in a different spirit (Trendelenburg 1877: 437). This is a long shot, and Rodier notes that it is hardly probable (Rodier 1900: 520). It is a very interesting suggestion, however, that fits nicely with the fact that Aristotle is after all a proponent of a (strongly revised) "like is known by like" theory of cognition. See below.

[8] See the argument in *An.* III 1 for the claim that our perceptual capacities cover everything that can be perceived, as well as the claim (introduced without argument) that *nous* can think all things, which, as we have seen, drives much of the argument in *An.* III 4.

III 7, 431a1, where *epistêmê* does not correlate with "beings" but with "things"—*pragmata*—as well), and observe that, from III 8, 432a3 onward, he returns to using *nous* to refer to the underlying capacity of the soul without showing any signs that he takes himself to be talking about something different. It is hard to say why Aristotle chooses to express himself in this way. Presumably, *epistêmê* here has the status of a paradigmatic intellectual state. If so, *epistêmê* and its corresponding objects can be employed in a *pars pro toto* way for all noetic states.

Having stated the distributive version of the identity claim, Aristotle announces an investigation with the goal of determining the *way* in which the identity between the object and the subject of cognition is supposed to hold. The question is this. *How—in which way—is the cognitive soul—that is to say, perception and thought—all beings*? If we include the first distributive restatement of the identity thesis, the answer takes the form of a five-step argument.

(i) DISTRIBUTIVE RESTATEMENT OF THE IDENTITY THESIS: All beings are either objects of perception or objects of knowledge, and knowledge is somehow identical with objects of knowledge, and perception is somehow identical with objects of perception.

(ii) DIVISION OF BEINGS AND COGNITIVE CAPACITIES: Thought and perception are each divided (*temnetai*) according to (*eis*) their respective objects. This is to say that they are divided both according to their objects and according to their objects' modality: that is, according to whether these objects are actual or potential. Thus, potential knowledge and potential perception correlate with potential objects, while actual knowledge and perception correlate with actual objects.[9] The division of beings and corresponding cognitive capacities shown in Fig. 5.1 results.

(iii) REFINED DISTRIBUTIVE RESTATEMENT OF THE IDENTITY THESIS: The cognitive capacities of perception and knowledge are their respective objects in potentiality; the capacity for knowledge is potentially the objects of knowledge, while the capacity for perception is potentially the objects of perception.[10]

(iv) THE FORM VS. THING ITSELF ALTERNATIVE: It is necessary that the capacity for perception and the capacity for knowledge each be potentially either their corresponding external objects themselves (i.e., the external objects of knowledge and the external objects of perception) or their forms.

(v) FORMAL IDENTITY THESIS: The capacities for knowledge and the capacity for perception cannot be potentially their corresponding external objects

[9] Hicks 1907: 543–544 offers a long discussion of the language of this passage. But the sense is clear: Aristotle speaks of a division of the cognitive capacities "according to" (*eis*) their corresponding objects.

[10] The singular expressions for the corresponding objects of the capacities "*aisthêton*" and "*epistêton*" should, I take it, be understood as "the perceptible object in each case" and "the object of knowledge in each case."

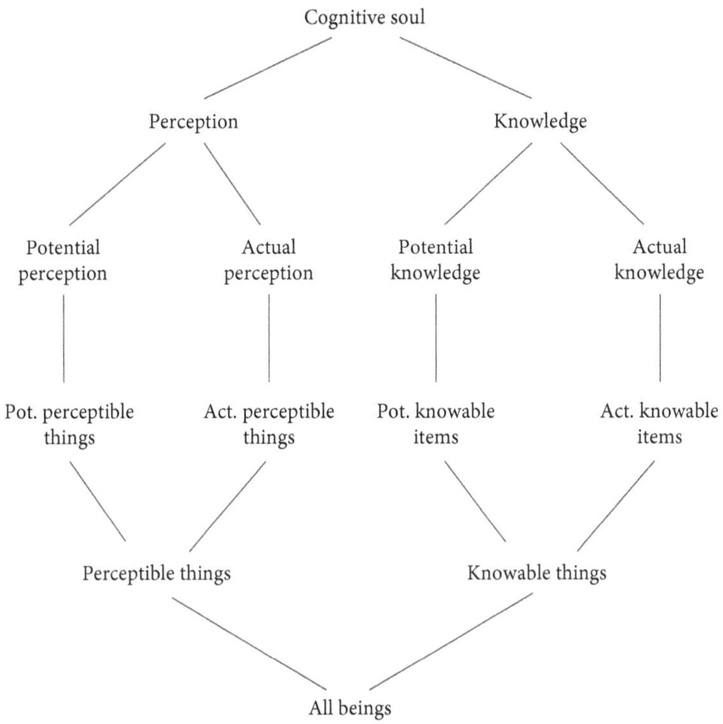

Fig. 5.1 Division of beings and cognitive capacities

> because when we actually perceive or actually think/know a stone (or anything else), it is not the stone itself that is in the soul but rather the stone's form.

Until and including step (iii), the argument merely unpacks the extension of the identity thesis, distributing it over a more fine-grained system of different kinds of beings with their corresponding cognitive capacities and according to different modalities (actuality or potentiality). This is no more than a restatement of the identity thesis, even if a more differentiated one. The statement in (iii) follows from (i) and (ii), but Aristotle does not state it as a conclusion. This is presumably because in this context he is less interested in the division of beings and cognitive capacities than in the resulting qualification of the identity claim to mere formal identity in (iv) and (v).

The whole argument outlined in (i)–(v) does not offer independent grounds that could support, or even justify, the main point of the identity claim, which is that the cognitive soul is somehow identical with its external objects. If the argument offers support for that claim, it does so only by giving a more detailed and refined formulation of it compared to the initial statement of the identity claim in *An.* III 8, 431b21. Step (iv) explicitly brings up the issue of identity, confronting us with the somewhat abruptly introduced exclusive alternative between full-blown identity on the one hand and formal identity on the other. Step (v) excludes the former and implicitly affirms the latter on the basis of one example for the perception of a particular object: namely, a stone. The idea here, of course, is that it could be any other object of perception as well.

At first blush, (v) may be interpreted as taking up one of Aristotle's arguments against those who proposed the materialist version of the LKL thesis advanced in *An.* I.[11] According to their version of the LKL thesis, cognitive agents come to be aware of things by virtue of the fact that their souls are made of the same basic material constituents as things. And, as both all things and the soul are composed from the elementary constituents, there is sameness on both sides of the cognition relation, and hence cognition. Aristotle's main objection to this view is that it is not going to be able to explain the cognition of the non-material features of things: that is, the proportions (*logoi*) and the combinations (*suntheseis*) of their material constituents. But if we added these features to the inventory of the materialist version of the LKL theory, our soul would have to consist literally of all things, which is of course absurd.[12] For, he continues, "who would puzzle over whether there is a stone or a human being in the soul?"[13] Here is the passage from *An.* I 5:

> It remains to be investigated how it is said that the soul is made out of the elements. For they say this for the soul to be able to perceive and cognize each of the things that exist. But this thesis must lead to many impossible consequences. For they assume that the like cognizes the like, *as if they were assuming that the soul is the things*. But there exist not only these things but also many other things (in fact, perhaps an infinite number), which are made out of them.[14]

By Aristotle's lights, the main flaw in the materialist version of the LKL theory is the reductivist assumption that the constitutive parts of things can, as it were, stand in for the things themselves. But since things are not identical with their material constituents, the materialist version of the LKL theory is unable to achieve its purpose. The modes of composition of the elementary constitutive parts are not their constitutive parts—their matter—but something else: namely, their form. Thus, what a thing is can only be adequately grasped if not only the matter but also the formal features are taken into consideration. Therefore, the auxiliary reductivist assumption of the materialist version of the LKL theory misfires. It cannot account for the cognition of things, apart from their material constituents. Aristotle's argument in *An.* I 5 certainly shows that he sees a connection between the identity claim

[11] For more on the LKL thesis, see Chapter 1 (Section 4).
[12] This only follows if there is no other way of combining material elements and the non-material features of things in the soul.
[13] *An.* I 5, 410a10–11.
[14] *An.* I 5, 409b23–29.

and the distinction between non-material and material aspects of things from early in the treatise. It also suggests that he takes the point about the stone not being in the soul as already established in *An.* III 8. The discussion of the materialist version of the LKL theory in *An.* I 5, then, provides us with at least *some* motivation for the "form vs. thing itself" alternative that Aristotle so abruptly introduces in step (iv), and which otherwise would somewhat hang in the air.

However, we should be careful not to confuse the distinction between the material components and their being, which Aristotle introduces not only in *An.* I 5 but also in certain passages of his *Metaphysics*, with the distinction between a thing itself—the "stone"—and its form in the soul at work here in *An.* III 8. There is a subtle but important difference. While the former distinction opposes matter and form ontologically in such a way that matter is conceived of as devoid of form and thus indeterminate, the distinction between things themselves (*auta*; 431b28: i.e., *ta pragmata*) and its form (*eidê*) in *An.* III 8 conceives of things themselves as being formally fully determined. It is a distinction between the hylomorphic compound and its form in the sense of the form that it already fully possesses. Things themselves in this sense are not the constitutive material parts of things, but the formally fully determined external hylomorphic objects. This is important because it is only if we conceive it in this way that we can see how Aristotle's identity thesis functions within his theory of cognition. Still, the distinction at work in *An.* I 5 between constitutive matter, on the one hand, and *logoi* and modes of composition (*sunthesis*) of matter, on the other, no doubt relates to the distinction between the things themselves and their forms in *An.* III 8.[15] It is strongly reminiscent of the distinction between what a thing is and what it is made of that we find, for example, in *Metaph.* VIII 3, where the expression "combination" (*sunthesis*) is moreover a term that figures prominently in the description of the form (*eidos*) of hylomorphic compounds.[16] The effect is that *sunthesis* and form (*eidos*) are treated as functionally equivalent in this chapter: namely, as standing for those features of the being of things that are not their material constituents, as they do in *An.* I 5 as well. Regarding intellectual cognition by *nous*, it moreover (and perhaps confusingly) seems that the form-part of the form–matter distinction fully coincides with the form-part of the thing itself vs. form distinction. For as we have seen, by thinking their essences, *nous* thinks "the cause of the being" of hylomorphic compounds, which *is* their essential form.[17] With regard to perception, however, the analogue does *not* hold. Perception does not take in the being, let alone the cause of being, of the external perceptible objects, but only their forms in the sense of their perceptual

[15] It could well be that Aristotle mentions *logoi* only because of the Empedocles quote that is going to follow and that the *kai* in the formulation *logoi tini kai sunthesei* in *An.* I 5, 410a2 is explicative. In that case the equivalent of the form–matter distinction in *An.* I is the constituent part–composition distinction.

[16] *Metaph.* VIII 2, 1043b4–13; cf. also *Phys.* II 3, 195a21 (*sunthesis kai to eidos*). See also next footnote.

[17] See *Metaph.* VII 17, 1041b9–33.

qualities. Perceptual qualities are not the being of hylomorphic compounds but physical aspects of them that, as we will see, rather fall on the matter side of the metaphysical form–matter distinction. The distinction between form and matter from Aristotle's metaphysics of physical objects, therefore, is to be sharply distinguished from the distinction between things themselves and their forms. *An.* III 8 uses the latter distinction.

The result of Aristotle's discussion above is a significantly qualified version of the initial formulation of the identity thesis. The cognitive soul, taken as the conjunction of the capacities of knowledge and perception, is only qualifiedly identical with its external objects—namely, in *potentiality* and in *form*—which is to say that it is identical with its objects in a way that excludes the external objects themselves. This is a statement about what the cognitive soul is as such and before it engages in any of its acts of cognition: the cognitive capacities, before they engage in acts of cognition, are potentially identical to all beings *in form*. This implies their actual formal identity in acts of cognition. The cognitive soul's actuality, then, will be identical to its objects' formal features. With this it is clear that Aristotle is a proponent of a qualified version of the LKL theory. The soul, in the act of cognition, is identical to the formal features of the things it cognizes. This is meant to explain what cognition most generally is: namely, formal identity between the objects and the subjects of cognition. However, as we have just seen and will also see below, what "formal" means is different in the case of the intellect and in the case of perception.

Aristotle's answer to the question advanced in *An.* III 8, 431b23–24, *how* the cognitive soul can be identical with all beings in (i)–(v), then, rehearses the most basic and important structural features of his previous treatment of the cognitive capacities in the stretch of text spanning from *An.* II 5 to *An.* III 4. They are mainly three:

(1) *Identity*. The process leading to perception is one of assimilation, which results in the likeness, or identity, of that which is capable of perceiving (*to aisthêtikon*) with the external object of perception (*An.* II 5, 417a20–21, 418a3–6; *An.* III 2, 425b25–426a1). This is parallel to the claim about intellectual cognition stating that the actual object of knowledge and knowledge itself are one and the same (see, e.g., *An.* III 4, 429a17–18, and 429a27–29). However, there is no indication that the identity of the cognitive subject and the cognitive object of thinking results from a *process* of assimilation. On the contrary, Aristotle's conception of *nous* as simple, impassible, and nothing in actuality before it thinks (*An.* III 4, 429a21–b5), precludes the possibility of gradual affection (as a process of assimilation would require it), due to the absence of a subject of assimilation or affection previous to the act of intellectual cognition. So, while there is formal identity in both perceptual and intellectual cognition, their respective identity with the cognized objects comes about in rather different ways. The act of perception is the

outcome of a process of assimilation in the perceiver; the act of thinking is not.[18]

(2) *Identity in potentiality.* The characterization of the perceptual and intellectual capacities as identical with their corresponding objects in potentiality is given in the context of the discussion of the different sense modalities in *An.* II (*An.* II 11, 424a7–16, and 12) and during the discussion of the thinking capacity in *An.* III 4 (429a15, 21–22, 28–29, 429b5–10).

(3) *Identity in form.* The claim that perception is the reception of the form of perceptible things is made in *An.* II 12, 424a17–25, and the claim that thinking is the reception of intelligible forms is made in *An.* III 4, 429a14–18.

To that extent, and to that extent *only*, it seems entirely appropriate to speak of *An.* III 8 as a literal and faithful summary of the previous discussion of the cognitive capacities. But it should be emphasized that the identity thesis ranges on a fairly high level of abstraction. Thus, while it is correct from Aristotle's point of view to say that the capacity for perception and the capacity for thinking are identical with their external objects formally and in potentiality, what it means for each of these two capacities to be potentially and formally identical with their objects is quite different. So, we may say that in *An.* III 8 Aristotle is more interested in bringing out what is common to thought and perception than in bringing out the differences between the two cognitive capacities. It is important to see this and to appreciate the high level of abstraction of the identity thesis in *An.* III 8. To this end, it is worth taking a closer look at the *differences* between the two cognitive capacities of the soul that the identity thesis, as it were, glosses over. But before we get to this, we shall add a further qualification to the identity claim, a qualification that Aristotle surely intends to apply, but apparently did not bother to make explicit in *An.* III 8.

The identity claim, as stated in the first part of the chapter, has it that the soul is identical with all beings in the highly qualified sense of being identical with them in potentiality and in form only. However, a further qualification must be added, even if Aristotle does not mention it explicitly. For surely, he does not wish to say that the cognitive soul is identical with all beings *at once* and it would be uncharitable to attribute such a view to him; it is much more likely that what he wishes to say is that the cognitive soul is identical with whatever given being it happens to cognize on any given particular occasion of cognition. Alexander of Aphrodisias,

[18] We have seen above that the presence of the essence in the cognitive agent while engaged in actual thinking happens instantaneously. See Chapter 2 (Section 4). See also *Phys.* VII 3, 247b1–248a6. This, as we will see below, is compatible with there being many processes involved in the coming about of episodes of human intellectual cognition. But Aristotle seems committed to saying that these processes are not part of the proper act of thinking, whereas by contrast he does seem to maintain that perception is the episodic actuality of the perceptual soul intrinsically involving (the right kind of) bodily affection.

in his *De anima*, sees the necessity of this additional qualification very clearly. He says:

> For to the extent that it receives their forms, it is these objects in a certain way, because they have being most of all in virtue of these [forms]. But as the soul is not these objects all at once but can become like each of them in a serial way, the soul thus is and becomes all beings in a certain way. For on each occasion, in a certain way it becomes what it perceives or what it thinks; and because it is some on some occasions and others on others, and every being is able either to be thought or to fall under the scope of perception, it becomes all things.[19]

What Alexander sees here—and he must be right in this—is that the cognitive soul's formal and potential identity with its objects can only be realized in a *seriatim* way (*kata meros*). In other words, identity is cashed out in terms of formal identity of the cognitive soul with one object of either perception or thinking at any given point in time, but with the qualification that this particular object can be *any arbitrary* object of thinking or perception. It follows that the cognitive soul is formally and potentially identical with all beings *by virtue of being able to become formally identical with any single arbitrary one of them at any moment of time.* I think we should, and are entitled to, understand Aristotle's identity claim in *An.* III 8 with this qualification in mind.[20]

2.1 The meaning of the identity claim when applied to the different cognitive capacities

(1) *In potentiality.* The stated commonality between perception and *nous*—namely, that they are identical with their external objects in form and in potentiality—is a rather abstract statement. On closer inspection, it turns out that what "potential formal identity" means in each case must be quite different, given that the two capacities and their corresponding objects are quite different from each other as well. The perceptual capacity is potentially and formally the objects of perception, and *nous* is potentially and formally the objects of thinking. And just as these objects are very different from one another, so are their corresponding

[19] Alexander of Aphrodisias, *An.* 91.16–21. Transl. Caston, slightly altered.

[20] This is confirmed by passages such as *Sens.* 6, 446b23–25 (cf. also *Sens.* 7, 447b24–26) and *Metaph.* XII 9, 1075a8, and it is implied in *An.* III 2, 426b24–427a9, as well as by the analogy with the wax-tablet in *An.* III 4, 429b31–430a2. Of course, what "one object of cognition at each time" means is likely to differ in thinking and in perception. I cannot engage in a full discussion of this issue here. Let me only say that Aristotle seems to allow for the simultaneous perception of various external objects (even if the cognitive object at any given moment of time would have to be unitary), while it is doubtful whether he allows for the simultaneous awareness of a plurality of essences. I thank Mike Arsenault for raising the issue.

potentialities.[21] This becomes clear as soon as we spell out what the two different capacities must be like, so as to be able to perform their respective jobs.

The capacity for perception, as it exists in living bodies prior to acts of perception, must correspond to actually existing physical (for Aristotle) properties, not only insofar as it has the organs that embody the perceptual capacity, but also because the capacity itself must in some way *be* a quality even before it perceives. More directly, Aristotle says that the perceptual capacity is a mean, a *mesotês*, and a *logos*, a proportion. By this he is referring not just to a mathematical mean and a mathematical proportion but to a qualitative proportion of values on a qualitative scale.[22] What is to receive the perceptual form (for instance, the hot and the cold in the case of the sense of touch, and the bright and the dark in the case of vision) ought to be neither of these contrary qualities in actuality but both potentially.[23] This entails that the perceptual capacity occupies a certain *position* on the relevant qualitative scale, which is also why there are blind spots in perception: that is, qualities that either match or are very close to the mean value on the scale and are for that reason imperceptible.[24] This makes the perceptual capacity itself something positively qualitative, even if only in potentiality. The capacity for perception, Aristotle says, is a qualitative *mesotês* (as it must be if it is to receive perceptual qualities). As such, it is not an embodied perceptible quality and it also has no extensional magnitude, but it still is a qualitative *something*. On Aristotle's way of thinking about the natural world, qualities are physical realities that are causally efficacious properties of physical things. This strongly suggests that the capacity for perception by Aristotle's lights is something physical even before it perceives, even if only in potentiality: it is a quality or, to be more precise, a *range* of potential qualities.[25] So much for the perceptual capacity.

The capacity for thinking, by contrast, is said to be "nothing at all in actuality" before it thinks (*An.* III 4, 429a24). This is required for it to be capable of receiving *all* intelligible forms. As the context makes clear, this is meant to contrast with the way the perceptual capacity is something actual in its own right, even if only in

[21] The definitional priority of the cognitive object over the corresponding cognitive capacity and act is made clear in *An.* II 4, 415a14–22. See Chapter 1 (Section 5).

[22] *An.* II 11, 424a4–6; *An.* II 12, 424a25–28; *An.* III 2, 426a27–b9. See Chapter 1 (Section 6) for my elaboration on this front.

[23] *An.* II 11, 424a1–15.

[24] *An.* II 11, 424a2–6; *An.* III 4, 429a24–27.

[25] Perceptual qualities are physical properties for Aristotle, and they are defined by *proportions* of extreme values on their respective qualitative scales (*An.* II 12, 424a417–24; *An.* III 2, 426b3–8; *Sens.* 3, 440a31–b25; *Sens.* 6, 445b20 ff.; *Metaph.* X 7). Aristotle seems to think of the capacity for perception as such a qualitative value, albeit of the very special character that it occupies the middle position on such scales where the two extremes "cancel each other out" (cf. Johansen 2012: 181). What is important in the present context is that this middle position is still a position on the scale which, even if only existent in potentiality, is something *physical*. Aristotle is just as much an ontological realist about capacities (cf. *Metaph.* IX 3) as he is an ontological realist about qualities as intrinsic and causally efficacious properties of natural things. For more on this point, see Chapter 1.

potentiality (namely, as just argued, a mean on a qualitative scale). The intellectual capacity is not of any given quality (*poios*; *An.* III 4, 429a25) before it thinks, not even in potentiality, which is also why this capacity, unlike the capacity for perception, has no bodily organ. The intellectual capacity "has no nature at all before it thinks, apart from being potentially" (*An.* III 4, 429a21–22). This is why it is said to be capable of thinking *everything* in a completely unrestricted way, including perceptible things and even itself: namely because, Aristotle argues, it is nothing determinate, not even potentially, but only an unrestricted potentiality for the essences of things. The perceptual capacity, contrary to this, is "not without body" (*An.* III 4, 429b4–5); it is of a certain quality, which makes it that it has a restricted domain—namely, the qualitative scale to which it belongs—so that it can also become only a certain determinate and limited range of qualities.[26] So, while the capacity for perception is potentially a given quality, the capacity for thinking is said to be an unrestricted potentiality for the essences of things. This has consequences *both* for the ways the two capacities are receptive of their corresponding objects *and* for the ways they are unaffected (*apathês*) prior to their respective acts of cognition (*An.* III 4, 429a29–b5). To be potentially a perceptual quality and to be potentially an object of thinking are very different kinds of being something in potentiality.

(2) *In form.* What does it mean to say that the two basic capacities of the cognitive soul are identical with the *forms* of their respective objects? Again, this means very different things for each of the two cognitive powers. In the case of perception, saying that one receives, and is identical with, the form of an external object is to put a *restriction* on one's identity. If *X* is identical in form with *Y*, and *Y* is a hylomorphic compound (as all perceptible objects are), then the formulation "identical in form" picks out just one aspect of *Y*, while *X* continues to be not identical with *Y* in other respects, most notably, as we have seen, when *Y* is taken unqualifiedly: that is, as *Y* "itself."[27] This is how Aristotle employs the notion of identity in form when

[26] In which sense is the perceptual capacity "not without body"? What exactly is the connection between perception and the body? Usually, the statement found in *An.* III 4, 429b5, is taken to mean that perception, unlike intellectual cognition, has an organ and that this organ is a bodily organ. This is certainly correct. But what must a natural *capacity* be like so as to require a bodily organ? The perceptual capacity is itself not "*chôriston*," separate or separable from the body, as *nous* is (cf. *An.* III 4, 429b5); for although it is not a magnitude, like that which perceives (the animal), it is still a capacity and proportion *of it* (*ekeinou*; *An.* II 12, 424a26–28). So, we may say that the capacity of perception is *essentially of* a body, which means that it has determinate physical existence even if in potentiality only (namely, as a qualitative proportion or *mesotês*).

[27] It is important to note that Aristotle's definition of perception as the capacity for receiving the objects of perception "without the matter" in *An.* II 12 says just that, despite the somewhat misleading expression. Aristotle uses the locution "without the matter" in a way that does not contrast color, or sound, or any of the other exclusive objects of perception with matter *per se* (constituent parts or even bare matter) but with matter in the sense of "things themselves" (*An.* III 8, 431b28) or "external object" (i.e., with the "things that have them"—namely, the perceptual special qualities, 424a22–24; for an argument that this is the meaning of "without the matter" in *An.* II 12, see Corcilius 2022: 148–150). Aristotle conceives of perceptual qualities as *properties* of things but that does not mean that he conceives of them as completely devoid of matter. Qualities are continuous and as such they have *extension*, which is a physical feature that Aristotle regularly associates with matter (see, e.g., *An.* I 1, 403a7–10, about

he applies it to perception: he *contrasts* it with the matter of the external object, not however with matter in the sense of "material constituents" but in the sense of the external object itself. Thus, when *X* is currently perceiving *Y* (an external hylomorphic compound), *X* is identical with *Y* in form but it is not identical with *Y* itself. Of course, *X* is also not identical with *Y*'s material constituents. But this does not mean that *X's perception* does not involve matter; on the contrary, all perceived qualities for Aristotle involve matter. This is different in the case of *nous*. There is at least one kind of thinking for which there seems to be no such restriction in the identity between the act of thinking and its object. Aristotle says that there is one kind of *per se* object of thinking introduced in *An.* III 4, 429b10–22—namely, separate substantial essences of type (1)[28]—the thinking of which amounts to nothing less than a full-blown and unqualified identity between the object and the act of intellection (*An.* III 4, 430a3–6; *An.* III 7, 431a1–2).[29] So, for separate substances, Aristotle clearly holds that the act of their thinking somehow *just is* a separate substance. There is no matter involved in it at all. This, by contrast, is not the case with the other two kinds of *per se* objects of thinking: namely, the essences of abstract objects and of perceptible things. To be sure, they are essences and so, like all essences, without matter; but since they are essences *of* some bodily or otherwise matter-involving object, they will contain some reference to matter. Consequently, our cognitive grasp on them, as we have seen in Chapter 2, requires the participation of, or a joint effort with, perception, which is the capacity responsible for the cognition of enmattered objects. Now the intelligible aspects (*noêta*) of matter-involving objects are said to be "in" these things in potentiality (*An.* III 4, 430a6–7). Again, this implies that becoming identical with these objects in thought amounts to a restricted kind of identity with the object, since, just as in the case of perception, the matter is excluded from identity with the object. As a result, "formal identity" seems to connote different things when applied to perception and the thinking of the intelligible aspects of hylomorphic compounds, on the one hand, and to the thinking of separate substances, on the other. Below I will discuss what it means to be an intelligible form of perceptible things, and how being such a form contrasts with being a perceptible form, when I discuss the claim that the objects of cognition are "in" perceptible magnitudes. For the time being, with respect to the

phantasmata which are qualitative changes). This has consequences for the meaning of "formal identity" between the object and the subject of perceptual cognition. The received object of perception is formal in a sense that does not contrast with matter as constituent material parts, but with matter in the sense of "external object." All qualities and with it all perceptual content include matter for Aristotle. This holds for "percepts" (*aisthêmata*) as it holds for "images" (*phantasmata*). The notion of form in the case of perception, therefore, does not exclude the material extension of the received form, and Aristotle indeed holds that the received perceptual qualities are (even if subtly) materially extended.

[28] See the three types of essences distinguished in Chapter 2.

[29] For more on the three types of essences, see Chapter 2 (Section 3) and the Glossary (*s.v.* NOÊTON) at the end of the volume.

thinking of separate substances, we find ourselves confronted with the question of whether the concept of "formal identity" can be applied to them in the first place. If the cognition of essences of type (1) amounts to a full-blown and unrestricted identity, the qualifier "formal" in "formal identity" seems out of place.[30]

Here, we face an interpretative problem. We can describe it with the help of the following questions. Does the talk of "formal identity" in *An.* III 8 capture a kind of identity between the object and the subject of cognition that is relevant for *all* kinds of intellectual cognition? Does Aristotle speak globally about *nous* here in such a way as to include the thinking of separate substances? *Or* does he restrict his claim to the thinking of things that are not separate from matter? This alternative prompts the even larger interpretative question of whether there is an intended *limitation* in the scope of the statements about *nous* in *An.* III 8 to the effect that Aristotle focuses on the embodied capacity for thinking present in human beings (the cognitive soul) to the exclusion of possible separate intellects.

Now, to start with, the thinking of separate (i.e., immaterial) substances was not excluded from the treatment of the thinking capacity offered in *An.* III 4–5. Aristotle mentions separate substances in his treatment of the objects of thinking where he says that they are identical with the thinking of them (*An.* III 4, 430a3–5), and *An.* III 5 is clearly concerned with separate, active, *nous.* But this broad scope, apparently ranging over all kinds of thinking in *An.* III 4 and 5, seems to be narrowed down to the treatment of the different kinds of embodied human thinking and other kinds of embodied cognition in the following two chapters. In these chapters, Aristotle is mainly concerned with propositional thinking (*An.* III 6) and with the different kinds of embodied cognition of the cognitive soul (*An.* III 7). The issue of separate substances is almost absent in these chapters, with three exceptions. He twice touches on separate substances toward the end of *An.* III 6 (430b24–26 and b29–31), and he makes a statement about separate substances at the very end of *An.* III 7 (431b17–19). But it would be an exaggeration to say that

[30] There seems to be no clear textual evidence for the thesis that Aristotle conceived of the thinking of separate substances as a thinking of *forms* (*eidê*). (For a brief survey of some arguments against the thesis that there can be forms without correlate matter, see Judson 2019: 281–282, especially footnote 49.) It is an open question even whether forms are the *per se* objects of thinking for Aristotle (i.e., whether forms are objects of thinking considered *per se* and in general). The term for the object of thinking in Aristotle's treatment of *nous* is *noêton* rather than *eidos*. Even though *An.* III 4–7 (up until 431b2) speaks of forms (*eidos*) as objects of thinking several times, this usage does not entail a clear commitment to the idea that the intellect is *per se* concerned with forms. *Eidos* occurs three times in *An.* III 4. It is found in 429a16 in the context of the comparison of thinking with perceiving. This use, due to the comparison, seems to be noncommittal with respect to thinking; *eidôn and eidê* in 429a28–29 seem to pick up the language preferred by a certain Platonic tribe (*hoi legontes*) which maintained that *nous* is the place of forms (cf. Plato, *Parm.* 132 B and perhaps Aristotle, *Top.* II 7, 113a25). So, there seems to be no clear commitment to forms as *per se* objects of thought in *An.* III 4. In *An.* III 7, 431b2, Aristotle speaks of *ta eidê* as referring to the forms of perceptible things, which the thinking part of the cognitive soul is said to calculate with by way of anticipation and preferential calculus. Again, this does not seem to be a reference to the *per se* objects of thinking. So, if *nous* is not *per se* related to *eidê*, it is likely that the locution of "form of forms" employed in *An.* III 8 may only refer to the objects of the embodied human intellect (i.e., of the cognitive soul) and not to the objects of the intellect *per se*. See below.

these chapters are concerned with separate substances as their subject: in *An.* III 6, 430b24–26, the remark on separate essences occurs in the context of the discussion of cognition of things by way of their opposites, where "opposites" includes their corresponding ("opposed") potentialities. Aristotle excludes essences of type (1) from having such opposites and remarks that in such cases we are dealing with separate and self-thinking "causes." Though no doubt important, this is a relatively isolated statement in the chapter. Second, Aristotle makes a statement at the outset of the chapter which he repeats at the end of *An.* III 6: namely, that there is no falsehood in uncombined simple thought (*An.* III 6, 430a26–27). The only difference with respect to the initial statement is that he now adds that things without matter fall into the class of uncombined thoughts (*An.* III 6, 430b29–30). While this is certainly a claim concerning the thought of essences generally, it may also include the thinking of separate substances of type (1). Third, there is the very last sentence of *An.* III 7. While it does mention separate substances, it does so only to raise doubt about the possibility that an embodied cognitive agent could ever think essences of type (1). Aristotle asks whether it is possible to think one of the separate objects—essences of type (1)—with a cognitive capacity that is not itself separated from magnitude. Quite tellingly, he does not answer the question in *An.* III 7.[31] So, it seems that none of these references to separate substances contradicts the thesis that *An.* III 6 and 7 are chiefly concerned with human propositional thinking and embodied cognition. Neither of these chapters is concerned with separate substances as its subject matter.[32] Rather, they are concerned with human intellectual thinking (*An.* III 6), and with the activities of what we have called the cognitive soul (*An.* III 7).[33] And this explains why they only very briefly mention the thinking of separate substances. Moreover, the fact that *An.* III 7 asks whether it is possible to think separate substances with a capacity that is not separate from magnitude seems to be strong evidence for the thesis that the chapter is *not* concerned with the thinking of separate substances.

So, the question at this point of the argument is whether or not Aristotle continues in *An.* III 8 with the same narrow focus on the cognitive soul adopted in *An.* III 6–7. The focus is narrow when compared with the perspective on all kinds of thinking adopted in *An.* III 4–5. Does Aristotle speak about the cognitive soul in *An.* III 8 in a way that disregards the thinking of separate substances perhaps as something alien to, or unreachable by, the embodied human intellect? *Or* does the chapter offer a summary of all things that have been said about *nous* in the previous chapters, including what was said about the separate intellect?

[31] For more on this question and why it is left unanswered, see Chapter 4 (Section 7).

[32] The statement in *An.* III 6, 430b24–26, that excludes separate substances from having opposites is discussed in Chapter 3 (Section 3).

[33] For an introduction to what is mean here by "cognitive soul," I refer the reader to the Glossary (*s.v.* COGNITIVE SOUL).

There is no room here to do full justice to all the implications of the two options outlined above. Still, I think the question can be decided. I start from Aristotle's otherwise well-attested commitment to the separation of the sciences. On that basis, it is not very likely that Aristotle envisages a full-blown theory of *nous per se* in a way that includes the separate divine intellect and the thinking of separate substances. The investigation offered in *De anima* is devoted to the project of defining the parts of the *soul*. This is what his explanatory essentialism and its application to the phenomena of living things requires, and it is also what Aristotle announces to do in *An.* I and *An.* II. Aristotle also gives us no reason to think that he changes his definitory goal over the course of the treatise's argument. Thinking separate substances seems to be no part of what the human embodied soul is designed to do for Aristotle (*An.* III 7, 431b17–19)—at least not *qua* such. And while there may be no universal agreement regarding the thesis that the separate intellect forms no part of the human soul, the simple fact that the separate intellect is a separate substance (an essence of type (1); *An.* III 5, 430a17–18) which is essentially actual/active (*energeia*), while the parts of the soul are capacities (*dunameis*), leaves us no other choice than to exclude the separate intellect from the parts of the human soul. This consideration gains additional support by the first sentence of the section on *nous* in *An.* III 4:

> Regarding the part of the soul by which the soul knows and understands—be it separate or separate not in extension but only in account—we must examine what distinguishes it and how thinking may ever come about.[34]

Aristotle here announces an examination of *nous* as a part of the human soul exactly as one would expect him to do from the general character, as well as from the methodology, of his investigation into the soul as the principle of his science of living things. Since we know that Aristotle does not believe that the human ensouled *nous* exhausts the possible range of intellectual activity in and outside of the universe, his announcement should be taken to announce a *limited investigation* into one specific kind of intellect: namely, the intellect as it is part of the human soul. However, if this is correct, it becomes a question why Aristotle discusses separate substances and the separate intellect in *De anima* in the first place, as he does in *An.* III 4 and *An.* III 5.[35] My suggestion is that Aristotle speaks of separate substances and active thinking in *De anima* because he thinks that one cannot speak of *nous* as a part of the human soul without saying something about

[34] *An.* III 4, 429a10–12.

[35] It is true that the first sentence of *An.* III 5 says that just as there is matter and potentiality and a corresponding cause and producer in nature, so these different factors (*diaphoras*) must also occur in the soul (*An.* III 5, 430a10). That, however, need not be taken to imply that active *nous* is a part of the human soul. See the discussion in Chapter 2 (Section 5).

nous per se, and talking about *nous per se* requires him to speak of the separate intellect (= active thinking). The methodology outlined in *An.* II 4, according to which the objects of psychic capacities have definitional priority over their activities, and the activities over their corresponding capacities, makes it mandatory that the objects of *nous* be dealt with first. Now, the *per se* objects of *nous*, as we have seen in *An.* III 4, are essences. Essences come in three kinds: essences separate from matter (type 1), essences of natural (hylomorphic) compounds (type 2), and essences that result from abstraction such as mathematical objects (type 3). This is why the specification of the *per se* objects of *nous* requires Aristotle to mention separate essences. This is so especially since he thinks that there is an important continuity among the different kinds of essences. They differ from each other by way of degrees of separateness from matter. Separate essences thus in a way structure the entire field of objects of thinking as the optimal case. And if a human being engages in actual thinking, this will be an exercise of *nous*, but it will be *nous* in a somewhat deficient, because not separated, mode. This continuity of all *per se* objects of thinking with, and their dependence on, separate essences makes it necessary for Aristotle to include separate substances in his discussion of the human capacity for thinking (*An.* III 4, 429b21–22, 430a3–7). *Nous* as a part of the human soul has a share in the features of separate *nous*.

If this is correct, Aristotle speaks of separate substances as objects of *nous* and of active thinking because defining human *nous* necessarily involves speaking of *nous per se*, and also because the account of the coming about of episodes of human thinking necessarily involves reference to active thinking as its actualizer. The conclusion of all of this is that the chapters on *nous* in Aristotle's *De anima* do talk of *nous per se* and of separate *nous*, but they do so only because the treatment of human *nous* requires them to do so. *De anima* is concerned with active thinking only to the extent that the treatment of human *nous* requires it. If this is correct, we should say that even though forms (*eidê*) are not the *per se* objects of *nous per se* (including separate thinking), forms are in some sense (to be discussed below) the *per se* objects of human *nous* (at least *qua* human). There are also other objects of thinking which do not have the character of forms: namely, separate substances and whatever else is devoid of matter.[36] The upshot of the above discussion is that *An.* III 8 *is a chapter that summarizes the main results of Aristotle's treatment of the*

[36] With all this in place, it cannot be completely ruled out that the thinking of separate substances is possible for human beings. But there is no clear textual indication that Aristotle thinks that this is the case. Based on what has been said so far about the workings of *nous*, such thinking would have to be free of *phantasmata*. This is strongly suggested by the last sentence of *An.* III 7. Aristotle says that the human capacity for thinking always thinks "in" the *phantasmata* (*An.* III 7, 431b2). The only conceivable scenario left for the possibility of a human thinking of separate substances, then, would be to say that when human thinking succeeds in thinking separate substances it thereby ceases (for the duration of that episode) to be an episode of *human* thinking (this is also what Johansen in his brief discussion of the issue seems to imply. See Johansen 2012: 240). But there is no clear indication in the text that Aristotle entertained such a scenario. For more on this, see Chapter 6.

cognitive soul. It does not discuss *nous per se*, nor does it discuss separate essences of type (1).

So far, then, Aristotle has stated his identity thesis regarding the cognitive soul and its objects. He imposes three restrictions on it: prior to engaging in an episode of cognition, the cognitive soul is identical with its objects, but it is so (i) in a serial way—that is to say, in virtue of being identical with any single given object of cognition at any given time (but not with all of them at the same time)—(ii) in form, either perceptual or intelligible, and (iii) in potentiality only. In acts of perceiving, the cognitive soul will be qualitatively identical with the perceptual form of its object, while actual human thinking will be numerically identical with the intelligible form of its object.

2.2 The analogy with the hand

Aristotle offers a vivid illustration of the account of the cognitive soul given so far. This is the memorable comparison of the cognitive soul with the hand, which is offered in the last section of this first part of the chapter (*An.* III 8, 432a1–3). As the language makes clear (*hôsper* combined with *kai*), the nature of the comparison is that of an analogy. Aristotle compares the soul with a hand, comparing the different *roles* they play in their respective domains. He seems to take it for granted that the hand is a (natural) tool that enables us to use all other tools which, unlike the hand, are not naturally attached to us.[37] The cognitive soul, then, is claimed to be analogically the same as the hand in the following respect: just as the hand is a tool for the use of (all) tools, so the cognitive soul is a form for the reception of either perceptible or intelligible objects: that is, the perceptual capacity is the form of perceptual objects and the intellectual capacity is the form of perceptible forms.[38] So much for the basic structure of the analogy.

The analogy makes good sense if we understand the comparison with the hand as a tool of tools in the sense of an illustration of the thesis, stated in the identity claim, that the cognitive soul is formally and potentially identical with all beings *by virtue of being able to become formally identical with any single arbitrary being at any moment of time.* It also seems plausible to call the hand "a tool of tools" in this way: that is, insofar as it is a tool that is naturally attached to us and that allows us to make use of any given arbitrary tool at any given moment of time. And maybe

[37] This is also how Trendelenburg takes the analogy (Trendelenburg 1877: 438). Crubellier 2020: 238 argues that the hand is actually *not* a tool and suggests on that basis that *nous* is not a form either. But see *Mot. An.* 8, 702a32–b5, which does seem to suggest a similarity between the tools that are naturally attached, such as the hand, and those that are not naturally attached. Regarding the claim that human *nous* and perception somehow are forms, there seems to be no room for disagreement, as Aristotle seems to be committed to it via his identity thesis.

[38] This also seems to be how Philoponus takes the analogy (*In An.* 567.33).

this is all Aristotle is getting at with his analogy. Among other things, this analogy would allow him to vindicate what seems to be the main goal of the argument in *De anima*, which is to define the basic capacities of the soul as principles for the scientific explanation of the phenomena of sublunary living things. With his definition of the cognitive soul as the set of two basic capacities allowing living things to cognize whatever there is at a given moment by becoming identical with any being in form, he seems to achieve his goal with respect to the cognitive functions of the soul.[39]

Still, even on that minimal reading there are a few lingering questions. For one, while we have at least a vague intuitive understanding of what tools are,[40] we have no such pre-philosophical understanding of what forms are supposed to be. In the case of perception, the capacity is supposed to be potentially the form of perceptible things. What this means emerges from Aristotle's treatment of the so-called exclusive objects of perception—color for sight, sound for hearing, and so on—in *An.* II 6–11, as we have seen above. These objects are said to correspond to perceptual affections (*pathêtikai poiotêtes*; *Cat.* 8, 9b2–9) and to consist in certain *logoi*: that is, proportions of values on given qualitative scales, which are physical properties for Aristotle. And it is in line with this idea that Aristotle describes the perceptual capacity as a qualitative mean value (*mesotês*, *logos*) in *An.* II 11, *An.* II 12, and *An.* III 2. The perceptual capacity is potentially a qualitative perceptual mean value, and the manifestation of this capacity during an episode of perception *is* an actual perceptual quality. The characterization of *nous* as the "form of forms," by contrast, cannot be fleshed out in terms of perceptual qualities. The objects of thinking are the objects of knowledge, and the objects of knowledge are not physical properties but, as Aristotle says, the outcome of either abstractions—that is, mathematical objects—or states ("havings," *hexeis*) and properties of perceptible things (*An.* III 8, 432a5–6). This is vague enough, and hence the characterization of *nous* as the form of forms may seem less informative than the characterization of the perceptual capacity as the form of perceptible objects (even if it is linguistically more fitting to the example of the hand as a "tool of tools"). But upon reflection this is probably

[39] Cf. *Probl.* XXX 5, 955b22–556a10, which uses the claim that *nous* is a tool as a premise for an argument as to why it is that we are better in using our *nous* at an older age. The chapter also compares *nous* as the tool of the soul with the hand as the tool of the body. Both are said to be natural tools that we possess for the usage of external tools (i.e., other tools or sciences). This goes beyond what our passage in *An.* III 8 claims about *nous*. Our passage does *not* say that *nous* is a natural tool (see also Shields 2016: 343); it only compares the *enabling relation* in which the hand stands toward the use of all other instruments to the enabling relation in which *nous* and perception (the cognitive soul) stands toward the cognition of all things. That latter enabling function is said to be exerted by the cognitive soul in virtue of being a *form*. See main text above.

[40] Crubellier's discussion of the hand example in *Part. An.* IV 10, 687a19–21 and 687b3–5, brings out this aspect rather nicely (see also *Juv.* 469b1–4). Rodier suggests—as he himself says—a more complicated reading of the analogy, according to which the perceptual soul is the tool of the intellect; Polansky follows him in this (Rodier 1900: 523–524; Polansky 2007: 496). This indeed complicates the analogy. And even though I agree that there is such an instrumental relation between the capacities of the soul for Aristotle, I do not think that this is the point of the analogy.

as it should be. The human capacity for thinking *qua* such is the matterless potentiality to think all the thinkable aspects of perceptual things. As such, it has to operate on the basis of the information that the perceptual capacity provides it with. As a result, the objects of human thinking *qua* such will be either mathematical abstractions from, or states and properties of, perceptible things, where states (or "havings") importantly include the essences of hylomorphic compounds. Because of this dependency on perception for its content, it makes good sense here for Aristotle to call human thinking the form of (perceptible) forms. And this dependency, in turn, must raise the question of whether the human capacity for thinking is *just* that: namely, just a capacity for picking out features (states, properties) of perceptual things without adding or contributing anything to them. This question will be relevant in the next passage, where Aristotle argues for what I here call the "empiricist claim." The "empiricist claim" states that all objects of thinking are "in" perceptible things, and that perception and *phantasmata* (which originate in perception) are therefore necessary for human thinking. In the final section of the chapter, Aristotle will answer the above question and argue that even the simplest human thoughts are irreducibly different from *phantasmata*, even if they depend on them as their necessary conditions.

3. Part II: the "empiricist" claim

The second part of *An*. III 8 falls into two sections: the argument for the "empiricist" claim and a short discussion of *phantasia* and its relation to thinking. I shall discuss the "empiricist" claim with a focus on the meaning of the statement that intelligible objects are "in" perceptible forms. Here is my reconstruction of the argument for that claim.[41]

3.1 The argument for the "empiricist" claim

(i) [The cognitive soul cognizes all beings: that is, perceptible and intelligible objects.]
(ii) There appears to be nothing separate beside perceptible magnitudes.
(iii) [Every being is somewhere.]
(iv) It follows that [ἐπεί; *An*. III 8, 432a3] the objects of *nous* are in the perceptible forms. This holds for objects said in abstraction and for the states and affections of perceptible things; they are all in the perceptible forms.
(v) [All cognition requires contact between the subject and the object of the relation of cognition.]

[41] For another reconstruction of the argument, see Shields 2016: 343.

(vi) It is for this reason [i.e., (iv) and (v)] that one who hasn't perceived anything, one who hasn't had contact with perceptual things, could neither learn nor understand anything, and that whenever one contemplates, one necessarily at the same time contemplates some *phantasma*; for *phantasmata* are just like perceptions, except that they are without matter.

Premise (i) is not in the transmitted text. But we need to supplement this (at this point, I think, entirely unproblematic) claim from the previous context if the argument is to get off the ground. Premise (iii) is necessary to yield the conclusion. I find it unproblematic as well. What it says seems to be a triviality for Aristotle. When he introduces his thesis that everything is somewhere in his *Physics*, he does not even argue for it but simply says that "all hold" (*pantes hupolambanousin*) that "beings are somewhere" (*pou*).[42] And without this thesis, or some such thesis, we could not see why Aristotle should locate the objects of *nous* in the first place. Now the sense of "locate" here is not the sense of Aristotelian *topos*.[43] One might object here that the "in-relation" Aristotle talks about in discussing how intelligible objects relate to perceptible forms and magnitudes may not be a spatial relation. But even if this were the case, it would still be *true* for Aristotle that everything that is—every being that is—is somewhere. And, furthermore, supposing that Aristotle were speaking here not of location but of something else, the transition from (ii) to (iv) as well as from (iv) to (v) would be somewhat mysterious. If this is correct, then what Aristotle is doing here is localizing the objects of *nous* in perceptual things and deriving an epistemological claim from it.[44] To do this, however, requires premise (v). Without it, we could not see why the fact that intelligible objects are localized in perceptible forms would allow us to infer (vi). But premise (v) seems unproblematic as well. It is true for all kinds of cognition for Aristotle that some sort of contact between the cognitive object and the cognitive subject is necessary for the cognition to come about. Aristotle offers an argument for this claim in *Phys.* VII 2 for perception in all five sense modalities, and also for the states of the intellectual part in *Phys.* VII 3 (247b1–248a9, as printed in the Ross edition, and similarly in *An.* III 7). With these additional premises in place, the argument seems valid, and we can turn to the discussion of its premises.

Thesis (ii) is certainly the most controversial, given that Aristotle is committed to the existence of separate substances both in and outside of his *De anima*. Recently, Michel Crubellier has argued that (ii) is trivial for Aristotle, on the grounds that

[42] *Phys.* IV 1, 208a29–31. See Morison 2002: 15–20.

[43] Aristotle does not assign a place, *topos*, either to the soul or to *nous*, as *topos* is intrinsically tied to extended magnitudes (cf. *Phys.* IV 4, 212a5–7). That, however, does not mean that soul and *nous* are not "somewhere" (*pou*) (i.e., that they do not have a *position* (*thesis*)). Aristotle locates the soul in the heart, while he at the same time distinguishes the soul from the magnitude in which it resides (*Mot. An.* 9, 703a1–3). This is important because, in Aristotle's physics, without a spatial position the soul could not have contact (*haphê*) with the body so as to act on it. See Primavesi and Corcilius 2018: cliv, footnote 13.

[44] About the meaning of the preposition "in," see below.

para + accusative expresses a very particular relation: namely, a relation between *X* and *Y*, where *X* and *Y* stand in an intrinsic relation to each other while there is no spatial overlap between them ("à côté de"). What (ii) says on this reading is not that there is nothing "beyond" or "over and above" perceptible magnitudes (which would be utterly false for Aristotle given his metaphysical commitments), but only that there is nothing in the universe that is somehow importantly *of* perceptible magnitudes (intrinsically related to them) and at the same time completely self-subsistent and spatially separate from them. The upshot of this, Crubellier argues, is that Aristotle here simply reminds us of his anti-Platonic commitment to the rejection of separate forms, and that therefore there is no conflict between (ii) and Aristotle's commitment to the existence of separate substances.[45] In other words, Aristotle merely denies the existence of forms *of* perceptible magnitudes that are separate from these very magnitudes, as some Platonists claimed.

This is an ingenious suggestion. It removes the cause of the uneasiness felt by previous interpreters with one stroke.[46] However, it raises the question whether such a reassertion of Aristotle's anti-Platonic ontological commitment does not affect the force of his main argument.[47] If premise (ii) does not exclude the existence of separate substances but only the existence of spatially separate forms *of* perceptible magnitudes, neither the conclusion in (iv) nor the conclusion in (vi) seems *obviously* to follow from the premises. For, on that interpretation, there are substances separate from perceptible magnitudes and the only premise in the argument that could prevent us from thinking that one could access them cognitively without perception is the claim (v) that all cognition requires contact between the cognitive subject and the cognized object. But (v) is a tacit background assumption and not something that Aristotle explicitly says. Furthermore, and more importantly, it is no longer clear why we are entitled to draw the conclusion that all objects of cognition are "in" perceptible things (provided one adds, as Aristotle would be happy to do, that separate substances are objects of cognition). So, on the interpretation under discussion, the force of the overall argument for the empiricist claim would be significantly weakened.

The alternative is to take (ii) at face value. The statement that it *appears* to be the case that there is nothing besides, and separate from, perceptible magnitudes

[45] Crubellier 2020: 241.

[46] Philoponus *ad loc.* must have felt particularly uneasy about (ii). He goes out of his way to undo the impression that Aristotle could say anything here that would contradict his belief in separate substances.

[47] There is also the further question (discussed in Crubellier 2020) of why, if his interpretation of (ii) is correct, Aristotle makes the epistemic qualification "as it seems" in (ii). Why should Aristotle epistemically qualify what he most probably takes to be one of the main points he was able to establish against the Platonist conception of forms as separate from the things they are the forms of? Crubellier (2020: 241–242) proposes that what gets epistemically qualified is the thesis that there is nothing besides *perceptible* magnitudes and that Aristotle adds this qualification on the grounds that this is common opinion, but that there may also be thinkers who believe in the independent existence of non-perceptible (e.g., mathematical) magnitudes.

is perfectly acceptable as a premise. It also makes an intuitive point if one argues not from the perspective of Aristotle's metaphysics, which arrives at the postulation of separate substances by way of complex philosophical argumentation, but rather *from the standpoint of the metaphysically unbiased person*. And as it stands—namely, with the proviso that it *appears* that there is nothing beside and separate from perceptible magnitudes—the thesis suffices to warrant the conclusion in (vi). For the fact that it appears to us, and quite naturally so, that there is nothing besides and separate from perceptible magnitudes allows one to establish that we could not learn or come to understand anything without the cognition of perceptible magnitudes. The mere appearance suffices in this case to exclude any *immediate cognitive access* to non-perceptible content, which is all that is needed to establish that perception is a necessary condition for all other kinds of human cognition. For if there was somehow an immediate and intuitive access to other objects of cognition available to us, it, due to its immediacy, would presumably appear to us as well. So, Aristotle need not be taken to say anything here that contradicts his philosophical claims regarding the existence of separate substances. All he needs for his argument is that it *seems* to be the case that there is nothing separate from perceptible magnitudes. This is therefore how I suggest we should understand the claim in (ii). The "as it seems" in *An.* III 8, 432a4, should not be taken as casting doubt on the claim that there is nothing beside and separate from perceptible magnitude; it should be made part of the claim.

On this hypothesis we can interpret the argument in a straightforward manner without saddling Aristotle with a view about separate substances that he manifestly did not hold, and also without making him cast doubt on an important premise of his own argument. The immediate and momentous upshot of this way of interpreting the argument is that Aristotle restricts the scope of human intellectual cognition to objects that *relate* to perceptible magnitudes in one way or another.[48] This, I take it, is confirmed by Aristotle's short list of the objects of thinking said to be "in" perceptible magnitudes. They are all the things said in abstraction, all the affections and qualitative properties (*pathê*), and all the states (*hexeis*) of perceptible magnitudes.[49] This list seems to exhaust all intelligible objects

[48] It is well known that Aristotle thinks that the first unmoved mover is located (i.e., has a position) somewhere at the outside of the outmost sphere. So, the first unmoved mover is not properly speaking *in* anything perceptible (*Phys.* VIII 10, 267b9; cf. *Mot. An.* 4, 699b32–35). The localization probably has to do with Aristotle's belief that there is no *actio per distans*, which commits him to the claim that *every* causal action and interaction requires *contact*, so that there must be a place in the universe where there is "nothing in-between" the first mover and the first moved thing. Does this view of the location of the first unmoved mover contradict (iii), the thesis that the objects of the intellect are in the perceptible forms? This depends on how one conceives of the cognition of separate substances in Aristotle. On the interpretation given, Aristotle seems to believe that if the cognitive soul can have access to the cognition of separate substances, it can have that access only *per aliud* (i.e., by somehow connecting it to perceptible substances, as is done, e.g., in *Metaph.* XII 6, where the connection is a causal one).

[49] See the *ta te en aphairesei legomena* corresponding to *kai hosa tôn aisthêtôn hexeis kai pathê*, in *An.* III 8, 432a5–6, which suggests exhaustivity.

that can be derived from perceptual forms by human *nous*. The list includes all abstractions from perceptible magnitudes (mathematical abstractions in the Aristotelian sense: i.e., abstract properties treated as separable from perceptible matter), all their states—that is, their relational properties in the broadest sense, including their virtues and the "having" of their essences—plus all their qualitative properties and affections. The states and affections are most plausibly interpreted as properties that are inseparable from perceptual matter, both the essential and the accidental ones. This gives us a clearer sense of what it means to be *contained* in perceptible magnitudes: namely, being either their states, or their properties, or abstractions from their properties. The list does not include separate substances. *An.* III 8 gives us no reason to suppose that Aristotle thought that the cognitive soul can grasp separate substances, at least not *per se*. Separate substances are neither perceptible magnitudes, nor states or affections, nor abstractions that are taken from perceptible magnitudes. This confirms the above thesis that Aristotle is limiting himself in *An.* III 8 to a discussion of the embodied cognition of the cognitive soul. This is also what we found him doing in the previous section and during the argument advanced in *An.* III 7, with the exception of the last sentence of the chapter, which however problematizes the *possibility* of grasping separate substances with a cognitive capacity that is not also separate from matter.[50] Hence, there is no sign that Aristotle returns to a discussion of the thinking of separate substances in *An.* III 8. Separate substances are a topic which was left behind at the beginning of *An.* III 6,[51] before Aristotle turned to propositional thinking (*An.* III 6) and embodied cognition (*An.* III 7). It is important to note, however, that the argument advanced in *An.* III 8 also does not rule out that the human intellect may come to think separate substances *per aliud*: namely, as principles and causes of perceptible magnitudes.

Let us now turn to the claim put forward in (iv). In which sense are intelligible objects "in" perceptual forms? First of all, it seems that the intelligible objects will have to be literally in the perceptible forms, in the sense of being *located* in them (because of the principle stated in (iii)). But this does not mean, I hasten to add, that they are spatial beings or even material constituents of perceptible things. From the previous arguments we learned that human *nous* (capacity) is the intelligible forms in potentiality (*dunamei ta eidê*; *An.* III 4, 429b29), that the intelligible objects are potentially in the things that have matter (*An.* III 4, 430a6–7), and that the intellectual part of the soul is in a way the locus of forms (*topos eidôn*; *An.* III 4, 429b27–28). This leaves us with no other option than saying that intelligible objects are "in" perceptible forms in virtue of the fact that the latter are potential objects of thinking (i.e., intelligible objects). One consequence of this reading is that when

50 I take this to be additional evidence for the thesis that the entire argument offered in *An.* III 7 is exclusively concerned with embodied cognition. See Chapter 4 (Section 7) and Corcilius 2020a: 185–220.

51 For the very short exceptions, see the discussion above.

their intelligible aspects are actually grasped by the cognitive soul, they will actually be in the cognitive soul (hence the intellectual soul is the "place of the forms"), but they will not actually (but only potentially) be in the perceptible objects. This is an attenuated sense of being "in" that corresponds to "being a potential object of a cognitive capacity." But it is a sense that seems well attested in Aristotle's discussion of the intelligibility of things with matter in *An.* III 4, where he says that "*in* things that have matter each of the objects of thought exists potentially" (*An.* III 4, 430a6–7). The intelligible aspects of enmattered things are "in" their perceptual forms in the sense that they are potential objects of thinking. Note that this does not mean that enmattered things do not actually *have* their essences; they do have them, but they do not have them *as* actual objects of thinking.[52] Perhaps this corresponds to the second example of a usage of "having" (*echein*), of which Aristotle says that it corresponds to "being in": namely, "having" in the sense of "being present as in something receptive, as for instance the bronze has the form of the statue, and the body has the disease" (*hôi an ti huparchei hôs dektikôi*; *Metaph.* V 23, 1023a11–13). Aristotle also speaks of potential objects of thinking (*to noêton*) as "present" (*huparchein*) in intelligible things (*An.* III 4, 430a6–9). This attenuated sense of "being in" is quite permissive. The way it is used in our case certainly does not suggest that the objects of the human intellect—essences—are contained in perceptible magnitudes *as* actual objects of thinking. What it suggests is rather that everything that can be thought in relation to perceptible magnitudes is "in them" in the sense that it can be thought as being true *of* them as *their* essential being (which being they, of course, actually have, albeit not as actual thoughts). This, I suggest, is confirmed by *An.* III 7, where Aristotle describes both practical and theoretical thinking (alongside the two kinds of enmattered essences distinguished in *An.* III 4, 429b10–22) as taking place "in *phantasmata*" (431b2–17). The objects of thinking are "in" the external objects as the intelligible being they "have," but which is not actually in them *as such*: that is, as actual objects of thinking. For instance, supposing for the sake of the argument that the intelligible being of a house is its structure, then that structure will no doubt be the structure of the house and it will actually be in it; but *as a universal intelligible object* the structure will be present in the house only potentially.

The conclusion advanced in (vi) follows from the foregoing on the basis of (v), the principle that all cognition requires contact between the subject and the object of cognition. This principle is a simple application of the general principle that all interaction in the universe requires contact between the agent and the patient of change. The conclusion in (vi), which I will refer to as the "dependency claim," applies the principle in two ways, diachronically and synchronically. *Diachronically*: to know or grasp anything by way of intellectual cognition

[52] I outlined in Chapter 2 what kind of preparation of their *phantasmata* is required to make them receptive of actual objects of thinking.

presupposes previous instruction, and instruction in turn presupposes previous experience with the perceptual world. Without having had contact with the perceptible world, we would be incapable of learning anything. *Synchronically*: thinking of *x* requires an occasion to think *x*, and that occasion is not identical with the thinking of *x*'s intelligible form; rather, *x* must be presented to our cognitive soul in some kind of perceptual way so that our intellect can have contact with it. *An.* III 7 is to some large extent dedicated to showing how contact between the subject and the object of cognition in all forms of embodied cognition comes about.[53] So contact by way of perception or *phantasia* is necessary for thinking because the intelligible objects are in perceptible forms in the sense of being *potentially* in them. Thinking could not latch onto them without the aid of perceptible forms. And it is for this reason that thinking cannot get a hold of its objects without simultaneously contemplating perceptible forms (if intelligible forms were actually present in perceptible forms, in the same way in which perceptible forms are actually present in perceptible magnitudes, we could probably carve them out somehow and contemplate them without their bearers). As a result, according to Aristotle's synchronic dependency claim, human thinkers have to think with the aid of mental representations (perceptual forms and their derivates), and necessarily so, because the objects of thinking are not available to us directly but only via perceptible forms—the objects of the intellect are in them, and they are *potentially* in them—meaning that without having contact with the bearers of their potentiality, we could not access them at all.[54] This is why the potential object of thinking, the perceptual bearer of an intelligible form, must be present in the soul of the cognitive agent as well. It is because of this contact requirement that human thinking necessarily requires *phantasmata*. This requirement, as we have seen, follows from the thesis that intelligible forms are *in* perceptible forms (iv) plus the further thesis that intelligible forms cannot be extracted from perceptible magnitudes and be stored in a cognitive agent's cognitive system *as thoughts*. Thoughts are not storable items for Aristotle. He is, as we have seen above, a staunch presentist about thoughts. The best we can do is to store the *phantasmata* that potentially contain them.[55] Now,

[53] In Corcilius 2020a: 185–220, I call this the "actuality principle." According to that principle, everything that comes to be *F* comes to be so by virtue of the agency of something that is actually *F*. *An.* III 7 shows how this principle holds in the various forms of embodied cognition and desire in a sequence of ascending cognitive demandingness. All these kinds of cognition need to be triggered by some kind of contact with the object in one way or the other.

[54] But this, to be sure, only regards the *occasion* to think essences or, if you will, only the triggering cause of thinking them which establishes the contact between the potential object of thinking and the cognitive soul. For, as I argued in Chapter 2, mere contact between the immediate potentiality of an object of thinking and the potentiality of thinking it in a thinking agent, both of which are passive potentialities, is not sufficient for actual thinking to come about; for that to happen it also requires the state-like presence of active thinking of type (1). Otherwise, there would be passive potentialities on both sides of the cognition relation and actual thinking could not take place.

[55] The contact requirement, I think, is referred to in *Mem.* 1, 450a7–9: "On account of what cause it is not possible to think anything without something continuous, nor [to think] the things that are in time without time, pertains to a different investigation (*allos logos*)."

in higher animals, and especially in humans, *phantasmata* can be used as a substitute for direct contact with perceptible things. The fact that Aristotle says on this occasion that *phantasmata* are without matter (432a10) need not confuse us. As already said, there is also no tension with the definition of perception as the capacity for taking on the perceptual form "without the matter" (*An.* II 12, 424a17–19; cf. also *An.* III 2, 425b24–25 with respect to *aisthêseis* and *phantasiai*). The expression "without the matter" in all these instances means the same thing: namely, "without the presence of the external objects of perception." What Aristotle says here, then, is that *phantasmata* are like percepts (*aisthêmata*), albeit without the presence of the external objects of perception. This repeats a point made earlier where it was said that *phantasmata* belong to thinking in the same manner as percepts (*An.* III 7, 431a14–15) and that this is the reason why the soul never thinks without a *phantasma* (*An.* III 7, 431a16–17). So, there is little reason to think that Aristotle is telling us something entirely new here.[56] If this is right, the so-called "empiricist claim" that we could not learn or come to understand anything without perception is not the most important message of our section of text.[57] Aristotle does not seem to be primarily interested in giving us an epistemological account of how we come to know; rather, he seems to be concerned with the dependency claim: that is, with establishing a causal thesis about the relation between the cognitive (embodied) soul and the physical world—namely, that perception and perception-like mental representations are necessary for human thinking both antecedently and simultaneously. We human thinkers are in this way bound to perceptible objects.[58]

3.2 *Phantasia* and its relation to thinking

In the last section of the chapter, Aristotle turns to the relation between *phantasmata* and basic thoughts (*prôta noêmata*), prompted by his discussion of *phantasmata* in the previous section (indicated by the *gar* in 432a9). He starts by distinguishing

[56] See *An.* III 3 429a4–6; *Mot. An.* 701b17–23 (cf. 702a5 ff.); *Phys.* 247a8 ff.; *Mem.* 452a1 ff.

[57] Apart, of course, from not being "empiricist" at all, if we understand empiricism in its classical usage as the thesis that *all* knowledge derives from sense perception and not, as "rationalism" in its classical usage has it, from innate ideas. To speak (as, e.g., Gasser-Wingate does) of Aristotle's empiricism, while at the same time maintaining that our perceptual knowledge is "deficient relative to our epistemic ideals" for Aristotle (Gasser-Wingate 2021: 156), is to use the term, as he himself admits, in a somewhat attenuated sense. And yet one would expect the "-ism" to indicate precisely the sufficiency of perceptual knowledge.

[58] There is still one important question. The fact that *phantasmata* act as causal substitutes for perceptible objects does not seem to warrant the claim that human thinking *never* takes place without *phantasma*. To deal with this issue properly would require a full account of Aristotle's views about the subconscious workings of the cognitive soul. But it may well be that Aristotle thinks that human thought requires highly processed complex mental (especially linguistic) representations that the senses as such could not possibly deliver. So even if he describes the simultaneous occurrence of the perception of something with the thinking of it, as he sometimes does (*Posterior Analytics* I 1, 71a17–24; II 2, 90a24–30), the corresponding thought for him may nonetheless involve *phantasmata* too.

phantasia from truth-apt propositional thought: that is, assertion and denial.[59] *Phantasia* here, I take it, stands generally for having *phantasmata* in the cognitive soul of a thinking agent. Aristotle says that the difference between *phantasmata* and affirmation and denial (propositional truth-apt thinking) is that what is true or false in this propositional way is an *interweaving* of thoughts (*noêmata*). These thoughts are the basic and uncompounded elements of truth-apt propositions. Now this analysis of affirmation and denial may give rise to the hypothesis that the simple *phantasmata* that correspond to simple and uncompounded thoughts just *are* these simple and uncompounded thoughts. So, on that basis, one may come to think that *phantasmata* may be just the same as the basic uncompounded thoughts and that therefore affirmation and denial are nothing but an interweaving of *phantasmata*.[60] Aristotle's reaction is to say that *phantasmata* are necessary but not sufficient for basic thoughts, because the basic thoughts that figure as constituents of propositions are not *phantasmata*, even if one considers them in isolation from the propositions of which they are components.[61] Why not? Here is what I take to be the most probable answer. *Phantasmata* taken as such are just what they are: perceptual stimuli stored in the body with causal powers to affect the perceptual capacity. As such, they have no intentional or otherwise conscious dimension. *Phantasmata* as such and on their own do not signify or represent anything, not even themselves. If they represent or causally substitute external perceptible objects, then they do so because *phantasmata* are part of *intentional contexts*. But such intentional contexts are never constituted by *phantasmata* alone. They require acts of the cognitive soul when it is engaged in thinking, or remembering, or in other intentional acts. Whether *phantasmata* signify and represent, and hence also whether they can be true or false, therefore, depends on the cognitive soul and the *use* it makes of them.[62] This is the difference between basic thoughts and *phantasmata*. Basic thoughts signify because they are *per definitionem* parts of intentional contexts (recall, Aristotle is a presentist about thinking; there are no stored *noêmata* in the soul); *phantasmata*, by contrast, can only have meaning in the derivative sense of *being made use of* as representational devices in intentional contexts which are governed by the activity of the cognitive soul. Thoughts, even the simple ones, then, are a class on their own and not to be identified with the material of mental representations (*phantasmata*).

[59] On propositional thought, see Chapter 3 (Section 3).

[60] Wedin discusses the hypothesis that one may see a form–matter relation between *phantasmata* and thoughts (Wedin 1988: 123). Shields asks whether the *prôta noêmata* are the thoughts that are "closest to sense perception" (Shields 2016: 347), which seems similar to the view that they are "lower universals," advocated by Torstrik (1862: 213–214), whereas Trendelenburg opted for the opposite view according to which they are the most fundamental thoughts (Trendelenburg 1877: 439). A full discussion of earlier interpretations can be found in Hicks' commentary (Hicks 1907: 547–548).

[61] I read, with most editors, *t'alla* and not *tauta* in *An.* III 8, 432a13. I do not see a major problem in taking "the other thoughts" as the basic uncompounded constituents of truth-apt propositions considered in isolation from the meaning of the proposition.

[62] Cf. *An.* III 2, 427a12–13.

The fact that *An.* III 3, 428b17–18, says that *phantasia* can be true or false does not conflict with this interpretation. For the way in which *phantasmata* are true or false is not the same as the way in which mental acts (thoughts) can be true or false. *Phantasmata* are true or false in the way in which representational objects can be true or false: that is, by bringing about an impression (*phantasia*) which in turn can be true or false (*Metaph.* IV 1025a4–6, 1024b21–26), if it occurs in an appropriate intentional context. So, if *phantasia* is true or false, then this is so only derivatively and in virtue of its capacity of causing, and being part of, mental acts.

Why does Aristotle discuss this issue here? It could be that the previous argument for the necessity of *phantasmata* for human thinking prompts him to bring out the difference between thinking and *phantasia* in order to emphasize the indispensable and irreducible role of the thinking soul. It may also be to forestall theories of cognition that try to reduce mental acts to the representational vehicles that enable their occurrence.[63] Against this, Aristotle insists on the *sui generis* character of thought proper. Aristotle is a realist about intellectual cognition: there are intelligible features of things and there are thoughts; both are real and both are nonphysical, even if their presence in nature involves physical enabling conditions.

4. Conclusion

An. III 8 tersely summarizes the basic points of the treatment of the cognitive soul from *An.* II 5 onward without mentioning the discussion of *nous per se*. This is in line with the idea that Aristotle discusses *nous per se* only insofar as, and to the extent to which, it is necessary and conducive to his project of defining *nous* as embedded in the (human) *cognitive soul*. The summary offered in Part I, at any rate, concentrates on the results achieved in the earlier chapters only insofar as the nature of the cognitive soul is concerned, reminding the reader only of the most fundamental results of the earlier discussions of the two cognitive parts of the soul in *De anima*. They are two: the perceptual capacity is identical with the forms of the objects of perception in potentiality, and the intellectual capacity is potentially identical with the intelligible objects it can cognize. From this *An.* III 8 draws the further and general conclusion that the cognitive soul *is* all things, on the grounds that things are either perceptible or intelligible, albeit in potentiality and in form only. From this the chapter draws the additional conclusions that the cognitive soul could not learn or come to know anything without having previously perceived, and that it could not engage in thought without an antecedent and simultaneously ongoing perceptual mental representation. In the last section of the chapter, Aristotle distinguishes his own view about the workings of the cognitive thinking soul from the reductive view

[63] See Torstrik 1862: 213–214.

that thoughts are just certain arrangements of mental representations. If applied to Aristotle himself, the famous Aristotelian dictum "*nihil est in intellectu quod not prius fuerit in sensu*" therefore has to be taken with a grain of salt. It pertains only to what *objects* thinking is concerned with, what it is about, and not to the features of thinking *qua* thinking: namely, (mainly) universality, objectivity, and necessity. And these features of thinking *qua* thinking, as has been argued in Chapter 2, directly depend on the presence of active thinking, which is neither a perceptible object nor a mental representation but an essence of type (1).[64]

The following general picture of Aristotle's theory of cognition results. Aristotle falls squarely within the camp of LKL theories. But his version of the LKL theory is complex and qualified. It is *qualified* because he combines the LKL theory with an assimilation thesis according to which cognition requires an assimilation of the cognitive agent who, previous to that assimilation, is other than (or different from) the cognitive object. The result of the assimilation (either in the form of a process as in perception, or instantaneous as in thinking) is the identity or likeness of the subject and the object of cognition, and this identity is an important element of the cognition (the other one is intentionality).[65] It is *complex* because Aristotle's application of the LKL theory to the two basic cognitive capacities yields different results for each of them. While the capacity for perception is potentially the qualities that the cognitive agent receives from the external objects of perception and hence itself is a *qualitative* potentiality, the capacity for thinking is not qualitative (explicitly stated in *An.* III 4, 429a25); it is "none of the beings at all," so as to be capable of receiving the essences of all things. The thinking capacity, therefore, should be able to become essences of all categories (including qualities, but of course only as intelligibles). This is not, or not entirely, the case with perception. Perception involves the production of an actual quality in the cognitive agent as a result of the affection by a perceptual object via a perceptual stimulus, which is qualitative as well. Moreover, that quality will be formally, but not numerically, identical with the perceptual quality of the perceptual object. Rather, it is the effect and outcome of the affection by the perceptual quality of the object. We may say, then, that on Aristotle's theory of perception, the quality of the external object is *reproduced* in the cognitive agent who is affected by it, albeit with the proviso that the reproduction is brought about by the causal agency of the external object itself. This is different in the case of thinking. The thinking of essences in a cognitive agent is *numerically identical* with the immaterial essences themselves.

This difference in the application of the LKL theory to the cognitive capacities has consequences for the ways in which we can speak of realism in Aristotle.[66] In the case of thinking, Aristotle is as direct a realist as one can be. In the thinking

[64] On these features of thinking *qua* thinking, see Chapter 2 (Section 6).
[65] For more on intentionality, see Chapter 1 (Section 3) and Corcilius 2022.
[66] On perceptual realism in Aristotle, see Broadie 1993, Broakes 1999, and Esfeld 2000.

of essences, which is the case Aristotle focuses on in *An.* III 4–5, the object of thinking is literally and unrestrictedly present in the cognitive agent.[67] This is not, or not entirely, the case with perception. First, the perceptual object is present in the perceiver only qualitatively. Second, it is not numerically *identical* to the external quality but only formally identical, even if the corresponding affection with the perceptual stimulus is the direct causal effect of the external object of perception. So, it is still true also in perception that the external object of perception partly constitutes the act of perceiving it, yet it does so in a mediated way, which is consequently not as direct as the case of the thinking of essences. But even in thinking we must understand the limitations of Aristotle's identity claim. The account of thinking in *An.* III 4–5 is an account of the thinking of essences only. These are simple thoughts without combination (even if their mental representation, definitions, and so on may involve all sorts of combinations). Such essences are very special items of thinking. The thinking of them can be classified neither as analytic nor as synthetic,[68] and while Aristotle holds that many, if not most, of us are not familiar with it, he still thinks that the capacity for thinking of essences is fundamental for the other kinds of human thinking. Propositional thinking (see Chapter 3), practical deliberation, and the like (see Chapter 4), depend on our capacity to engage in this kind of thinking.

On the interpretation advanced here, it is a core feature of Aristotle's theory of intellectual cognition that it is based on what I referred to above as the bifurcated ontology. The bifurcated ontology distinguishes between things that involve matter (and, hence, are objects of perception), on the one hand, and immaterial objects of thinking, on the other, and it distinguishes between them in such a way that this distinction is exhaustive. I have argued that Aristotle's account of human thinking is based on the idea that there can be a qualified matterlessness in a cognitive agent with regard to a given domain of beings. This qualified matterlessness is the outcome of suitably prepared mental representations of the features that hold of that domain insofar as it is such. Given the bifurcated ontology, this qualified matterlessness, due to its absence of matter, will be the immediate potentiality for the presence of the corresponding essence; however, it will be so *only to the extent to which it is free from matter* (*An.* III 4, 429b21–22). Now, given the presence of active thinking, which is an essence of type (1), the fact that the immediate potentiality for the presence of the essence in the cognitive agent is not devoid of matter should result in some sort of screening that issues in the less than full presence of type (1) thinking in the cognitive agent. This less than full presence, in combination with the domain-specific matterlessness, I have argued, can explain the actual presence of the essence of the domain in the cognitive agent. Hence, when the required qualified matterlessness in a given domain of things is brought

[67] See, e.g., *An.* III 5, 430a19–21 and *An.* III 7, 431a1–3, and *Metaph.* XII 8, 1074b38–1075a5.

[68] See Oehler 1962: 247.

about by a suitably prepared thinking agent, both the immediate potentiality of the object of thinking and the immediate potentiality of the subject of thinking are present in her. Since both potentialities are passive, it takes the presence of active thinking "like a state" to make them actual so that the act of thinking the relevant essence comes about. On the basis of his bifurcated ontology and his other theoretical commitments—most notably his commitment to the existence of immaterial essences of things, and especially of entirely transcendent essences of type (1)—it seems that Aristotle *succeeds* with this account of thinking. He is able to offer an account of human thinking capable of *explaining* some of the most distinctive features of human thinking: namely, its objectivity, universality, and necessity. In this way, Aristotle is able to make good on his promise to render an account of the capacity of thinking as a cognitive capacity "concerned with the truth" (*An.* I 2, 404a31), and (almost) without cognitive restriction. The only restriction human thinking faces in Aristotle's account springs from the fact that he seems to conceive of human thinking as *to some residual extent* representational. All human thinking, as he says many times, involves *phantasmata*. This prevents human thinking from thinking essences of type (1), the self-thinking and separate substances, as they are in themselves. Humans are prevented from thinking these substances *per se*, since that would require the absence of *phantasmata*, which however is the very vehicle that enables human thinking of hylomorphic essences to occur in the first place. But it is possible for humans to think them *per aliud*: namely, as principles and causes for other things (more on this in Chapter 6, Section 5).

Hence, Aristotle can still claim that in a way the human capacity for thinking can think all beings. It also seems that with his account of human thinking Aristotle meets the criteria he himself formulated in the course of his critique of the predecessors' theories of the soul (see Chapter 1). His account is *commensurately universal* as it applies to all human beings; it can account for the *cognition of both the material and the formal features* of things (jointly with perception); and it can explain the *cognition of items in all categories*. Perception is qualitative, as we have seen, but the capacity for thinking can cognize items in all categories, even if only one at each time, and even then, as we have seen as well, these thoughts will have a qualitative aspect to them insofar as they involve *phantasmata*. So, all in all, and by his own methodological standards and ontological commitments, Aristotle's theory of intellectual cognition is a success.

6
Nous and nature

1. Introduction

At the outset of *De anima* Aristotle promised that knowledge of the soul would "contribute in the greatest extent to truth as a whole, and especially [truth concerning] nature (*phusis*); for the soul is like the principle of living things."[1] In the introduction to this volume (Chapter 1) we have seen in what sense the soul is "the principle of living things" and what this claim implies for both the structure and the status of *De anima* in the context of Aristotle's science of living things. In Chapters 2–5 we have followed step by step how Aristotle's account of *nous*, as one of the three canonic parts of the soul, is developed in *An.* III 4–8. The present chapter is intended to answer the following question: *in what way exactly has Aristotle's account contributed to truth concerning nature?*

This question is complicated due to a peculiarity of *nous* brought up—implicitly—right after Aristotle's promissory note about truth and nature: among the attributes of the soul we are about to explore, "some appear to be affections exclusive to the soul, while others belong by means of the soul also to the living thing."[2] The appearance of exclusivity (much emphasized by Plato) turns out to be, by Aristotle's lights, a mere appearance in all cases but one: namely, thinking (*noein*) in the technical sense of grasping essences with respect to which the thinking part of the soul is to be defined in *An.* III 4–5. Unlike all other life-activities, thinking *is*—in a sense that is yet to be properly understood—an affection exclusive to the thinking part—that is, *nous*—of the soul. This idea turns out to be directly connected to Aristotle's repeated claim that unlike other capacities of the soul, *nous* is *not* a part of nature in the sense defined in the *Physics*.[3] If this is true, then knowledge of *nous* cannot contribute to truth concerning nature in any

I wish to thank Klaus Corcilius, Michel Crubellier, and Andrea Falcon for stimulative discussions and valuable feedback on earlier versions of this chapter. The material was presented at Humboldt University in Berlin and Charles University in Prague: many thanks to audiences for helpful comments, especially to Jonathan Beere and Jaroslav Rytíř. The chapter is dedicated to the memory of Sarah Broadie.

[1] *An.* I 1, 402a4–7.

[2] *An.* I 1, 402a9–10.

[3] Nature is famously defined in *Phys.* II 1 as each thing's proper "principle of motion and rest" (192b13–14, 20–23; cf. *Metaph.* V 4, 1014b18–20, 1015a13–19). It seems to be this concrete notion of nature that Aristotle has in mind at *An.* I 1, 402a5. That needs to be emphasized because Aristotle also uses the notion of nature in a more abstract way as basically synonymous with essence (this seems to be the case right at 402a7–8). For an instructive analysis of how important this difference between the concrete and the abstract uses of nature can be, see Rapp 2021 on Aristotle's alleged political naturalism.

Aristotle on the Essence of Human Thought. Klaus Corcilius, Andrea Falcon, and Robert Roreitner, Oxford University Press.
 DOI: 10.1093/9780198921820.003.0006

straightforward way, as presumably knowledge of other capacities of the soul does. Knowledge of *nous* is not a part of the knowledge of nature.

This complication is rarely taken seriously by interpreters. And that seems at least partly due to the fact that those who did take the complication seriously usually ended up ascribing views to Aristotle that seem hardly compatible with his other commitments: above all, the view that human *nous* (if not the human soul as a whole) is something supernatural which can exist separately from the human body, and which thus falls under the scope of Aristotle's theology rather than natural philosophy. The aim of this chapter is to show why both the divinization and the naturalization of human *nous*—which have seemed to be the only two available options—in fact seriously distort Aristotle's view.

2. Exclusive affections and the explanatory project of *De anima*

In Chapter 1, we have seen that in *An.* I 3–4 Aristotle charges his predecessors with the fallacy of isomorphism of *cause* and *effect*: in the case of self-motion, typically, the idea is that the soul, as what ultimately moves the animal body, must itself be in motion. Aristotle extends this charge *mutatis mutandis* to cognition, insofar as it can be conceived as a kind of motion (*kinêsis*): it is wrong to infer, for example, that since (P1) perception is a kind of motion and (P2) soul is what makes animals perceptive, (C) soul itself must be the subject of this motion.[4] While perception is the primary focus of this complaint, Aristotle thinks it can be further extended, for example, to discursive thinking (*dianoeisthai*).[5] But, significantly, Aristotle never extends this kind of objection to thinking (*noein*) proper. The reason is surely not that, by Aristotle's lights, his predecessors were more cautious when talking about thinking. On the contrary, his view is that they mostly failed to properly distinguish it from perception.[6] And even Plato, who distinguishes sharply between sensation and thinking, conceives of the latter in the *Timaeus* in terms of a circular motion.[7] When criticizing this conception,[8] Aristotle, significantly, does not attack the idea (C*) that thinking belongs to the soul or *nous* itself. Rather, he attacks the assumption (P1*) that thinking can be described as a motion; for "thinking resembles being at rest and coming to a stop rather than motion."[9] Later on, right after criticizing the fallacy of isomorphism of *cause* and *effect* in the case of perception and discursive thinking,[10] Aristotle makes the following observation that may help explain why the objection *cannot* be extended to thinking:

4 *An.* I 4, 408b12–18.
5 See *An.* I 4, 408b5–12.
6 See, e.g., *An.* III 3, 427a17–b27; cf. *Metaph.* IV 5, 1009b11–39.
7 See *An.* I 3, 406b25–407a2.
8 *An.* I 3, 407a2–b12.
9 *An.* I 3, 407a32–33.
10 *An.* I 4, 408a34–b18.

> Thinking (*noein*) and theorizing (*theôrein*) fade away when something else inside is corrupted: it is, however, itself impassive. Discursive thinking (*dianoeisthai*), loving, and hating are not affections of it, but of that which has it insofar as it has it.[11]

Aristotle, effectively, returns here to the issue of the so-called affections of the soul from *An.* I 1: "are all of them common to that which has [the soul], or is any of them exclusive to the soul itself?"[12] The only serious candidate for an affection exclusive to the soul was thinking (*noein*).[13] The quoted passage confirms that something like this option is still in play after *An.* I 1: while discursive thinking is described as something belonging to *that which has* thinking or *that which has nous*[14] and not to *nous* itself, thinking is an activity that, so to speak, stands on its own or constitutes an affection exclusive to *nous*.

Prima facie, the idea of thinking as an affection exclusive to the soul or its *nous* may seem to be at odds with the very nature of Aristotle's inquiry into the soul.[15] As a part of the soul, *nous* should be the ultimate *explanans* for the phenomena of our intellectual life, such as solving a math problem or understanding a historical fact. It should not be itself *doing* something, such as thinking, because that would seem to only make a further *explanandum* from it.

This idea informs not only Aristotle's critical discussion of predecessors in *An.* I, but also his positive account. At the end of his preliminary outline of soul in *An.* II 1, Aristotle concludes, in line with his general hylomorphism, that the soul can by no means be separable in existence from the body—it is no more separable from it than a shape is from the wax on which it is impressed.[16] The soul, or rather the capacities that are constitutive of the soul (its parts), are inseparable from the body because their "actuality is the actuality of the [bodily] parts themselves."[17] For example, seeing, for which the perceptive soul is responsible, *is* the actualization of eyes (and other perceptive bodily parts) themselves, so that it makes *no sense* at all to talk about the perceptive soul (the ultimate *explanans* of seeing) as existing apart from the body or "doing" something on its own.

This finding is, however, qualified at the end of *An.* II 1—in a way that would hardly be intelligible were we to forget the issue about thought being an exclusive

[11] *An.* I 4, 408b24–27.

[12] *An.* I 1, 403a3–4.

[13] See *An.* I 1, 403a7–11. Aristotle speaks of thinking here as an affection "exclusive to the soul" (rather than to *nous*), and he takes it to imply that the soul (rather than *nous*) can be separated (*An.* I 1, 403a10–11). What he most probably means, however, is that thinking is a candidate for an affection exclusive to the soul *or a part of it*—namely, the so-called *nous* of the soul—and that if this were so, then *something of the soul*—namely, its *nous*—can be separated. More on the notion of separation below in Section 5.

[14] Cf. *An.* I 4, 408b29–30.

[15] As described in Chapter 1.

[16] See *An.* II 1, 412b6–9 and 413a4–5.

[17] *An.* II 1, 413a5–6.

affection. The conclusion reached about inseparability only applies to *some* parts of the soul;[18] in the case of other parts, "nothing prevents" their being separable from the body, "because they are *not* actualizations of a body."[19] Although Aristotle speaks in the plural here, he clearly has just *nous* and thinking in mind. Indirect confirmation that the option mentioned here in fact expresses Aristotle's considered view comes from the account of human embryology offered in *Gener. An.* II 3, where we are told, among other things, that *nous* alone "comes from without," and that this is so "because the bodily activity takes no part in its activity": that is, in thinking which thus turns out to be an affection exclusive to *nous*.[20]

We will see that this idea continues to inform Aristotle's reflections about *nous* in the subsequent chapters down to *An.* III 4–5. But before further following this idea and attempting to better understand its significance and consequences, it is worth stepping back and asking whether it can fit at all within the framework of Aristotle's inquiry into soul.[21] The first thing to notice in this respect is that the idea of thinking as an affection exclusive to *nous* does not necessarily imply that the present inquiry will have nothing to say about it.

The famous metaphor of the sailor and the ship at the end of *An.* II 1 may be intended exactly at assuring the reader that this need not to be the case.[22] The perceptive and the nutritive parts of the soul will be defined as the ultimate *explanantia*, respectively, for the fact that animals can orient themselves in their surroundings by discerning objects around them and for the fact that all living beings can sustain themselves, grow, reproduce, and preserve their bodily form while shrinking. It would be a serious categorical mistake (amounting to a kind of reification) if we wanted to ascribe these activities—or, indeed, any other activity—to these parts of the soul themselves as affections exclusive to them. Similarly, *nous* as the thinking part of the soul is the ultimate *explanans* for the fact that human beings play board games, reflect about their past, and the like, and it would be equally wrong to ascribe any of these activities to *nous* itself. *But* Aristotle does not think it is wrong to ask whether *nous* as the ultimate *explanans* of the wide range of human intellectual activities is—or, indeed, must be—itself something active, involved in, or perhaps identical to, an activity which is *not* an activity of the body, as for example seeing or growing is.[23] The relevant activity would be the grasping of essences as analyzed in *An.* III 4–5.

[18] *An.* II 1, 413a4–5.

[19] *An.* II 1, 413a6–7. Besides the quoted passage from *An.* I 4 (408b18–30), compare also Aristotle's assertion in *An.* I 5 to the effect that not all parts of the soul can be conceived as "holding together" some bodily parts: "This seems impossible, for what [bodily] part and how *nous* would hold together is difficult even to imagine" (411b17–19).

[20] *Gener. An.* II 3, 736b28–29, cf. 737a9–11. For a detailed analysis of this claim, I refer the reader to Roreitner 2024; the meaning of "coming from without" is briefly spelled out below in footnote 94.

[21] For which, see Chapter 1.

[22] *An.* II 1, 413a8–9 (cf. *An.* I 3, 406a4–12).

[23] Precisely in this respect *nous* would resemble the sailor who also causes the ship to sail by exercising an activity of his own which is *not* an activity of the ship.

The main point now is that Aristotle intentionally leaves the option open that his inquiry into soul may arrive at such a principle which is active in itself or identical to activity that is not an activity of the body. The primary motivation for this move is not a moral concern (e.g., the aim to defend some version of personal immortality, as the move was often interpreted). Rather, it is Aristotle's conviction that only such a principle, active in itself, can play the role of the ultimate *explanans* of the respective phenomena.[24] What must be stressed is that this claim is very different from, and does not commit Aristotle to, a view of *nous* as "the mind" in the sense of the subject of our intellectual life. Thinking, as the activity exclusive to *nous*, is none of the phenomena that we normally *experience*; rather, it falls on the side of the ultimate *explanans* that must be posited if we are ever to *understand* these phenomena.[25]

If this is true, then the inquiry into *nous* in *An.* III 4–8 can be seen as an integral part of Aristotle's endeavor to define the ultimate *explanantia* of life—even if thinking turns out to be an affection exclusive to *nous*. This anomaly notwithstanding, the inquiry into soul would be seriously incomplete if it left *nous* aside. But that does not mean there is a perfect fit between the account of *nous* and the rest of *De anima*. Aristotle tends to conceive the inquiry into soul as a part of his *natural* philosophy; the mentioned anomaly, however, is one of the reasons why he is inclined, nevertheless, to think that natural philosophy cannot on its own comprehend *nous*. This produces a tension at the heart of *De anima* and it is not obvious whether Aristotle intended to resolve this tension, or indeed how it can be done.

This will be the leading question of the following two sections. In Section 3, I explore how Aristotle's inquiry into *nous*, as an integral part of *De anima*, relates to his program of natural philosophy. In Section 4, I attempt to spell out in a nutshell what kind of contribution the Aristotelian inquiry into nature can make toward explaining the phenomena of human intellectual life for which *nous* is the ultimate *explanans*. In Section 5, I tackle what may have been historically the most controversial question, concerning the sense in which human *nous* is, and the sense in which it isn't, separable from the other parts of the soul and from the body. The claim will be that the idea of *nous* not being a part of nature needs to be sharply distinguished from the view, informing most commentaries in late antiquity and the Middle Ages, that human *nous*, as defined in *De anima*, can survive bodily death and exist separately from the human body.

[24] See *An.* III 4, 429a18–27, for Aristotle's argument that *nous* can have no bodily organ.

[25] The point is that even when we are blessed enough to arrive at a genuine act of grasping some essence, what we experience will always be a way more complex phenomenon with the act of grasping an essence as its primary, defining constituent.

3. The inquiry into *nous* and Aristotle's natural philosophy

In *An.* I 1 Aristotle famously argues that because the *explananda* under consideration are "enmattered formulae" (*logoi enuloi*),[26] "it belongs to the natural philosopher (*phusikos*) to study the soul . . ."[27] This is so because natural philosophers in Aristotle's account are those who neither limit their attention—in a reductive manner—to the material side of phenomena, nor focus on forms abstracted from matter as the mathematician (or Platonist dialectician) does; rather, they understand forms as the ultimate *explanantia* of phenomena that are essentially enmattered.[28] And most phenomena of life are such (although that doesn't need to be immediately obvious): anger, for instance, is to be understood as a motion of such and such a body caused by this for the sake of that.[29] Soul can then be approached as the formal *nature* of living beings: that is, the "principle and cause" of their typical ways of "being moved and being at rest," including self-motion, perception (i.e., a way of being moved by perceptible objects), and growth.

One may think that this notion of nature is broad enough to accommodate *all* the phenomena of living things. After all, as we have seen, even thinking is said to "resemble being at rest and coming to a stop."[30] But Aristotle's caution here is significant: he only says that thinking *resembles* being at rest and coming to a stop *more than* it resembles motion, and although he is not always so cautious, it seems that in his considered view being at rest or coming to a stop constitute at most a necessary condition for thinking, as we will see.[31] Thinking itself is neither a motion nor a being at rest, and so *nous* is not a nature.[32] Thinking as such is not an enmattered formula, and so it is not the task of the natural philosopher to study it. This seems to be why Aristotle qualifies the above-mentioned inference: "it belongs to the natural philosopher to study the soul—either the whole of it *or the soul of this kind*."[33] The same limitation is imposed more openly in *Metaph.* VI 1: "it belongs to the natural philosopher to study the soul *to some extent*: namely, [to study] all [the parts of] the soul that are not without matter."[34]

[26] *An.* I 1, 403a25.

[27] *An.* I 1, 403a27–28.

[28] See also *Phys.* II 2 (with Lennox 2008).

[29] *An.* I 1, 403a25–27. This passage seems to contain a schema of what the full explanation of a phenomenon like anger would have to provide. Aristotle's *De anima* clearly does not aim at filling this schema, on its own, for any phenomenon.

[30] *An.* I 3 407a32–33.

[31] See, e.g., *Phys.* VII 3, 247b11–12, *Int.* 3, 16b21–22, and *Posterior Analytics* II 19, 100a5–7, 12–16; cf. *Phaed.* 96b6–8.

[32] In contrast to *An.* II 5–III 3 and, obviously, *An.* III 9–11, the *kinetic* language is entirely absent from *An.* III 4–8 (except for passages in *An.* III 7 where Aristotle is concerned with perception and action). If thinking is indeed an affection exclusive to *nous*, and *nous*, as a part of the soul, cannot be itself the subject of motion or being at rest (i.e., the privation of motion) as argued in *An.* I 3–4, then clearly thinking can be neither motion nor being at rest.

[33] *An.* I 1, 403a27–28.

[34] *Metaph.* VI 1, 1026a5–6.

The opening sentence of *An.* III 5 (430a10–13) has sometimes been read as if Aristotle was here subordinating the entire soul, including *nous*, to nature.[35] But when correctly understood, the passage only confirms what has just been said. Far from situating soul together with *nous* within "the whole nature," nature here only represents one subdomain of a larger domain that also includes human arts and artifacts.[36] It is not entirely clear how large this domain is (perhaps it is the domain of all things that *come to be*, or all things that undergo *transition* from potentiality to actuality),[37] but it surely includes both natural and non-natural items. Since human soul, including *nous*, falls into this larger domain (apparently because human thoughts, unlike divine thinking, come to be), there must be two causal factors in it:

> Since (*epei*), just as (*hôsper*) in all nature, there is something which is matter for each kind of object (this is what is potentially all these things) and something else which is the cause and producer because it makes them all, as art stands in relation to its materials, it is necessary that there be these different [factors] in the soul as well.[38]

Rather than subordinating *nous* to nature, Aristotle signals that the relevant domain under which human *nous* falls is larger than nature.[39]

It is significant in this context that, in his introductions to two large projects that fall within his natural philosophy—namely, the so-called *Parva naturalia*[40] (in *Sens.* 1) and the inquiry into the parts of animals (in *Part. An.* I 1)—Aristotle reminds the reader that, for methodological reasons, *nous* as such lies beyond the reach of the present investigation.[41]

[35] See references in footnote 38 below.

[36] For a classical contrast between natural beings and artifacts, see *Phys.* II 1.

[37] For nature as the paradigmatic (but not exclusive) domain of coming to be, see *Phys.* II 1, 193b12–17.

[38] *An.* III 5, 430a10–14. Ross 1961 (followed, e.g., by Shields 2016) excises the word *hôsper*, making it sound as if the whole soul, including *nous*, was classed here under "the whole nature" (see already Alexander, *An.* 88.17–23, and Themistius, *In An.* 98.12–20). Caston 1999: 205–207 (followed by Polansky 2007 and Segev 2017: 189; cf. Caston 1996b: 189–190) retains *hôsper* (on the cost of tacitly suppressing *epei* in his translation) and confronts us with a dilemma: either Aristotle is treating *nous* (at least the human, "material" *nous*) as a case of nature (the option Caston seems to prefer), or his inference appears to be based on a mere analogy (and his talk of "necessity" doesn't seem to be justified).

[39] So *An.* III 5 is very far from being "stubbornly naturalistic" (*pace* Wedin 1988: 161, 194). Notice that the proposed interpretation, unlike those mentioned in the previous footnote, makes good sense of the transmitted text as it stands: both *epei* and *hôsper* have important roles here (without implying that "Aristotle lost control of his syntax," as Menn 2020: 125n33 complains), and the *anankê* of Aristotle's inference is a genuine inferential necessity.

[40] Aristotle also seems to have *De motu animalium* in mind.

[41] It is worth stressing that there is no clear-cut line in Aristotle's thought between natural philosophy and natural science as we might tend to draw it from a modern perspective. The investigation which starts from a treatment of the principles of nature and motion in Aristotle's *Physics* and continues with inquiries into motions of the heavenly bodies (*De caelo*), the elements of earthly compounds and their coming to be and perishing (*De generatione et corruptione*), and the meteorological phenomena (*Meteorologica*), passes continuously into an investigation of animals (*Historia animalium*, *De partibus*

In the opening chapter of *Part. An.* I, Aristotle makes a claim very similar to the one made in *An.* I 1 and *Metaph.* VI 1: "It will belong to the natural philosopher to treat the soul and to have knowledge about it."[42] This is directly relevant in the context of *Part. An.* I 1 because Aristotle wants to insist against Democritus and other reductionists that every animal part is what it is only on account of the soul.[43] But, again, Aristotle makes it clear that this holds for the soul only under a certain description: namely, as the *nature* of the living being in the sense of its essence—that is, the primary moving and final cause.[44] "Such," Aristotle adds, "is *either* the whole soul of the animal *or* a part of it."[45] This disjunction, familiar from *An.* I 1 and *Metaph.* VI 1, is now said to contain a puzzle:

> Having considered what we were just saying, one might raise a difficulty as to whether natural philosophy ought to treat the soul as a whole, or [just] some [part of it].[46]

Strictly speaking, Aristotle does not develop a full puzzle here, for he pays no attention to what might seem problematic about the second disjunct (I return to that question below). His objection against the first disjunct, in any case, is known as his Correlatives Argument:[47]

> For if [natural philosophy is to treat] the soul as a whole, there will remain no philosophy beyond the scientific knowledge of nature. The reason is that *nous* is concerned with objects of thought; and so it would follow that natural philosophy is knowledge of everything. [This would be so] because it belongs to one and the same [discipline] to study *nous* and the object of thought, since they are correlative and the study of correlatives is always one and the same, as is also the case with perception and perceptible objects.[48]

The methodological principle behind this argument is the one outlined in *An.* II 4: as a capacity of the soul, *nous* can only be defined on the basis of its corresponding manifestation—namely, the activity of thinking which is prior to it in account; however, since this activity is object-related, its definition presupposes

animalium) and their generation (*De generatione animalium*). For an outline of this project (also including an investigation of plants), see *Mete.* I 1, 338a20–339a10. The thoroughly *philosophical* nature of this project as a whole is emphasized in Falcon and Lefebvre 2017. We refer, accordingly, to this whole project as Aristotle's natural philosophy.

42 *Part. An.* I 1, 641a21–22.
43 *Part. An.* I 1, 641a17–21.
44 *Part. An.* I 1, 641a22–27.
45 *Part. An.* I 1, 641a28.
46 *Part. An.* I 1, 641a32–34.
47 This conventional label goes back to Broadie 1996: 169.
48 *Part. An.* I 1, 641a34–b4.

an understanding of the corresponding objects.[49] When we reflect on this principle and the way it is invoked in the Correlatives Argument, this will bring us to a more satisfying understanding of this argument than the one adopted by most interpreters.

Most often Aristotle's reason for excluding *nous* from the reach of natural philosophy in the Correlatives Argument is understood along the following lines: if natural philosophy were to treat *nous*, then the scientific knowledge of nature would "swallow up" all other disciplines like mathematics, ethics, and rhetoric.[50] Interpreted in this way, the argument has often been found dubious by Aristotle's own standards: it was criticized for confusing "the mathematical study of [mathematical] objects" and "a philosophical study of mathematical reason,"[51] and for ignoring Aristotle's insight that the same object can be considered both "*qua* enmattered" (by natural philosophy) and "*qua* separable from matter" (by mathematics).[52] But, in fact, none of this is implied by Aristotle's claim that "it belongs to one and the same [discipline] to study *nous* and the object of thought."

If the Correlatives Argument is, in line with *An.* II 4, primarily concerned with the question of how to *define nous*, as suggested above, then this is the context in which we should understand what Aristotle means by the "study of the object of thought (*to noêton*)."[53] What is needed for the definition of *nous*, as we can see in *An.* III 4, are not theorems of individual sciences or disciplines, such as mathematics; just as for the definition of the perceptive capacity one does not need theorems of harmonics (not to mention, e.g., biology as a different kind of study of perceptible objects). Rather, for the purposes of defining *nous*, one needs to have a general grasp of what it is to be an object of thought.[54] And such a grasp, at least by Aristotle's lights, essentially involves an understanding that there are three irreducible classes of objects of thought and that the natural objects represent just one of them.[55] So, if someone is to define *nous*, she must not stick to natural objects as

[49] See Chapter 1 (Section 5).

[50] See Broadie 1996: 168–171. See also Charlton 1987: 411; Caston 1996b: 182; Lennox 1999: 3, 14 (cf. Lennox 2001: 142–143); Frey 2018: 165; cf. Le Blond 1997^2: 89–90n58.

[51] See Lennox 1999: 3 and 14.

[52] See Frey 2018: 165. Compare also Caston's remark that "the intellect is something of a fifth wheel" in the argument (Caston 1996b: 182). The argument had already been severely criticized by its first Latin commentator, Pietro Pomponazzi: see Perfetti 1998.

[53] Charlton describes the Correlatives Argument as "defective" because, he says, the objects of thought are related to *nous* in a different way than the perceptible objects are related to the perceptive capacity (Charlton 1987: 411). But this objection seems to miss the generality of the methodological principle laid down in *An.* II 4.

[54] Indirect confirmation that Aristotle has this kind of general understanding of what the objects of thought are like, rather than particular theorems about them, comes from the fact (often disregarded in translations) that he speaks of studying *nous* and "the object of thought" (*to noêton*) in the singular: the study he has in mind, apparently, is concerned with what it is to be an object of thought in general rather than treating particular objects of thought one by one.

[55] For the tripartition, see *An.* III 4, 429b10–22. Kullmann 1974: 41 sees the importance of the mathematical objects and the objects of metaphysics for the argument; but he takes these to be only examples.

a natural philosopher would be obliged to do. It is necessary also to understand the thinkability of mathematical objects, and—perhaps most importantly for the Correlatives Argument—the thinkability of objects that exist separately from matter.[56]

This tripartition is something that necessarily escapes natural philosophy. So, if a natural philosopher as such were to define *nous*, this would imply—since *nous* is able to think everything[57]—that there is just one kind of object: namely, natural objects composed of matter and form. No other philosophy would be needed or indeed possible.[58] There would remain no place for a philosophy that is not an integral part of the project of acquiring scientific knowledge of nature. But, as Aristotle also emphasizes in *An.* I 1, this is not how things are.[59] Or to put it more cautiously: if somebody wanted to treat *nous* as a natural philosopher, assuming that there are no other objects than natural objects, this would mean overstepping her competences, for a natural philosopher cannot as such decide the question of whether there are other kinds of objects besides natural objects;[60] it would be, in other words, a sign of erroneous naturalism. If interpreted in this way, the Correlatives Argument is in no way dubious; on the contrary, it spells out an insight which is at the heart of Aristotle's treatment of *nous* in *De anima*.[61]

If we want to prevent the naturalistic error exposed by the Correlatives Argument, Aristotle continues, we need to acknowledge that natural philosophy cannot study and define the soul as a whole, but only the parts of the soul which constitute the nature of the living being—that is, those that play the role of a moving cause[62]—and that means *de facto* all the parts except for *nous*:

> Or is it that (*ê*)[63] not the whole soul is a principle of motion, nor every part [of it]; rather of growth the principle is that which is also present in plants, of alteration the perceptive part, and of locomotion yet something else, but not the thinking part? [It cannot be the thinking part,] because locomotion also belongs to other kinds of animals [besides humans], but discursive thinking to none. It is therefore clear that natural philosophy ought not to treat the soul as a whole,

[56] Under this interpretation, it is no surprise that at *Part. An.* I 1, 641b10–15, Aristotle explains why natural philosophy is unable to understand the "abstract" mathematical objects.

[57] Cf. *An.* III 4, 429a18.

[58] Natural philosophy would be the wisdom sought in *Metaph.* I 2 under the descriptions of a "knowledge of everything" (see *Metaph.* I 2, 982a8–10, 982a21–23).

[59] See *An.* I 1, 403b14–16. Cf. *Phys.* II 2, 194b9–15; *Metaph.* VI 1, 1026a27–30.

[60] In fact, Aristotle seems to believe (most clearly in *Phys.* VIII) that the natural philosopher is led to recognize the existence of such objects even from within her philosophical project, and thus to recognize the limits of this project.

[61] It has already been explained why this insight is *not* contradicted by the opening sentence of *An.* III 5 (*pace* Caston 1996b: 190). It should also be clear by now why the Correlatives Argument cannot be read as concerning the divine rather than human *nous* (*pace* Frede 1992: 105).

[62] See again *Part. An.* I 1, 641a27.

[63] This is Aristotle's standard way of introducing the solution to a problem.

> for not the whole soul is a nature, but [only] some part of it, be it [just] one part or more.[64]

What seemed implied in *An.* I 1 is here asserted without any ambiguity: *nous*, unlike the other parts of the soul, is not a nature; it is not as such the principle of *any* motion or rest (Aristotle duly enumerates all the three main kinds of motion), and so the inquiry into soul cannot as a whole belong to natural philosophy.[65] This does not mean just that the inquiry into *theoretical nous* does not belong to natural philosophy. Aristotle makes no such qualification and seems to have practical *nous* in mind as well: practical *nous* is the principle of human action, but not directly a cause of motions in or of the human body.[66]

As flagged above, Aristotle has not fully developed the puzzle in the quoted passages from *Part An.* I 1, for he has not explained why the second disjunct, which situates *nous* beyond the reach of a natural philosopher, might seem problematic. But that can readily be gathered from the larger context. In his polemic with the reductive materialists that prompted Aristotle's stress on the need for knowing the soul, which in turn led to our puzzle, the human hand was offered as a prominent example of an animal part.[67] But it will later turn out that in order to understand what a hand is, one must take into account the exceptional level of practical intelligence in humans;[68] and that seems to be the result of their having *nous*. Moreover, the human upright posture (which determines the overall order in which Aristotle proceeds in *Part. An.*) is even more openly explained as a way of facilitating human thinking (*noein*) that makes us god-like.[69] And there are other bodily parts whose constitution can only be understood with a teleological reference to *nous*: human lips[70] and human tongue[71] are exceptionally soft, for only as such can they allow for the unparalleled level of articulation required by human speech; and human front teeth have a special shape which serves the same function.[72] We also learn

[64] *Part. An.* I 1, 641b4–10.

[65] This conclusion is not contradicted by *EN* X 7, 1178a2–8 (*pace* Segev 2017), describing "life in accordance with *nous*" as that which is appropriate to human beings *têi phusei*. First, *physis* may mean just essence (the being of each thing: see 1178a2, cf. *An.* I 1, 402a7–8). Second, it is possible to say that life in accordance with *nous* is most natural to human beings—it is the highest realization of human nature teleologically directed to *nous* (cf. *Pol.* VII 15, 1334b15)—and still insist that *nous* as such is no part of nature.

[66] For Aristotle's claim that *nous*—including practical *nous*—is not as such the principle of motion, not even in human action, see Corcilius 2008a: 160–207, 224–235, cf. Lennox 1999: 4–5, Lennox 2009: 14–17, Lennox 2019: 103–107, and Lennox 2021: 193–198. Contrast, e.g., Charlton 1987: 411. Cf. Balme 1972: 92. See also Cooper 2020, interpreting *Mot. An.* 6–7 as ascribing to thought the role of "the fundamental causal factor" in animal locomotion. Contrast this reading with Corcilius 2020a.

[67] See *Part. An.* I 1, 640b21, 35; 641a5, 6.

[68] See *Part. An.* IV 10, 687a6–21.

[69] See *Part. An.* IV 10, 686a27–32; cf. *Part An.* II 10, 656a7–13 and *Inc. An.* 5, 706b3–16.

[70] See *Part. An.* II 16, 660b29–661a14.

[71] See *Part. An.* II 17.

[72] See *Part. An.* III 1, 661b13–15. For articulation as the characteristic feature of *dialektos* pertaining also to birds, see *Hist. An.* IV 9. For the specific kind of articulation unique to human speech (*logos*), see *Poet.* 20. For the difference between bird and human articulation, see Labarrière 1993.

that the qualities of the blood determine not only how well the animal perceives, but also its intelligence: thinner and cooler blood is more conducive to thinking (*noerôteron*) than thicker and hotter blood.[73] And similar remarks are made about the qualities of the flesh, the size of the brain, and the thinness of the skin.[74] All this suggests that if Aristotle's natural philosopher is to include the human being in her inquiry (or, indeed, make it the paradigm of it),[75] she will *have to* treat *nous* to some extent; for many key aspects of the human body and its functioning can only be properly understood as teleologically determined by *nous*.

That is why Aristotle's puzzle above is a genuine one: it seems, on the one hand, that natural philosophy must treat *nous* (for it cannot succeed without taking it into account), and, on the other hand, that it cannot treat *nous* (because that would presuppose an account of what it is to be an object of thought which escapes the purview of natural philosophy). Any attempt at solving this puzzle will have to start from distinguishing different senses of "treating *nous*."[76] Aristotle's point seems to be, roughly, that while natural philosophy needs to *know about nous* as a crucial determinant of the phenomena which it studies, it cannot *know nous as such* and provide its definition.[77] It is vital for the natural philosopher to be aware of this delicate situation, in order neither to leave a key explanatory factor out of her considerations, nor to overstep her competences with respect to it.

4. How can natural philosophy contribute to the explanation of human intellectual life?

It would be wrong to infer from what has been said that natural philosophy has nothing to contribute to the study of human intellectual life. As stressed in Chapter 1, Aristotle's inquiry into *nous* in *An.* III 4–5 is two steps removed from a study of phenomena like solving a math problem or designing a machine. The part of the soul called *nous* is defined primarily as the principle of thinking in the technical sense of grasping the essences of things, and this activity is neither a motion nor a being at rest; as a result, unlike other life-activities, thinking is not *natural* and seems to be *exclusive* to *nous*. But, as we have seen, this "thinking" (*noein*)

[73] See *Part. An.* II 2, 648a2–14; cf. *An.* II 4, 650b18–24.

[74] See *An.* II 9, 421a22–26, on a correspondence between the softness of the flesh (differing even within the human species) and the level of intelligence (cf. *Part. An.* II 16, 660a11–13); *Gener. An.* II 6, 744a26–31, where the largeness of the human brain is connected with the purity of the heat in the human heart, which is said to be manifested in the exceptional level of human intelligence; and *Gener. An.* V 2, 781b17–22 (cf. V 5, 785b8–9) for a connection between the exceptional human perceptivity to differences and the peculiar thinness of human skin.

[75] Cf. *Hist. An.* I 6, 491a14–26 or *Gener. An.* II 4, 737b25–27.

[76] See also Lennox 1999: 13–15; cf. Lennox 2019.

[77] That is why (*pace* Frey 2018: 169) one *cannot* infer that "if the study of a human's nature demands that we study the intellect, then the intellect will be included in natural science's domain."

must not be mistaken for the mental phenomena; rather, the phenomena of our intellectual lives ought to be explained as somehow grounded in it.[78]

A full Aristotelian account of these phenomena would surely involve a great deal of work that pertains directly to natural philosophy. For instance, it would involve an account of *phantasia* and memory and the specific ways they are put to use, which would all need to be duly analyzed as motions of certain bodily parts with their proper moving and final causes. Moreover, a full explanation of the phenomena of our intellectual lives would certainly involve an account of human language, including its robust natural underpinning, and how it determines what we "think" in the everyday sense of "thinking."[79] Without all this there would be no "mental" phenomena of the kind mentioned above, and indeed there would be no human thinking at all, not even in the narrow technical sense of *An.* III 4–5, for our *nous* could never develop and be actualized without the contribution of all these factors. While we might regret that Aristotle did not make more progress in explaining individual phenomena of human intellectual life, he can hardly be blamed for underestimating these factors. And, indeed, he has interesting things to say about the bodily aspects of human thought.[80] All this notwithstanding, the main point stands: natural philosophy cannot *know nous* as such, but it must *know about* it; accordingly, it cannot treat thinking as such, but it can, and indeed should, explore the *enabling conditions* of thinking. These necessary (but not sufficient) conditions would constitute a large part of any full account of a mental phenomenon. Still, Aristotle relentlessly warns us against mistaking them for a part of the account of thinking itself.

Many of Aristotle's observations about the bodily aspects of human intellectual life are to be found in short treatises falling under the traditional label of *Parva naturalia*.[81] Thus it is significant that the introduction to these short essays—namely *Sens.* 1—contains an explicit statement to the effect that the natural factors, as important as they are, can constitute nothing more than enabling conditions of thinking.

Toward the end of *Sens.* 1 Aristotle compares the ways in which sight and hearing, respectively, contribute to the self-preservation and the well-being of animals.[82] While sight "is more important [than the other senses] with respect to the necessities [of life] and is so *per se*," hearing "is more important [than the other senses] with respect to *nous* and is so incidentally."[83] Sight contributes to the necessities of life because the common, cross-modal perceptible objects, such as

[78] For how propositional thought is (teleologically) grounded in the grasping of essence, see Chapter 3.
[79] See Labarrière 2004; cf. Wedin 1993.
[80] See van der Eijk 1997 and now Connell 2021.
[81] The other most important source is *Part. An.*, whose first chapter was briefly discussed above.
[82] For the details of this passage, see Roreitner (forthcoming a).
[83] *Sens.* 1, 437a3–5.

shape, size, or motion, are best perceived by it and that helps the animal more than anything else to identify, for example, a predator or a prey in its surroundings. The contribution is *per se* because common objects are *per se* perceptible.

> Hearing, by contrast, announces only the differences of sound, and to a few [kinds of animals] also the differences of voice; but incidentally hearing contributes the most to understanding, for speech is the cause of learning, being audible not *per se*, but incidentally; for speech is composed of words and each of the words is a symbol.[84]

The reason why hearing contributes the most to understanding (*phronêsis*, covering here both the understanding of practical and the understanding of theoretical objects)[85] is that most understanding is in fact acquired by listening to someone else. The contribution of hearing, though, is not *per se* but incidental, because speech (*logos*), unlike common objects of perception, is not *per se* but only incidentally perceptible. What is perceptible *per se* are only the differences of voice[86] which serve as the matter of human speech,[87] which in turn stands in a *symbolical* relation to human thought.[88] Importantly, the reason why hearing contributes only incidentally to *nous* is not that speech only mediates knowledge which originally derives from experience. Even where this is the case, it will be no less true for the original experience—such as noticing some commonality in the bodily structure of certain kinds of animals—that perception only contributed incidentally to *nous*. It is so because the proper contents of *nous* can never be *per se* objects of perception. What perception, and indeed any natural phenomenon, including *phantasia*, memory, and experience, can provide is only *an occasion* for *nous* to be developed and actualized. That development and actualization itself is no longer a natural phenomenon: natural capacities are used here for non-natural goals.

Sens. 1 is not the only place in *Parva naturalia* where Aristotle insists on the difference between the enabling conditions of thinking and thinking itself. When discussing memory, as another enabling condition of thinking, Aristotle repeats the same point. On the one hand, memory is clearly indispensable for any dispositional knowledge which presupposes a kind of "remembering of objects of thought."[89] On the other hand, just as we cannot perceive the objects of thought as such, we cannot, properly speaking, remember them either. What we remember *per se* are perceptual contents, retained by means of *phantasmata*:

[84] *Sens.* 1, 437a9–15.
[85] See *Sens.* 1, 437a2–3.
[86] For the difference between sound and voice, see *An.* II 8, 420b5–33; cf. *Gener. An.* V 7.
[87] See *Gener. An.* V 7, 786b18–22; cf. *Metaph.* VII 12, 1038a5–9.
[88] See *Int.* 1, 16a4–9; cf. *Int.* 2, 16a26–29; *Int.* 14, 24b1–4.
[89] *Mem.* 1, 450a11–12; cf. *An.* III 4, 429b5–10.

> Thus it [i.e., memory] will pertain to *nous* incidentally, while pertaining *per se* to the perceptive capacity.... And it is the contents of *phantasia* that are remembered *per se*, while all that which cannot be without *phantasia* is remembered incidentally.[90]

By now it should be clear that Aristotle's thought would be gravely misunderstood if we took "incidental" here to mean "irrelevant."[91] The natural phenomena that incidentally contribute to *nous*, like hearing, are anything but irrelevant for it. They are indispensable, and *nous* is a true goal for them. Thus, "incidental" is also very far from meaning just "fortuitous."[92] Indeed, calling natural phenomena "enabling conditions" of thinking might be an understatement: a full account of these phenomena would apparently involve a full causal account of thinking in the contemporary sense of "causal," including its triggering causes.[93] When characterizing the contribution of perception or memory as "incidental," Aristotle is very far from denying this deep embeddedness of human thinking in nature; his point is rather that the realm of human thinking is *sui generis* and not itself a natural phenomenon or something supervening on natural phenomena.[94] Human thinking can only be enabled and triggered by natural phenomena, but it cannot be necessitated by them. A right constellation of memories and *phantasmata* provides all that is needed for an act of human thinking—except for the object of thought itself; the grasping of such an object by human *nous* is an irreducible, non-natural event.

5. The separability of *nous*

So far, we have seen, in a brief outline, the reasons why *nous* is apt for serving as the ultimate *explanans* of various mental phenomena that are all immensely more complex than thinking itself and whose explanation will have to take many other

[90] *Mem.* 1, 450a13–14, 23–25. See also *Mem.* 2, 451a25–31.

[91] This is how "incidental" can be paraphrased in some, but certainly not all contexts: e.g., when a house is built by a flute player (cf., e.g., *Phys.* II 5, 196b26–27, 197a14–15).

[92] In contrast, e.g., to the case of finding treasure while digging a well (cf. *NE* III 3, 1112a27, and *Phys.* II 5, 197a5–8; cf. *Phys.* II 8, 199b18–25). Unlike here, there is a genuine teleological link between the natural phenomena and *nous*. For a use of the phrase *kata sumbebêkos* closer to our context, see, e.g., Aristotle's account of incidentally pleasurable smells at *EN* III 10, 1118a9–23, and *Sens.* 5, 443b18–30.

[93] For the triggering causes of thinking, see *An.* III 7 with Chapter 4 in this volume and Corcilius 2020a. The triggering causes do not replace the account of objects of thought as being themselves the efficient causes of thinking from *An.* III 4–5, but that account would apparently not count as "causal" in the contemporary sense. The same holds for the interpretation on which it is the agent *nous* of *An.* III 5 that "acts on" the *nous* of the soul whenever we think (cf. Chapter 2).

[94] Cf. *An.* III 8, 432a12–14. This seems to be directly connected to Aristotle's famous claim in *Gener. An.* II 3 that *nous* alone "comes from without" (cf. footnote 20): the principle (*archê*) of this part of the soul cannot be produced by "concoction" and it cannot be actualized by the process of embryogenesis or any other natural process; it can only be actualized by culture and learning, and it is only very rarely developed into its proper form of a power for truly grasping essences.

factors into account which will directly involve the body, even though *nous* is not a nature and thinking is an activity exclusive to it. We have also seen hints suggesting that *nous* depends for its development in us directly on such natural factors, although it is not itself a part of our nature and does not develop naturally. What remains to be addressed is the notorious question of its separability.

One reason why this question was, and indeed remains, highly controversial is that by saying that *X* is *chôriston* Aristotle means different things in different contexts, depending on (1) whether *chôriston* is used in the sense of "separable" or "separate" (both being linguistically possible), (2) what *X* is separable/separate *from* (the body/matter/magnitude, motion, the other capacities of the soul), and (3) *in what respect* it is separable/separate (in place, in account, in existence).[95] Accordingly, there are at least three senses in which it is relatively safe to speak of human *nous* as separate/separable. First, *nous* seems to be separable in account from all other capacities of the soul: this means that the thinking capacity (i.e., *nous*) of the soul can be defined without any reference to other capacities of the soul and their acts. This is not a special feature of *nous*: the nutritive and the perceptive capacities are equally separable in account.[96] Second, as argued above, the *nous* of the soul is separable in account from motion and from the body, for its defining activity—that is, thinking (*noein*)—is not an activity of the body or a motion.[97] This characteristic already singles out the thinking capacity from all other capacities of the soul, for these are inseparable in account from motion and from the body in the sense that their defining activities are bodily activities: that is, motions.[98] Finally, *nous* is taxonomically separable from other capacities of the soul, which is a special case of separability in existence: there are instances of *nous*—namely, divine *nous*—whose existence is independent from the other capacities of the soul, and, indeed, from the soul as such, and *a fortiori* from the body and from motion.[99] A similar kind of separability is to be found in the case of the nutritive capacity because it is instantiated in plants independently from other capacities of the soul; unlike divine *nous*, though, the nutritive capacity of plants remains, of course, to be a soul which is inseparable both in existence and in account from the plant body.

These three ways in which *nous* can be safely claimed to be separable/separate need to be distinguished from the issue of whether human *nous* is unqualifiedly separable from the other parts of the human soul, and so from motion and from the body: that is, whether the very *nous* that we know primarily as a part of the

[95] See the Glossary (*s.v.* SEPARABLE/SEPARATE, TO BE SEPARATED) for an overview.

[96] Cf. Corcilius and Gregoric 2010 and Johansen 2012: 47–72.

[97] See *An.* II 1, 413a6–7; cf. *An.* III 4, 429a24–27, b5, and *Gener. An.* II 3, 736b28–29, 737a9–11.

[98] See *An.* II 1, 413a4–6; cf. *Gener. An.* II 3, 736b21–26.

[99] See *An.* III 4, 430a3–5; *An.* III 5, 430a17–25; *Metaph.* XII.7–9; cf. *An.* II 2, 413a31–32. The importance of the notion of taxonomical separability was emphasized by Caston 1999. It is also listed by Miller 2012: 308–314. We will see below that this notion can in fact only be applied to *nous* with a grain of salt (footnote 132).

human soul (namely, the ultimate *explanans* of human embodied intellectual life) can also exist independently from the soul and the body. Aristotle clearly found this to be an important question. His observation at the end of *An.* II 1 to the effect that "nothing prevents" a part of the soul (i.e., *nous*) from being "separable from the body" seems to be intended to raise exactly this question. And the following reflection in *Metaph.* XII 3 is unambiguously doing so:

> Whether something also continues existing later [i.e., after the composite has perished as such] ought to be explored. For in some cases, nothing [from the general hylomorphic considerations outlined in the preceding lines] prevents [this from happening], for instance when we take the soul to be such, not the soul as a whole, but *nous*, for it is surely impossible for the whole soul.[100]

To be sure, Aristotle is not claiming in any of these passages that human *nous* can exist apart from the body (when the rest of the soul perishes); what he does is rather to point out that the reason why other parts of the soul can never exist independently from the body does not pertain to *nous*. Roughly, in the case of the other parts of the soul, the fact that they are not unqualifiedly separable from the body is entailed by their inseparability in account from motion and from the body; but since *nous* is separable in account from motion and from the body, the question of unqualified separability needs to be decided on other grounds.

And Aristotle does not drop this question with *An.* II 1. He returns to it in the chapter that immediately follows, although here the language of *chôriston* is especially tricky. Several different meanings of it are explicitly in play in *An.* II 2, which has led some scholars to read Aristotle's remark quite differently. What he says is this:

> About *nous* and the theoretical capacity nothing is clear as of yet, but it seems to be a different genus of soul,[101] and this alone can be separated, as the eternal from the perishable. But it is clear from what has been said that the other parts of the soul are not separable, as some say. What is clear is that they are different in account.[102]

Since antiquity, Aristotle's assertion about *nous* here has occasionally been read along the lines of taxonomical separability, with a reference to his application of

[100] *Metaph.* XII 3, 1070a24–27.

[101] *Prima facie* Aristotle's expression *psuchês genos heteron* could be equally well understood as "a genus different from the soul." But Aristotle seems to be addressing here the question raised at *An.* I 1, 402b1–3, as to whether souls which are not uniform in kind (*homoeidês*) differ in species (*eidei*) or in genus (*genei*). The two meanings are, in any case, closely interrelated: if *nous* as a different genus of the soul turned out to be unqualifiedly separable from motion and the body, it would have to become, upon its separation, a genus different from the soul.

[102] *An.* II 2, 413b24–29.

that notion to the nutritive capacity earlier in the same chapter.[103] But Aristotle's specification of *nous* in terms of a theoretical capacity already makes this reading difficult, for *nous* is clearly not instantiated in separate substances as a capacity. And even more importantly: if Aristotle had taxonomical separability in mind, he could hardly be saying that *nous alone* can be separated, for he has already made clear twice that the nutritive soul is taxonomically separable, too.[104] Moreover, the immediate context suggests that Aristotle is speaking of something different. In what precedes he argued, roughly, that no part of the soul constituting the nature of an animal can be unqualifiedly separated from other parts—for instance, by cutting the body of the animal—and this suggests that these parts of the soul are only separable from each other in account, but they are not separate from each other in place (as Plato would have it).[105] Nothing like that is clear as of yet about *nous*, for—Aristotle explains—it is a different genus of soul: that is, it is not a nature.[106] Aristotle surely does not want to suggest that *nous* has a special bodily organ with which it could be cut out from the body or in which it could exit the body as if in a cart—in fact, he will later argue that *nous* has no bodily organ whatsoever.[107] But it is not yet clear whether it can perhaps be unqualifiedly separated from the other parts of the soul in some other way. And this observation about *nous* makes perfect sense given that in *An.* II 1 Aristotle has left the question of its unqualified separability from the body open: if *nous* turned out to be unqualifiedly separable from the body, it would obviously also be unqualifiedly separable from the other parts of the soul (since we know these for sure to be inseparable from the body by their very definition).

The quoted passage was often approached with the assumption that if Aristotle is speaking here of unqualified rather than taxonomical separability, it implies an individual *post mortem* existence. That is why this passage was cheered by some and it also seems to be why Alexander of Aphrodisias argued to the contrary that the passage must rather be talking about taxonomical separability.[108] But we will see that there is no need for making this choice: reading the passage as concerned with the unqualified separability of human *nous* does not imply that it refers to individual *post mortem* existence, for which there seems to be, indeed, little room

[103] See *An.* II 2, 413a31–b1; cf. already *An.* I 5, 411b29–30 (and again *An.* II 3, 415a2–3). There is a tradition of reading the quoted passage in this way that goes back to Alexander's (lost) commentary on Aristotle's *De anima* (see Philoponus, *In An.* 261.10–19; cf. *In An.* 241.28–242.11). Cf. Broadie 1996: 163, Caston 1996b: 186, and Caston 1999: 210. Contrast Polansky 2007: 181, Miller 2012: 313, or Shields 2016: 187–188.

[104] *An.* I 5, 411b29–30; *An.* II 2, 413a31–32.

[105] See *An.* II 2, 413b13–24; cf. *An.* I 5, 411b19–27.

[106] Cf. also *An.* II 3, 415a11–12.

[107] *An.* III 4, 429a18–27.

[108] Cf. footnote 103 above. For a more detailed discussion of both strategies, see Roreitner 2021a and Roreitner 2021b.

in Aristotle's mature thought.[109] It is worth emphasizing at this point that the question of unqualified separability of human *nous* is not external to the project of *De anima*.[110] It is not, as is sometimes thought, motivated primarily by Aristotle's moral concerns, such as qualms about denying personal immortality.[111] As we have seen, Aristotle is defining the ultimate principle of human intellectual life and he finds that this principle is very different from the principles of nutritive and perceptive life, for *nous* does not belong to our nature and thinking is an affection exclusive to it. This leads directly to the question of how exactly *nous* relates to the body and its natural form, and the issue of unqualified separability is perhaps the most obvious aspect of that question—especially in an intellectual *milieu* akin to Plato's Academy where arguments from performances of *nous* to unqualified separability of the soul seem to have enjoyed considerable popularity.

In fact, in *An.* I 1 Aristotle had already flagged this question as something he would need to deal with: "If this [i.e., thinking] is (a) a *phantasia* or (b) not without *phantasia*, it will not be possible even for this to be without the body."[112] If (a) were true, *nous* would be a nature inseparable from the body in the same way as the other parts of the human soul are. It would be inseparable in account from motion, for one could define it only as the principle of a bodily motion caused by this for the sake of that. But we know that this is not Aristotle's considered view.[113] What remains in play is option (b), which would also imply that human *nous* cannot exist in separation from the body, but (as emphasized in *An.* II 1) not in the sense that its activity is an activity of the body: namely, a motion (or rest). The question of affections exclusive to the soul itself, thus, turns out to be more complicated than it might first appear: thinking can be an affection exclusive to *nous* in the sense that it is the activity of the *nous* itself, or identical with it, in which "the bodily activity takes no part," but not exclusive to it in the sense that it could take place without being supported by *phantasia*, which itself is an affection (a motion) of the body. The latter would imply that the definitory acts of *nous* are essentially constituents of more complex activities of the cognitive soul.[114] The question of whether the human *nous* is separable from the other capacities of the human soul unqualifiedly or in account only is flagged again at the outset of *An.* III 4: initially Aristotle

[109] Contrast the surviving quotes from and references to Aristotle's early dialogue *Eudemus*: Proclus, *In Tim.* 323.31–324.4, *In Pol.* 349.14–26; Ps.-Plutarch, *Consolatio ad Apollonium* 115b10–e9; Themistius, *In An.* 107.3–4; Elias, *In Cat.* 114.32–115.3; Augustine, *Contra Iulianum* 4.78.

[110] As described in Chapter 1.

[111] Although it is certainly not unconnected to ethics: when one is encouraged to immortalize (*athanatizein*) oneself (*EN* X 7, 1077b26–1078a8; cf. *EN* X 7, 1177a13–17), one may reasonably ask what kind of immortality can and cannot be attained by the human *nous* understood as that which each of us is in the most proper sense.

[112] *An.* I 1, 403a8–10.

[113] Option (a) is most explicitly denied at *An.* III 3, 427b14–27 and *An.* III 8, 432a10–14.

[114] See the Glossary (*s.v.* COGNITIVE SOUL).

suggests leaving the question open as to whether the thinking part of the soul is "[unqualifiedly] separable or not separable in magnitude but only in account."[115]

So, what is Aristotle's answer? He returns to the test from *An.* I 1 in *An.* III 7–8 and makes a strong case here for the view that the thinking of natural and mathematical objects always depends for its existence on *phantasia* and so, indirectly, on the body:[116] the grasp of the essence of such an object, it turns out, can only exist as a constituent (namely, the defining constituent) of a more complex activity of the cognitive soul inseparably bound to the body. In fact, at *An.* III 4, 429a21–22, Aristotle has already suggested that the level of separateness of the acts of *nous* directly corresponds to the level of separateness of their objects: since neither natural nor mathematical essences are unqualifiedly separable from matter, neither are the acts of thinking them. If this is true, it implies that human *nous* could only be unqualifiedly separable if and as far as it can think a separate substance. This consideration seems also to be behind the question flagged by Aristotle at the end of *An.* III 7:

> The question whether or not it is possible for it [i.e., human *nous*] to think any of the separated entities, while not being itself separated from magnitude, must be investigated later.[117]

At first sight, it could seem that Aristotle is here rhetorically suggesting a negative answer (in line with the correspondence established at *An.* III 4, 429b21–22). In combination with Aristotle's conviction that human *nous* can think separate substances (an epistemological assumption behind the project of "first philosophy"), the implication would, then, seem to be that human *nous* must be unqualifiedly separable from the body. But the issue is more complicated due to the fact that there are two different ways in which the thinking of separate substances can in principle take place: either a separate substance can be thought on its own and purely as it is in itself (*per se*), or it can be thought in relation to something else (*per aliud*)—namely, as the unmoved mover of the uttermost heavenly sphere and the ultimate cause of the order of the universe, in line with *Phys.* VIII 10 and *Metaph.* XII 6–10. From all we can gather from the texts, only the latter option is clearly attested. And to the extent that we are limiting our focus to the thinking of separate

[115] *An.* III 4, 429a11–12. The second option, I take it, boils down to being a distinct but inseparable part of an individual soul as the form of a body: a part which is as inseparable in place from the other capacities as these are from each other (cf. *An.* II 2, 413b13–24). The first option need not be understood in terms of separability *in magnitude* as is often done (see, e.g., Themistius *In An.* 93.32–94.4; Hicks 1907: 476; Ross 1961: 291; Polansky 2007, 435; Shields 2016: 295–296): rather, Aristotle seems to have unqualified separability from other capacities of the soul in mind (cf. *An.* II 2, 413b24–27), which in combination with the separability in account from motion and from the body would entail unqualified separability from the body. Contrast also Broadie 1996: 163–164, interpreting the first option in terms of taxonomical separability.

[116] See *An.* III 7, 431a14–17, b2–5, and *An.* III 8, 432a3–10; cf. *Mem.* 1, 449b30–450a7.

[117] *An.* III 7, 431b17–19.

substances as causes, it can be argued that this thinking depends no less for its existence on *phantasia* than the thinking of natural and mathematical essences does. And that provides another, complementary reading of the final lines of *An.* III 7: human *nous* can think separate substances even as an inseparable part of an individual soul, but it can only think them as causes of motion and the order in the universe.[118] If it turns out that this is the only way human *nous* can think separate substances, it will follow that this *nous* is not unqualifiedly separable from the soul and the body. Aristotle's claim at *An.* III 5, 430a24–25, that "the passive *nous* is perishable" is very suggestive of that outcome.

Now how is this compatible with the claim of *An.* II 2 according to which "*nous* and the theoretical capacity . . . can be separated, as the eternal from the perishable"?[119] One clue is provided by the following consideration about the ontology of the soul's thinking of separate substances. To think (*noein*) means for the soul to receive the essence of something in *nous.*[120] And Aristotle is committed to two striking claims concerning immaterial substances: (1) any such substance will not only be a potential object of thought for us, it will also be an actual object of thought for itself, because it always thinks itself;[121] (2) for such a substance there is no difference between it and its essence.[122] So what I have in *nous* when I know and think such a substance (as the cause of motion and order) must, in some sense, be this self-thinking substance itself: the act of thinking that substance is, in a strong sense, identical to it. If this is right, then we can better understand what Aristotle may mean when he says that a *nous* in us can be unqualifiedly separated as the eternal from the perishable. Clearly, no part of my person is eternal (since I have surely not existed before I was conceived and born), so this can hardly be what Aristotle means; but if I have acquired the knowledge and thought (*nous*) of an immaterial substance, and so there is in me *nous* identical to it,[123] I have something eternal in me which seems indeed unqualifiedly separable: even when it ceases to be thought and known by me (when it ceases to be my thought or my *nous*) it continues to be thought by itself—as it has ever been.[124]

Under this interpretation, what is unqualifiedly separable is nothing other than the thinking of a separate substance itself, which, upon its separation, ceases to be my, and, indeed, a human, act of thinking ("it is only what it really is"):[125] in this way a *nous* in me can be described as unqualifiedly separable, without conflicting

[118] For details, see Roreitner 2021a: 262–267.

[119] Assuming we are satisfied with saying that *An.* III 5, 430a24–25, simply contradicts the claim of *An.* II 2 (cf. Menn 2020: 135, 136n50).

[120] See *An.* III 4, 429a15–16, 27–29; cf. *Metaph.* XII 7, 1072b22.

[121] See *An.* III 4, 430a3–5.

[122] See *An.* III 4, 429b11–12.

[123] Cf. *An.* III 4, 429b5–10.

[124] This consideration is akin to what Alexander says at *An.* 90.11–91.6 about the separability of the thought of a separate substance taking place "in us."

[125] *An.* III 5, 430a22–23.

with the claim that human *nous* (i.e., the passive *nous*) is perishable due to its inseparability from the cognitive soul. Yet this may still be capturing only a part of the truth. Why does Aristotle specify the *nous* that can be unqualifiedly separated as "the theoretical capacity"—that is, apparently the human *nous* itself—in *An.* II 2?[126] What did he mean before when he insisted that *nous* comes to be present in us as a substance and that it does not perish?[127] And how should we understand Aristotle's exhortation to immortalize ourselves (as far as possible), supported by an emphasis on the fact that *nous*—apparently even when thinking divine *nous* and so identical to it—is what each of us most truly is?[128] These texts seem to be jointly pointing to a certain kind of unqualified separability, imperishability, or immortality of the human *nous* itself.[129] But does the account of *De anima* leave any room for it? One upshot of *An.* III 4–8, as interpreted in this book,[130] is that such an imperishability or immortality could only be granted to human *nous* as far as it can think a separate substance, not only as the cause of motion and order in the universe, but on its own and as it is in itself.

But does it make sense to say that the very *nous* existing as a part of an individual human soul can think a separate substance on its own and so become unqualifiedly separate from the soul—at least for a while during one's life, and maybe forever after the biological death? What makes this question difficult to answer is exactly the fact that when doing so the *nous* in question would cease to be a part of the soul: it seems that in such a case it could not but perfectly coincide with the self-thinking act of the separate substance itself, so that the label "human" could hardly apply to it anymore.[131] Still, there are reasons to insist that rather than being a case of perishing, this is the ultimate fulfilment of human *nous*: that is, the very *nous* that existed as a part of an individual cognitive soul. This is so because as the *nous* of the soul—that is, the principle of human intellectual life—*nous* is already nothing personal: what each of us most truly is consists essentially in transcending one's individual, and even human, perspective toward pure objectivity; and this calling is most perfectly realized in the thought *of a god* where the objective and the subjective genitive come to coincide. If this is so, then the idea of human *nous*

[126] The reading proposed in the preceding paragraph can ascribe a reasonable meaning to *dunamis* here: namely, that of an *acquired capacity* for thinking a separate substance at one's will (cf. the Glossary, *s.v.* Nous). But one can insist that the whole expression "*the* theoretical capacity" is more naturally read as referring to the human *nous* as such.

[127] *An.* I 4, 408b18–19 (assuming that the passage does express Aristotle's view, *pace* Cohoe 2018). This passage can be interpreted along the lines proposed in the preceding paragraph as concerning, at the end of the day, specifically the human thought of separate substances. But one can insist again that Aristotle's claim that "*the nous* comes to be present" in us seems at least *prima facie* more general.

[128] *EN* X 7, 1077b26–1078a8; cf. *EN* X 8, 1178a22, about the "separated" happiness of the human *nous*, and also *Metaph.* XII 7, 1072b23–26.

[129] Many thanks to Klaus Corcilius for insisting on this point.

[130] And in Roreitner (forthcoming b).

[131] Cf. again *An.* III 5, 430a22–23: "Once separated, it is only what it really is, and this alone is immortal and eternal."

coming to think a separate substance on its own as it is in itself does not appear inconceivable after all: it is true that this thinking act will leave no room for any difference between human and divine *nous*; but that is exactly the point, for the difference was primarily a difference between a capacity and the most perfect fulfilment of it—which happens to be an eternal self-subsisting activity devoid of any potentiality.[132] Aristotle's inquiry in his *De anima* seems carefully constructed so as not to exclude these kinds of considerations. But it is also very clear about the fact that they are beyond its scope, for as far as *nous* becomes unqualifiedly separated from the human soul it also becomes irrelevant to the question about the principle of human intellectual life.

This having been said, it must be stressed that human *nous* can certainly not be reduced to being a capacity for thinking a separate substance or separate substances. It is exactly *qua* human—as a part of the human cognitive soul—that *nous* becomes capable of thinking not only separate substances (as causes), but also natural and mathematical essences and anything that derives from them. As such, human *nous* is an inseparable capacity of the human soul; but this makes it capable of immensely more than divine *nous*. Hence the importance for the project of Aristotle's *De anima* of insisting that—although there may be a good sense in which human *nous* can be unqualifiedly separated (albeit not *qua* human) in coinciding with a separate substance—*it is perishable.*[133] When a human cognitive soul perishes, *nous* perishes with it exactly as a *capacity for thinking everything*—that is, as a passive *nous*—for as such *nous* cannot exist apart from the human soul.

6. Concluding remarks: the status of Aristotle's inquiry into *nous*

If we return to Aristotle's tripartition of the objects of thought and the fields of knowledge with these results in mind, we can better understand what is methodologically so difficult about human *nous*. The problem is that it does not fall under any one of these three classes: it is neither a natural object, for it is separable in account from motion, nor a mathematical object, for it is not a mere abstraction, nor an object that could, as such, exist separately from matter as the substances that the first philosophy is primarily concerned with.[134] This exceptional status

[132] This finding (anticipated in Chapter 2, Section 3, under the heading of "the problem of the subject of thinking"), if true, problematizes the notion of taxonomical separability as applied to *nous*, for my human *nous* seems to be more intimately related to the divine *nous* than as just another numerically distinct instance of the same kind of thing. The notion of taxonomical separability does capture an important truth insofar as separate substances are instances of *nous* independent from perception and nutrition; but we should not be misled by it into understanding one's human *nous* as being numerically distinct from divine *nous* in the way in which one's nutritive capacity is numerically distinct from the nutritive capacity of a plant. The plant's growth can hardly become our own fulfillment.

[133] Cf., again, *An.* III 5, 430a24–25. For more on the relation between human and divine *nous*, see Roreitner (forthcoming b).

[134] Cf. the tripartition at *An.* I 1, 403b9–16.

clearly has to do with the unparalleled versatility and plasticity of *nous*: it is predisposed for everything but for nothing in particular; there is no limit to its receptivity. As such, it is the only "thing" in the universe that can understand all the three kinds of objects (i.e., natural, mathematical, and immaterial) and so embrace all the three fields of knowledge (i.e., natural philosophy, mathematics, and first philosophy)—unlike divine *nous* which is literally incapable of both mathematics and natural philosophy.[135] But it is extraordinarily difficult to understand the principle of all understanding. It is extraordinarily difficult because none of the three major disciplines of thought seems on its own adequate for this understanding.[136]

This finding excludes one easy way of resolving the apparent tension at the heart of Aristotle's inquiry into soul, sometimes adopted by interpreters who, commendably, want to resist the dominant tendency to naturalize Aristotle's inquiry into *nous*.[137] The idea is that Aristotle's inquiry into soul should be understood as a combination of natural philosophy (for all parts of the soul except for *nous*) and first philosophy *qua* theology (for *nous*).[138] One of the aims of this chapter has been to show that the position ascribed by Aristotle to human *nous* in the universe and in the realm of knowledge is much more complicated, and interesting, than that. Aristotle's focus throughout his *De anima* is on natural beings and the primary principles of their lives. What complicates the situation is the fact that humans are natural beings that are teleologically directed to *nous*, and that means determined in what they essentially are by a principle that is not a nature. This,

[135] This plasticity seems not to be appreciated by McCready-Flora 2019: 44–45 when he writes that we cannot search for the "rational-making feature" in humans "among high-level *perfections* of reason," such as "grasping essential definitions," because we "share with god the comprehending soul (*nous, to noêtikon*, etc.) that enables such achievements," and so we should "set our sights lower" and concentrate on "belief" (*doxa*). The reply is that human *nous* is very different from divine *nous* (which is *not* a soul) and is distinguished from it exactly by its plasticity; we should, thus, emphatically not set our sights any lower when searching for the ultimate "rational-making feature" in humans. A similar objection pertains to Cagnoli Fieconni 2019: 69–74 when she identifies the peculiarity of human rationality in its being "aided and hindered by non-rational cognition and desires."

[136] Not even first philosophy will do, not at least in the way in which it is developed in Aristotle's *Metaphysics*. First, it is introduced as an inquiry into all beings *qua* being, not *qua* thinkable. And second, it is governed by the goal of finding separate substances as the ultimate *archai* of all beings (and excluding false candidates). For the aim of Aristotle's *Metaphysics*, see Menn (forthcoming). While something like the resulting *theologikê* seems indispensable for an adequate understanding of human *nous* insofar as separate substances are among its objects, first philosophy does not as such lead to that goal, for the question about the principle of human understanding is bypassed in its program as set down by Aristotle. In sharp contrast to this, the question can by no means be bypassed in natural philosophy.

[137] For such a naturalization, see, e.g., Frede 1992, Caston 1996b, and Caston 1999 (cf. Caston 1997: 338). See also Johansen 2012: 245, concluding that "Aristotle's psychology is of a piece with his physics." Cf. McCready-Flora 2014: 426: "Human cognition is not special, on his view, in virtue of possessing some non-natural characteristic that would render it inaccessible to scientific inquiry;" Connell 2021: 225 ascribing a "broadly naturalistic account of human thinking" to Aristotle: "the human intellect is part of the study of the natural world" (238); and Frey 2018: 172: "Aristotle makes the strongest case he can for the intellect's exclusion from natural science. But . . . we must, and Aristotle does, reject these arguments." Cf. footnotes 38 and 65 above.

[138] See, e.g., Reeve 2017: xxvii–xxix, Kietzmann 2019: 25, 36–42, or Carter 2019: 227.

however, does not make human *nous* a separate substance, and so its treatment cannot be simply delegated to theology. Aristotle cannot, as it were, interrupt his natural inquiry at the end of *An.* III 3, put on the hat of a theologian for the next five chapters, and then take it off again as he continues with *An.* III 9.

His procedure is rather that of starting from natural philosophy as the basic framework for the inquiry into soul, and then showing step by step how we need to transcend and transform that framework if we are ever to understand the phenomena of human intellectual life and the place of man in nature. This procedure is riskier than acknowledged by either of the two mentioned approaches (i.e., the naturalization and the divinization of human *nous*), because it leads to a territory that none of the established fields of knowledge can cover on its own. But it seems to be the only way to an understanding of the peculiar sphere of human thinking that transcends nature by its non-kinetic character, but that falls short of the divine due to its lack, as such, of unqualified separability from motion and body. This understanding is emphatically not a goal that natural philosophy could achieve on its own, for while the sphere of human thinking is deeply embedded in nature, it is not natural. But an understanding of this sphere is vital for natural philosophy because some of the most significant natural phenomena cannot be properly understood without taking *nous* into account as their final goal; and these natural phenomena (pertaining to the structure and the workings of the human body) are to a great extent paradigmatic for how the scientific knowledge of nature ought to be structured as a whole, at least according to Aristotle. That is why Aristotle's inquiry into soul must transcend and transform the framework of natural philosophy in which it is set, in order to gain insight into the principle of all human insights. It must do so exactly because natural philosophy, although it can never understand *nous* on its own, cannot do without drawing on such an understanding.

7

Conclusion: Aristotle on *nous*

Separatism, embeddedness in a cognitive soul, rationalism

An. III 4–8 is a single textual unit. It is also one of the densest and most difficult stretches of text in the entire Aristotelian corpus. Part of the difficulty lies in the argumentative strategy adopted in these chapters, which is anything but straightforward. This strategy is especially opaque in *An.* III 6–8. Quite tellingly, these chapters have often been treated by scholars as a set of mere appendices or even piles of scraps. To fully appreciate the overall argumentative strategy, we must return to Aristotle's main goals in *An.* III 4–8 and recall how he hopes to achieve them. The key goal is definitory. Aristotle wants to define the human capacity for thinking by giving a definition of the principle, or ultimate source, of that capacity: namely, *nous*. But the task of defining *nous* as the ultimate *explanans* of the phenomena related to human thinking turns out to be inseparable from other tasks. First, if *nous* really is what Aristotle takes it to be, how can thinking ever come about? This question is announced, together with the definitory question, right at the outset of *An.* III 4.[1] Second, if *nous* is defined in the remarkably narrow way in which Aristotle defines it (see Chapter 2, Section 6), how can it play the role of the ultimate *explanans* for the entire range of our mental phenomena?

The second subtask is not singled out by Aristotle at the beginning of *An.* III 4, but it emerges as we read on. Throughout *An.* III 4–5 Aristotle is narrowly focused on a highly specialized form of thinking: namely, grasping essences. It does not take long to see that Aristotle cannot stop here if he wants to provide a theoretical framework for a full account of the phenomena related to human thinking. *An.* III 6–8 goes a long way toward fulfilling this goal. Here Aristotle goes beyond what he takes to be the fundamental case of thinking by showing how propositional thinking is possible, and, indeed, why it can only be explained with reference to *nous* as the capacity for grasping the essences (*An.* III 6). He also provides the resources to understand how the capacity for thought works as part of the integrated system of cognitive powers we have called "cognitive soul" (*An.* III 7–8).[2] When we look at *An.* III 4–5 and *An.* III 6–8 in this way, we see that they are two steps in a single argument whose goal is to provide the conceptual foundation for a study of specifically human mental phenomena. Aristotle is not directly concerned with the

[1] *An.* III 4, 429a12–13.
[2] For an introduction to this terminology, see the Glossary.

Aristotle on the Essence of Human Thought. Klaus Corcilius, Andrea Falcon, and Robert Roreitner, Oxford University Press.
 DOI: 10.1093/9780198921820.003.0007

explanation of mental phenomena in *An.* III 4–8. *Rather, he is focused on providing the explanatory starting point from which to understand them and on showing that this is indeed the explanatory starting point for all of them.* More directly, and more boldly: what we nowadays would call a theory of the human mind is nowhere to be found in *An.* III 4–8. What Aristotle offers here is the theoretical framework in which we can usefully pursue such a project.[3]

In *An.* III 4–8 Aristotle is centrally concerned with the essence of human thought, which he takes to be part of our essence as human beings. Moreover, this essence is to be defined with respect to the essences of things broadly conceived. By his lights, the capacity for thinking, defined as the capacity for grasping essences, is what distinguishes human from non-human animals. In *An.* III 4–8, Aristotle establishes what this capacity is, how it can account for the entire range of the respective phenomena, and how it works. His definitory and explanatory efforts are based on a sharp distinction between what Aristotle takes to be this capacity, on the one hand, and its preconditions, on the other. Among the latter it is possible to count (without pretense of exhaustiveness) the unique structure of our human body, our ability to speak a language, and our ability to form and use *phantasmata*.[4] While our capacity for thinking crucially depends on the fulfillment of these preconditions, it is conceptually separate from all of them—just as it is from our volition to exercise this capacity, which, too, is regarded by Aristotle as external to an act of human thinking. In the end, *nous* understood as the principle or source of the human capacity for thinking is the pure and immediate potentiality to think every thinkable aspect of reality. That is a truly optimistic finding. But we should not mistake what Aristotle is saying here. While every human being is *qua* such endowed with this remarkable capacity, the conditions of its proper actualization are rarely fulfilled in an act of grasping an essence. Indeed, according to Aristotle, in most of us *nous* remains at an embryonic level throughout our lives. That, however, does not prevent Aristotle from insisting on his answer to the *ti esti* question when raised in connection with the human capacity for thinking.[5] We can restate his answer by saying that human *nous* is the readiness to think every thinkable aspect of reality—every essence—while being nothing at all in actuality before thinking.[6]

[3] See Chapter 1 for our attempt to disabuse the reader from thinking of Aristotle's treatment of *nous* as a straightforward contribution to a theory of the human mind.

[4] A brief introduction to the Aristotelian account of *phantasmata* can be found in the Glossary. On *phantasmata* as one of the enabling conditions of human thinking, see Chapter 1 (Section 7), Chapter 4 (Sections 5 and 7), and Chapter 5 (Section 2). For an idea of what a full account of human thought, including its preconditions, would involve, see Chapter 6 (Section 4).

[5] The rationale for Aristotle's confidence is spelled out in Chapter 3. See also Aristotle's qualifications of the identity thesis set out in Chapter 5 (Section 2).

[6] The strategy adopted to answer the *ti esti* question with respect to *nous* is further discussed in Chapter 2, Section 5.1. For an attempt to spell out how this intellectual blank is to be understood, see Chapter 5 (Section 2(a)).

Nous so understood turns out to be a very special kind of entity to the extent that it is unmixed with the body, has no dedicated bodily organ, and is separate from the body. As a result, *nous* cannot be assimilated to any of the other parts of the soul. While the definition of the latter always requires reference to motion and to a certain kind of body, *nous* does not: it is separate from motion and body in account, and so it cannot be a part of nature. We can refer to this aspect of Aristotle's account of *nous* as *separatism*. Separatism implies that *nous*, while it belongs to our essence as human beings, is not part of the form or the nature of a human being and is not to be equated with the first actuality of a human body that is potentially alive. Separatism so understood does important work in the explanation of intellectual cognition by Aristotle.[7]

At the same time, *nous* as the principle of human thought is always embedded in a cognitive soul. But a cognitive soul only occurs in an embodied cognitive system since the soul is the form of a living body. Among other things, this means that the distinctive activity of human *nous*—thinking—takes place in the context of a larger set of activities which are common to body and soul. While Aristotle sharply distinguishes the non-bodily activity of *nous* from those other activities, he also seems to think that our ability to engage in both practical and theoretical thinking crucially depends on their support. But if our capacity to engage in practical and non-practical thinking requires the full functioning of the cognitive soul, and the cognitive soul is by definition an embodied cognitive system, it follows that human *nous*, while definitionally separable from the human body, is ontologically inseparable from it. In line with Aristotle's methodology, this inseparability seems to be grounded in the dependence of human thinking on *phantasia*. And this dependence is, in turn, due to the fact that the objects of human thought are such that they can only be thought "in *phantasmata*."[8]

Separatism and *embeddedness in the cognitive soul* may seem to pull us in opposite directions. And yet, Aristotle develops an account of *nous* in which both ingredients feature in a conspicuous way. But there is a third salient aspect of his treatment of *nous* that calls for a few words of elaboration. We can refer to this aspect as *rationalism*. A clear, and indeed central, message of Aristotle's *De anima* is that we come to know the world around us via two fundamentally different cognitive powers: *nous* and perception. *Nous* and perception are fundamentally different cognitive powers because the nature of their corresponding objects is fundamentally different. This way of drawing the distinction between *nous* and perception is at the very heart of Aristotle's theory of cognition. They remain fundamentally

[7] For more on this front, we refer the reader to Chapter 2 and Chapter 6. SEPARABLE/SEPARATE (the Greek term is *chôriston*) is defined in the Glossary.

[8] *An.* III 7, 431b2. For the relevant methodological principle, see Chapter 1 (Section 5). The embeddedness of *nous* in a cognitive soul is extensively discussed in Chapters 4 and 5. For the difficult question of how human thinking of immaterial substances fits within this picture, see Chapter 6 (Section 5).

separate ways of knowing the world around us even when they are jointly involved in thinking matter-involving essences. Aristotle envisions two such cases: our thinking of the essence of hylomorphic compounds and our grasping of mathematical essences.[9] In both cases, *nous* avails itself of perception in the sense that *nous* co-opts our perceptual capacity to access the relevant object of thought. But this does not mean that perception has itself access to these objects of thought (e.g., the matter-involving essence of flesh) or that *nous* is to be assimilated to, or derived from, perception when it comes to the cognition of matter-involving essences. By Aristotle's lights, *nous* alone cognizes them even if it gets help from the perceptual capacity to the extent that these two different kinds of essences cannot be thought in isolation from their respective matter since they are matter-involving essences.[10]

This puts strictures on the kind of empiricism that can be ascribed to Aristotle. Human thought is surely dependent on perceptual experience in the sense that the former could not exist without the latter. But that is a rather trivial claim. What is more significant is that, according to Aristotle, thought cannot be epistemically derived from perception and experience (*empeiria*), for no amount of experience can fully justify the grasp of an essence. Nor can such a grasp be psychologically derived from experience. The content of thought is *sui generis*: it is something over and above the content of any possible perception and experience, and it cannot be arrived at simply by leaving out some aspects of the latter (in an abstractionist manner). Some passages, most famously in *Metaph.* I 1 and *Posterior Analytics* II 19, have often been read as implying some such derivation. If the proposed interpretation of *An.* III 4–8 is on the right track, however, what Aristotle says in these passages should be understood against the background of the contrast between thought itself and its enabling conditions. With this contrast in mind, we can see that what has often been taken as a sign of Aristotle's empiricism, speaks in fact of the enabling conditions of thought alone.

That having been said, we hasten to add that Aristotle is not a Platonist in the sense of believing that the contents of our thoughts have an otherworldly nature. By his lights, there are no separate Forms of material or mathematical objects. And while Aristotle is firmly convinced about the existence of a separate, transcendent thought, this thought is remarkably thin in the sense that it can never have any matter-involving essence for its object, for the reasons spelled out in *An.* III 4–8. That is why human thought of these essences can no more "emanate" from transcendent thought, or be completely backed by it, than it can derive from experience. The realm of human thinking, whose ultimate *explanans* is studied in *An.* III 4–8, stretches between experience (*empeiria*) and transcendent thought without being reducible to either.

[9] *An.* III 4, 429b10–22.

[10] For more on the collaboration between *nous* and perception, see Chapter 2 (Section 2).

Greek Text and Translation

Sigla and Abbreviations

The Greek text and critical apparatus are taken from Aurelius Förster's still unsurpassed 1912 Budapest Academy of Letters edition. We hope that this edition will soon be substituted by the critical edition under preparation by Justin Winzenrieth (TIDA). For the reader's convenience, we inserted some notable textual decisions from other editors in the apparatus. The few places where our text departs from Förster's are noted there as well. The translation is ours. What follows here is a list of sigla and abbreviations used in Förster's apparatus. A description and *stemma codicum* can be found in Förster's *praefatio* viii-xiv.

Manuscripts

E	Codex Parisinus 1853 (10th century[1])
E^1	Corrections by the scribe in E
E^2	Corrections or additions by a reviser in the margin of the text in E (10th century).
E^3	Interlinear corrections in E (15th century)
E^x	Places where no clear distinction can be made between E^1 and E^3 (and only very rarely E^2)
C	Codex Parisinus Coislinianus 386 (11th century)
C^2	Corrections in Codex C (12th century)
C^3	Later corrections in C
L	Codex Vaticanus 253 (14th century)
S	Codex Laurentianus 81.1 (13th century)
S^2	Later corrections in S
U	Codex Vaticanus 260 (13th century)
U^2	Corrections by various hands in U
V	Codex Vaticanus 266 (14th century)
V^2	Later corrections in V
V^3	Very late corrections in V
W	Codex Vaticanus 1026 (13th/14th century)

[1] The original part of Codex E contains Books I and III more or less completely. However, in the third book 430a24-431b16 and then again 434a31-435b25 are missing from the original part of E. The pages that contained the second book of *De anima* have been replaced by a text belonging to a different branch of the tradition. The original version of the second book E is only preserved in fragments. They are printed in the modern editions since Torstrik (1862).

W^2	Later corrections, different from the first hand, in W
X	Codex Ambrosianus H. 50 (12th/13th century)
X^2	Scholia and interlinear corrections in X (by a similar hand, 12th/13th century)
X^3	Very late corrections in X
Y	Codex Parisinus Bibl. Nat. 2014 (13th/14th century)
y^2	Later corrections in y
P	Codex Vaticanus 1339 (14th/15th century)
o	All manuscripts except P in the second book, and L in the third book. Note that for III 5, 430a24 – 7, 431b16, the siglum **o** does *not* include E as these parts of the manuscript have been lost.
a	Family formed from manuscripts E and L
b	Family formed from manuscripts CSUVWXy

In order to express himself concisely, Förster uses the minus sign in the following way, for example:

o-y	All ms (**o**) except one, y

Ancient testimonies

Si	Simplicius
Si^l	Simplicius lemma
Si^c	Simplicius citatio
Si^p	Simplicius paraphrasis
Ph	Philoponus
Ph^l	Philoponus lemma
Ph^c	Philoponus citatio
Ph^p	Philoponus paraphrasis
Th	Themistius
Th^c	Themistius citatio
So	Sophonias
Prisc	Priscian
Alex	Alexander Aphrodisiensis
Asclep	Asclepius Trallensis
Theophr	Theophrastus

Where a commentator's entry is accompanied by a letter (e.g. Si^lA), this indicates the manuscript from which the commentator's wording is taken.

DE ANIMA III 4–5

[429^{a}10] Περὶ δὲ τοῦ μορίου τοῦ τῆς ψυχῆς ᾧ γινώσκει τε ἡ ψυχὴ καὶ φρονεῖ, εἴτε χωριστοῦ ὄντος εἴτε μὴ χωριστοῦ κατὰ μέγεθος ἀλλὰ κατὰ λόγον, σκεπτέον τίν' ἔχει διαφοράν, καὶ πῶς ποτὲ γίνεται τὸ νοεῖν.

[429^{a}13] εἰ δή ἐστι τὸ νοεῖν ὥσπερ τὸ αἰσθάνεσθαι, ἢ πάσχειν τι ἂν εἴη ὑπὸ τοῦ νοητοῦ ἤ τι τοιοῦτον ἕτερον. ἀπαθὲς ἄρα δεῖ εἶναι, δεκτικὸν δὲ τοῦ εἴδους καὶ δυνάμει τοιοῦτον ἀλλὰ μὴ τοῦτο, καὶ ὁμοίως ἔχειν, ὥσπερ τὸ αἰσθητικὸν πρὸς τὰ αἰσθητά, οὕτω τὸν νοῦν πρὸς τὰ νοητά. ἀνάγκη ἄρα, ἐπεὶ πάντα νοεῖ, ἀμιγῆ εἶναι, ὥσπερ φησὶν Ἀναξαγόρας, ἵνα κρατῇ, τοῦτο δ' ἐστὶν ἵνα γνωρίζῃ· παρεμφαινόμενον γὰρ κωλύει τὸ ἀλλότριον καὶ ἀντιφράττει· ὥστε μηδ' αὐτοῦ εἶναι φύσιν μηδεμίαν ἀλλ' ἢ ταύτην, ὅτι δυνατόν. ὁ ἄρα καλούμενος τῆς ψυχῆς νοῦς (λέγω δὲ νοῦν ᾧ διανοεῖται καὶ ὑπολαμβάνει ἡ ψυχή) οὐθέν ἐστιν ἐνεργείᾳ τῶν ὄντων πρὶν νοεῖν.

[429^{a}24] διὸ οὐδὲ μεμεῖχθαι εὔλογον αὐτὸν τῷ σώματι· ποιός τις γὰρ ἂν γίγνοιτο, ἢ ψυχρὸς ἢ θερμός· ἢ κἂν ὄργανόν τι εἴη, ὥσπερ τῷ αἰσθητικῷ· νῦν δ' οὐθὲν ἔστιν.

καὶ εὖ δὴ οἱ λέγοντες τὴν ψυχὴν εἶναι τόπον εἰδῶν, πλὴν ὅτι οὔτε ὅλη ἀλλ' ἡ νοητική, οὔτε ἐντελεχείᾳ ἀλλὰ δυνάμει τὰ εἴδη.

[429^{a}29] ὅτι δ' οὐχ ὁμοία ἡ ἀπάθεια τοῦ αἰσθητικοῦ καὶ τοῦ νοητικοῦ, φανερὸν ἐπὶ τῶν αἰσθητηρίων καὶ τῆς αἰσθήσεως. ἡ μὲν γὰρ αἴσθησις οὐ δύναται αἰσθάνε-

429^{a} 10 τοῦ$_{2}$ ESV *Th 93,32*: om LCUWX *Si*^{l} *bis, Ph*^{l} ^{c}*517,33; 520,21*: om et μορίου post ψυχῆς ponit y τε **o**–CW *Si*^{l} *bis, Ph*^{l} ^{c}*517,33; 520,21.25*: τί C: om W **11** εἴτε **a** *Si*^{c}*222,10*: εἴτε καὶ **b** *Si*^{l} *Ph*^{l} ^{c}*520,30* **12** (κατὰ τὸ μ. W) (κατὰ τὸν λ. W) **13** (τὸ νοεῖν γίνεται W) **14** τὸ **o**–SV *Si*^{lc}*225,14 Ph*^{l}: om SV τι **b** *Si*^{lc}*264,17* ^{p}*223,39 So 124,19 cf Ph*^{p}*522,10*: ὅτι **a** **15** (δὲ] sscr γὰρ V) **16** (ἔχειν om X, ins X^{2}) **17** (τὸ νοοῦν V) **18** ἐπεὶ **a** *Si*^{l}: ἐπειδὴ **b**, ins δὴ E^{2} *Ph*^{l} *Th 94,18* **20** κωλύσει W *Th 94,23*) ἀντιφράττει **a** *Ph*^{p}*523,15 So 124,26*: ἀντιφράξει UW *Ph*^{l} *Th 94,23*: «ἀντιφράττοντος ἢ ἀντιφράξοντος» *Si*^{p}*226,8*: ἀντιφράζει SVXy, C [ζ corr in ττ C^{2}] **21** (εἶναι φύσει y: φύσιν εἶναι W) μηδεμίαν **a** CWXy: τινὰ μηδεμίαν SUV *Si*^{l} **22** δυνατόν **o**: δυνατός *Si*$^{l\,p}$*227,7 cf. Th 94,25* Ross **25** τις [τι y] γὰρ ἂν Ey *Si*^{l}: γὰρ ἄν τις **o**–Ey γένοιτο *Si*^{l} ἢ ψυχρὸς ἢ θερμὸς E: ψυχρὸς ἢ θερμὸς L *So 124,32*: ἢ θερμὸς ἢ ψυχρὸς y *Si*^{l}: θερμὸς ἢ ψυχρὸς **b**–y *Ph*^{p}*524,1* **26** ἢ κἂν **a** y: κἂν CW *Si*^{l} *So 124,33*: καὶ SUVX: ᾗ κἂν scripsit Förster **27** δὴ **o** *Si*^{l} *Ph*$^{l\,c}$*165,25; 307,31 Ph*^{c} *in phys 516,10 So 125,36*: γε *Ph*^{c}*93,4 Si*^{c} *in phys 540,9 Asclep*^{c} *in metaph 69,19; 167,30* οἱ τὴν ψ. εἰρηκότες *Asclep l.c.* εἶναι **o** *Ph*^{l} *So 125,36*: om *Si*^{l} *Ph*^{c}*93,4; 165,26; 307,32 Asclep l.c. Si*^{c} *in phys l.c.* **28** ἀλλ' ἡ **a** CWy *So 125,36*: om SUVX **29** (ὅμοια ἡ ἀπαθεία S) **30** αἰσθητικοῦ **a** CWy, corr U^{2}V^{2} *Si*^{l} *Th 104,31 So 124,37*: αἰσθητοῦ SUVX τοῦ$_{2}$ **o** *Si*^{l} *So 124,38*: om *Th 104,32*

DE ANIMA III 4–5

Introduction

Regarding the part of the soul by which the soul knows and understands—be it [429a10] separate or separate not in extension but only in account—we must examine what distinguishes it and how thinking may ever come about.

From the analogy between thinking and perception, it follows that the thinking part of the soul is nothing in actuality

So, if thinking is like perceiving, it should either be an affection of a certain kind by [429a13] the object of thinking or [15] something else like that. Therefore, it has to be impassive but able to receive the form, and the capacity for thinking has to relate in the same way to the objects of thinking as the perceptual capacity relates to the objects of perception. It must therefore, since it thinks all things, be without any admixture, as Anaxagoras says, "in order to rule," that is to say, in order to know; [20] for the clouding from an external admixture would be hindering and standing in the way. Thus it must have no nature of its own but this: to be capable. What therefore is called the thinking [part] of the soul—by "thinking [part]" I mean that by which the soul thinks and forms opinions—is not in actuality any of the things that are before it thinks.

Thinking must be separate from the body

This is why [25] it makes no good sense that it be mixed with the body, because then [429a24] it would become of a certain quality, either hot or cold, or there may even be an organ [for it], just as [there is an organ] for the perceptual capacity; but this is not the case.

And indeed, those who said that the soul is the place of forms were right—except [429a27] that it is not the soul as a whole but the thinking soul, and the forms are not in it in actuality, but in potentiality.

That the impassivity [30] of the perceptual capacity and that of the capacity for [429a29] thinking are not of the same sort is evident in the case of the sense-organs and

[429^{b}1] σθαι ἐκ τοῦ σφόδρα αἰσθητοῦ, οἷον ψόφου ἐκ τῶν μεγάλων ψόφων, οὐδ᾽ ἐκ τῶν ἰσχυρῶν χρωμάτων καὶ ὀσμῶν οὔτε ὁρᾶν οὔτε ὀσμᾶσθαι· ἀλλ᾽ ὁ νοῦς ὅταν τι νοήσῃ σφόδρα νοητόν, οὐχ ἧττον νοεῖ τὰ ὑποδεέστερα, ἀλλὰ καὶ μᾶλλον· τὸ μὲν γὰρ αἰσθητικὸν οὐκ ἄνευ σώματος, ὁ δὲ χωριστός.

[429^{b}5] ὅταν δ᾽ οὕτως ἕκαστα γένηται ὡς ὁ ἐπιστήμων λέγεται ὁ κατ᾽ ἐνέργειαν (τοῦτο δὲ συμβαίνει ὅταν δύνηται ἐνεργεῖν δι᾽ αὑτοῦ), ἔστι μὲν οὖν καὶ τότε δυνάμει πως, οὐ μὴν ὁμοίως καὶ πρὶν μαθεῖν ἢ εὑρεῖν· καὶ αὐτὸς δὲ αὑτὸν τότε δύναται νοεῖν.

[429^{b}10] ἐπεὶ δ᾽ ἄλλο ἐστὶ τὸ μέγεθος καὶ τὸ μεγέθει εἶναι καὶ ὕδωρ καὶ ὕδατι εἶναι, οὕτω δὲ καὶ ἐφ᾽ ἑτέρων πολλῶν, (ἀλλ᾽ οὐκ ἐπὶ πάντων· ἐπ᾽ ἐνίων γὰρ ταὐτόν ἐστι). τὸ σαρκὶ εἶναι καὶ σάρκα ἢ ἄλλῳ ἢ ἄλλως ἔχοντι κρίνει· ἡ γὰρ σὰρξ οὐκ ἄνευ τῆς ὕλης, ἀλλ᾽ ὥσπερ τὸ σιμόν, τόδε ἐν τῷδε. τῷ μὲν οὖν αἰσθητικῷ τὸ θερμὸν καὶ τὸ ψυχρὸν κρίνει, καὶ ὧν λόγος τις ἡ σάρξ· ἄλλῳ δέ, ἤτοι χωριστῷ ἢ ὡς ἡ κεκλασμένη ἔχει πρὸς αὑτὴν ὅταν ἐκταθῇ, τὸ σαρκὶ εἶναι κρίνει. πάλιν δ᾽ ἐπὶ τῶν ἐν ἀφαιρέσει ὄντων τὸ εὐθὺ ὡς τὸ σιμόν· μετὰ συνεχοῦς γάρ· τὸ δὲ τί ἦν εἶναι, εἰ ἔστιν ἕτερον τὸ εὐθεῖ εἶναι καὶ τὸ εὐθύ, ἄλλο· ἔστω γὰρ δυάς. ἑτέρῳ ἄρα ἢ ἑτέρως ἔχοντι κρίνει. ὅλως ἄρα ὡς χωριστὰ τὰ πράγματα τῆς ὕλης, οὕτω καὶ τὰ περὶ τὸν νοῦν.

[429^{b}22] ἀπορήσειε δ᾽ ἄν τις, εἰ ὁ νοῦς ἁπλοῦν ἐστι καὶ ἀπαθὲς καὶ μηθενὶ μηθὲν ἔχει κοινόν, ὥσπερ φησὶν Ἀναξαγόρας, πῶς νοήσει, εἰ τὸ

429^{b} **1** *ψόφου ἐκ* LW *So 125,1*: *τοῦ ψόφου ἐκ* **b**–W: *ἐκ τοῦ ψόφου* E *Th 104,34*   *τῶν μεγάλων* **o** *So 125,1*: *τοῦ μεγάλου* [*ἢ*] *τῶν μικρῶν Th 104,34*   **2** (*ἐκ*] *ἐπὶ* W)   **5** (*αἰσθητὸν* X)   (*ὁ δὲ*] sscr *νοῦς* W: *ὁ δὲ νοῦς* y)   **6** (*ἕκαστα*] sscr *ἑκάστῳ* V: ante *οὕτως* W)   *ὁ*$_{1}$ **a** CUVX *Si*^{l}: om S, [ins W^{2}]Wy *cf Theophr ap Prisc 31,8*   *ὁ*$_{2}$ **a** Cy *Si*^{l}: om SUVWX *cf Theophr ap Prisc 31,9* **7** (*ἑαυτοῦ Ph*^{l})   **8** (*ἔσται* V) *οὖν* LW *Theophr ap Prisc 31,10 Ph*^{l} *Th 95,16*: om **o**–LW *καὶ τότε* **a** W *Theophr ap Prisc 31,10*: *γὰρ καὶ τότε* y: *καὶ τότε ὁμοίως* C, ins *ὁμοίως* E^{2}: *ὁμοίως καὶ τότε* SUVX *Ph*^{l} *Th 95,16* *ὁμοίως* **a** CWy *Si*^{c}*230,8 Ph*$^{l\,p}$*524,27 Th 95,16*: om SUVX   (*καὶ*$_{2}$ om y)   *ἢ*] *καὶ Theophr ap Prisc 31,11*   **9** *δὲ αὐτὸν* **o**: *δι᾽ αὑτοῦ* Bywater Ross   **10** *τὸ*$_{1}$ **o**–Wy *Ph*^{l}: om W *Si*^{l} *Ph*^{c} *528,33*: *τό τε* y   (*τὸ*$_{2}$ om C, exp E^{2}: *τῷ* S)   **11** *ὕδωρ* **o** *Ph*^{l}: *τὸ ὕδωρ Si*^{l}*A Ph*^{c}*528,33*   *ὕδατι* **b** *Ph*^{l}: *τὸ ὕδατι* [*τὸ* exp E^{2}] **a** *Si*^{l} *Ph*^{c}*528,34* [*τῷ Dt*, sed *τὸ* ^{p}*528,37*]   (*εἶναι*] *ἐστιν* X)   (*οὕτω δὲ* om C: *δὲ* om V)   (*ἑτέρων δὲ πολλῶν* CV)   **12** *οὐκ* **o** *Si*^{l} *Th 96,5*: *οὐ καὶ Ph*^{l} (*γὰρ*] *μὲν γὰρ* W)   (*ταὐτὸ* E, *ν* ins E^{3})   **13** *ἢ*$_{1}$ **b**–y *Si*^{l} *Ph*^{l}: *καὶ ἢ* **a** [*καὶ* exp E^{2}]: *καὶ* y   *ἔχοντι* CWXy *Si*$^{l\,p}$*232,13 Ph*^{l} *Th 94,14 cf Ph 259,25 So 126,25*: om **a** SUV, ins E^{2} *κρίνει* **b**: *κρίνει ὁ νοῦς* **a** [exp *ὁ νοῦς* E^{2}, E^{3}] **14** (*σιμόν*] *σιμ-* in ras E^{3}: *σημεῖον* y, U [eras, in ras *σιμόν*])   (*τόδε* om V)   **15** *τὸ θερμὸν καὶ τὸ ψυχρὸν* **b**–V *Si*^{l} *Ph*^{l}: *τὸ θερμὸν καὶ ψυχρὸν* **a**: om V   (*καὶ*$_{2}$ om C, ins C^{3}: exp E^{2})   **16** (*ὁ λόγος* E)   (*δὲ* om V)   *ἡ*$_{2}$ **a** Cy *Si*^{c}*232,31 Ph*^{l}: om SUVWX   (*κεχωρισμένη* X)   **17** *αὑτὴν* SU, corr V^{2}: *ἑαυτὴν Si*^{c}*232,32 Ph*^{l}: *αὐτὴν* **o**–SU   (*εἶναι καὶ κρίνει* L)   **18** (*ἐν* om X)   **19** (*εἰ* om L)   (post *ἔστιν* ins *δ᾽* V^{2})   **20** (*τὸ*$_{1}$ in *τῷ* X^{x})   *ἄλλο* CSVX: *ἄλλῳ* **a** UW [sscr **o** W^{1}], y *Si*^{l} *Ph*^{l} **21** (*ἑτέρω* X)   *ὅλως* LCSUVX *Si*^{l} *Ph*^{c}*532,12*: *καὶ ὅλως* EWy   (*ἄρα* om E, ins E^{2})   **22** (*καὶ* corr ex *τε* V^{1} **23** (*ἁπλοῦν* corr *ν* in *σ* V^{x})   (*ἀπαθὴς* E, corr in -*ὲς* E^{3})   **24** *ἔχει* **a** CWy *Si*^{l}: *ἔχειν* X: *ἔχων* SUV   (*φασιν ὁ Ἀ.* X)   (*εἰ* … 25 *ἐστιν* om W, ins W^{2})

perception. For perception is unable to [429b1] perceive after an [affection by a] too intense object of perception—for instance, it is not able to hear a sound after a loud noise, or to see or smell after strong colors or smells—whereas the capacity for thinking is no less capable of thinking lesser objects whenever it thinks something highly intelligible, but rather even more [capable]. This [5] is due to the fact that the perceptual capacity is not without a body, whereas the capacity for thinking is separate.

The capacity of thinking as first actuality

When it [i.e., the capacity for thinking] becomes each [object of knowledge] in [429b5] such a way as the actual knower is said to be—this is the case when he is capable of being active by his own effort; and then it is still in potentiality in a way, not however in the same way as it was before learning or discovering; and then it is also capable of thinking itself.

Different types of objects of thought

Since magnitude and what it is to be a magnitude are not the same, and water and [429b10] what it is to be water, and so in many other cases (but not in all, since in some cases it is the same), one discriminates flesh and what it is to be flesh either with some other [capacity] or with [the same capacity] in a different state. For flesh does not exist without its matter, but is, like the snub, a this in a that. Now, [15] one discriminates the hot and the cold, and the qualities of which flesh is a given proportion, with the perceptual capacity; but one discriminates what it is to be flesh with something other, which is either separate [from perception] or with something [which is not separate from perception and] that stands in the same relation [to perception] as a bent line stands to itself when it has been straightened out. Again, in the case of objects that are by abstraction, the straight is like the snub, for it is connected to a continuum, whereas its essence, if what [20] it is to be straight is something other than the straight, is something else—say, the two. Therefore, one discriminates [it] with another [capacity] or with [the same capacity] in another state. On the whole, therefore, just as its objects are separate from matter, so also what pertains to thought.

Difficulties

Someone might raise a difficulty: if the capacity for thinking is simple and impas- [429b22] sive and has nothing in common with anything whatsoever, just as Anaxagoras

νοεῖν πάσχειν τί ἐστιν; ᾗ γάρ τι κοινὸν ἀμφοῖν ὑπάρχει, τὸ μὲν ποιεῖν δοκεῖ τὸ δὲ πάσχειν.

[429b26] ἔτι δ᾽ εἰ νοητὸς καὶ αὐτός, ἢ γὰρ τοῖς ἄλλοις νοῦς ὑπάρξει (εἰ μὴ κατ᾽ ἄλλο αὐτὸς νοητός, ἓν δέ τι τὸ νοητὸν εἴδει), ἢ μεμειγμένον τι ἕξει, ὃ ποιεῖ νοητὸν αὐτὸν ὥσπερ τἆλλα.

[429b29] ἢ τὸ μὲν πάσχειν κατὰ κοινόν τι διήρηται πρότερον, ὅτι δυνάμει πώς ἐστι τὰ νοητὰ ὁ νοῦς, ἀλλ᾽ ἐντελεχείᾳ οὐδέν, πρὶν ἂν νοῇ· δεῖ δ᾽ οὕτως ὥσ-
[430a1] περ ἐν γραμματείῳ ᾧ μηθὲν ὑπάρχει ἐντελεχείᾳ γεγραμμένον· ὅπερ συμβαίνει ἐπὶ τοῦ νοῦ.

[430a2] καὶ αὐτὸς δὲ νοητός ἐστιν ὥσπερ τὰ νοητά. ἐπὶ μὲν γὰρ τῶν ἄνευ ὕλης τὸ αὐτό ἐστι τὸ νοοῦν καὶ τὸ νοούμενον· ἡ γὰρ ἐπιστήμη ἡ θεωρητικὴ καὶ τὸ οὕτως ἐπιστητὸν τὸ αὐτό ἐστιν. τοῦ δὲ μὴ ἀεὶ νοεῖν τὸ αἴτιον ἐπισκεπτέον. ἐν δὲ τοῖς ἔχουσιν ὕλην δυνάμει ἕκαστον ἐστι τῶν νοητῶν. ὥστ᾽ ἐκείνοις μὲν οὐχ ὑπάρξει νοῦς (ἄνευ γὰρ ὕλης δύναμις ὁ νοῦς τῶν τοιούτων), ἐκείνῳ δὲ τὸ νοητὸν ὑπάρξει.

[430a10] Ἐπεὶ δ᾽ ὥσπερ ἐν ἁπάσῃ τῇ φύσει ἐστὶ τι τὸ μὲν ὕλη ἑκάστῳ γένει (τοῦτο δὲ ὃ πάντα δυνάμει ἐκεῖνα), ἕτερον δὲ τὸ αἴτιον καὶ ποιητικόν, τῷ ποιεῖν πάντα, οἷον ἡ τέχνη πρὸς τὴν ὕλην πέπονθεν, ἀνάγκη καὶ ἐν τῇ ψυχῇ ὑπάρχειν ταύτας τὰς διαφοράς· καὶ ἔστιν ὁ μὲν τοιοῦτος νοῦς τῷ πάντα γίνεσθαι, ὁ δὲ τῷ πάντα ποιεῖν, ὡς ἕξις τις, οἷον τὸ φῶς· τρόπον γάρ τινα καὶ τὸ φῶς ποιεῖ τὰ δυνάμει ὄντα χρώματα ἐνεργείᾳ χρώματα.

[430a17] καὶ οὗτος ὁ νοῦς χωριστὸς καὶ

25 ᾗ **o**–L *Si*^{l} *cf Ph*^{p}*532,24*: ἢ L: εἰ Ald *Ph*^{c}*532,23 Dt* **26** (δ᾽ om E, ins E^{2}) **27** γὰρ **o**–y *Ph*^{c}*532,34*: γὰρ καὶ y *Si*^{l} νοῦς **a**: ὁ νοῦς **b** *Si*^{l} *Ph*^{c}*532,34* ὁ αὐτὸς *Si*^{l} *A* **28** (τι$_{2}$] τῇ S) **29** (πάσχειν om V) **30** διήρηται LCUWXy *Si*^{lc}*236,10 Ph*^{l}: διείρηται SV, ut v E [corr ει in η E^{3}] **31** (οὐδὲν . . . 430a1 ἐντελεχείᾳ om L) ἂν C, ins E^{2} *Th 97,20*: ἄν μὴ SUVWy, [eras μὴ] X: om E *Si*^{l} ^{c}*236,17 Prisc 35,33* νοῇ **o**[–L] *Th 97,20*: νοεῖν *Si*^{l} ^{c}*236,17 Prisc 35,33* δεῖ δ᾽ **o**: δυνάμει Cornford Ross

430a **1** γραμματείῳ ᾧ W: γραμματείῳ ESUVXy, ut v C [ins C^{x}] *Si*^{l} ὑπάρχειν SUVXy, [eras ν] C *Si*^{l}: ὑπάρχει EW: ἐνυπάρχει Ross γεγραμμένον **b** *Si*^{l} *Th 97,22* καταγεγραμμένον **a** [κατα exp E^{2}] **2** (ὥσπερ S) (δὲ eras X) **3** (ἐστι καὶ τὸ y) **4** ἡ$_{2}$ **b** *Si*^{c}*237,24.31 Th 97,36 Prisc Lyd 36,26*: om **a** *Ph*^{c}*534,2* καὶ τὸ **o** *Si*^{c}*237,24.31 Th 97,36*: τὸ δὲ *Ph*^{c}*534,2* **5** ἐπιστητὸν LSUVWX, γρ. E^{3} *Si*^{c}*237,24.31 Ph*^{c}*534,2 Th 97,36*: ἐπιστον E, exp E^{2}: θεωρητικὸν Cy, ins E^{2} **6** δυνάμει **o**–y: δυνάμει μόνον y *Si*^{l} **7** ὑπάρξει **o**–V *cf Si*^{p}*239,4*: ὑπάρχει V *Si*^{l} *A* **8** δύναμις **a** *Si*^{l}: δύναμίς ἐστιν **b**, ins E^{3} ἐκεῖνο L: ἐκείνοις X [οις in ras X^{2}] *Si*^{l} *cf* ^{p}*239,29.31* (ἀνόητον y) **10** (δ᾽] δὴ W) ὥσπερ **o**: om *Th 98,12, Alex DA 88,17* Ross ἁπάσῃ **o**–Wy *Ph*^{l} ^{c}*539,13 Th 103,1 So 125,15*: πάσῃ Wy *Theophr ap Th 108,20 Si*^{l} *240,1* ἁπάσῃ τῇ φ.] πᾶσιν *Si*^{l} *241,17* τι **o**: om *So* Ross **11** ἑκάστῳ **o** *Ph*^{c}*539,14*: ἐν ἑκάστῳ *Si*^{l} *A So 125,15*: ἑκάστῳ τῷ *Ph*^{l} *D* ὃ **a** SUVW, corr C^{x} *Si*^{l} *Ph*^{l} ^{c}*539,14 So 125,15*: τὸ CX, corr E^{2}: τὸ ὃ y: ὅ τε *Ph*^{c}*539,14t* (ἐκεῖνο E, ο in α E^{3}) **12** ποιητικὸν **o**–LW *Si*^{l} *Ph*^{l}: τὸ ποιητικὸν LW τῷ ESUVWy *Si*^{l}: ὃ τῶ LC [τῶ ex τὸ], X [ὅτω], *Ph*^{l} (ἡ om V) **13** (πέπονθε πρὸς τὴν ὕλην S) **14** (τῷ] τὸ S) **16** (καὶ om V) (ὄντα om *Th 106,4*) **17** (ἐνεργεία ὄντα χρώματα W) (οὗτος corr ex οὕτως C^{x}V^{2}: οὐχ ὡς S)

says, how will it think, if [25] thinking consists in some kind of being affected? For it seems that it is insofar as there is something common to both that one thing acts and the other is acted upon.

Again, if the capacity for thinking is itself an object of thinking, then (granting [429b26] that it is not an object of thinking in virtue of some of something else, and that "object of thinking" is some one thing in kind) either thinking will belong to all other objects as well, or it will have something mixed with it, which will make it an object of thinking like any other.

Answer to the first difficulty: the writing tablet

Or is it rather that we have previously made a distinction about "being acted upon [429b29] in virtue of something common"—namely, that the capacity for thinking is potentially in some way the objects of thought, but it is none of them in actuality before it thinks? [430a1] It must be just as on a writing tablet, in which nothing is written in actuality, which is exactly what happens in the case of the capacity for thinking.

Answer to the second difficulty: asymmetrical identity

And it [i.e., thinking] is also itself an object of thinking just like the [other] objects [430a2] of thinking. That is to say: in the case of objects without matter, that which thinks and that which is thought are identical, because theoretical knowledge is [5] identical with what is known in this way. (We will have to inquire into the reason why it does not always think.) In [the domain of] things that have matter, however, each thing is [only] potentially an object of thinking; so that the capacity for thinking will not belong to them (for the capacity for thinking is a capacity for such objects without matter), but it will belong to it [i.e., to the capacity for thinking] to be an object of thinking.

There must be a productive principle of thinking

Since, just as in all nature, there is something which is matter for each kind of ob- [430a10] ject (this is what is potentially all these things) and something else which is the cause and producer because it makes them all, as art stands in relation to its material, it is necessary that there be these different [factors] in the soul as well: and there is one such kind of thinking on account of becoming [15] all things and another [such kind of thinking] on account of making all things, like a state, as light does: for in a way light makes potential colors colors in actuality.

ἀπαθὴς καὶ ἀμιγής, τῇ οὐσίᾳ ὢν ἐνέργεια. ἀεὶ γὰρ τιμιώτερον τὸ ποιοῦν τοῦ πάσχοντος καὶ ἡ ἀρχὴ τῆς ὕλης. τὸ δ' αὐτό ἐστιν ἡ κατ' ἐνέργειαν ἐπιστήμη τῷ πράγματι (ἡ δὲ κατὰ δύναμιν χρόνῳ προτέρα ἐν τῷ ἑνί, ὅλως δὲ οὐδὲ χρόνῳ), ἀλλ' οὐχ ὁτὲ μὲν νοεῖ ὁτὲ δ' οὐ νοεῖ. χωρισθεὶς δ' ἐστὶ μόνον τοῦθ' ὅπερ ἐστί, καὶ τοῦτο μόνον ἀθάνατον καὶ ἀΐδιον. οὐ μνημονεύομεν δέ, ὅτι τοῦτο μὲν ἀπαθές, ὁ δὲ παθητικὸς νοῦς φθαρτός· καὶ ἄνευ τούτου οὐθὲν νοεῖ.

18 *ἀπαθὴς καὶ ἀμιγής* **a** *Si*^{l} ^{p}*243,14 Si*^{c} *in de coelo 279,21 Th 99,35; 105,5*: *ἀμιγὴς καὶ ἀπαθὴς* **b** *Ph*^{l} ^{p}*540,4 So 125,22* (*ὢν*] *ὡς ὢν* y) *ἐνέργεια* Uy, corr C^{x} *Theophr ap Prisc 28,12; 29,25 Si*^{c} *in phys 1162,3A Si*^{l} ^{c}*243,37* ^{p}*245,21; 248,12 Si*^{c} *in de coelo 279.22 So 125,23A cf Ph*^{p}*534,24*: *ἐνεργείᾳ* **o**–Uy *Ph*^{l} ^{c}*540,6 Th 106,5 So 125,23BC* **19** (*τὸ δ' αὐτὸ . . .* 22 *οὐ νοεῖ* suspexit Ross) *τὸ δ' αὐτὸ* **a** *So 125,24*: *τὸ αὐτὸ δ'* CUVWXy *Ph*^{l}: *αὐτὸ δ'* S: *ἡ αὐτὴ δὲ Si*^{l} **21** *οὐδὲ* **b** ins *δὲ* E^{2}W *Si*^{l} *So 125,25*: *οὐ* **a** *Ph*^{c}*540,30*: *οὐδὲ ἐν Th*^{c}*101,23.28* **22** *οὐχ* **o**–Wy *Ph*^{p}*540,21 Th*^{c} *101,24* ^{p}*99,35 Alex Plotinus Marinus ap Ph 535,26.29.33*: om Wy *γρ.* mg U^{x} *Si*^{l} ^{p}*245,34* ^{c}*263,8 Plutarchus ap Ph 535,13 So 125,26* (*ὅτε δ' οὐ νοεῖ* W) (*ἐστὶ* om V: post *μόνον* W) **23** (*ἀΐδιον καὶ ἀθάνατον* W) **25** (*οὐδὲ* X)

On the nature of the productive principle of thinking

And this kind of thinking is separate, unaffected, and unmixed, it being an actuality by its essence. [430a17] For that which acts is always more valuable than what is acted upon, and the principle is more valuable than the matter. Actual knowledge is identical with its object, and potential knowledge is prior in time in the individual, however, on the whole [it is] not even [prior] in time; but it is not at one time thinking and at another time not thinking.

When it is separated, it is only what it really is, and this alone is immortal and [430a22] eternal. But we do not remember, because this is unaffected, whereas passive thinking is corruptible; and without the latter, it does not think anything.

DE ANIMA III 6

[430^{a}26] Ἡ μὲν οὖν τῶν ἀδιαιρέτων νόησις ἐν τούτοις, περὶ ἃ οὐκ ἔστι τὸ ψεῦδος. ἐν οἷς δὲ καὶ τὸ ψεῦδος καὶ τὸ ἀληθές, σύνθεσίς τις ἤδη νοημάτων ὥσπερ ἓν ὄντων, καθάπερ Ἐμπεδοκλῆς ἔφη "ῇ πολλῶν μὲν κόρσαι ἀναύχενες ἐβλάστησαν," ἔπειτα συντίθεσθαι τῇ φιλίᾳ, οὕτω καὶ ταῦτα κεχωρισμένα συντίθεται, οἷον τὸ ἀσύμμετρον καὶ ἡ διάμετρος· ἂν δὲ γενο-
[430^{b}1] μένων ἢ ἐσομένων, τὸν χρόνον προσεννοῶν καὶ συντιθείς. τὸ γὰρ ψεῦδος ἐν συνθέσει ἀεί· καὶ γὰρ ἂν τὸ λευκὸν μὴ λευκὸν τὸ μὴ λευκὸν συνέθηκεν· ἐνδέχεται δὲ καὶ διαίρεσιν φάναι πάντα. ἀλλ' οὖν ἔστι γε οὐ μόνον τὸ ψεῦδος ἢ ἀληθές, ὅτι λευκὸς Κλέων ἐστίν, ἀλλὰ καὶ ὅτι ἦν ἢ ἔσται. τὸ δὲ ἓν ποιοῦν, τοῦτο ὁ νοῦς ἕκαστον.

[430^{b}6] τὸ δ' ἀδιαίρετον ἐπεὶ διχῶς, ἢ δυνάμει ἢ ἐνεργείᾳ, οὐθὲν κωλύει νοεῖν τὸ ἀδιαίρετον, ὅταν νοῇ τὸ μῆκος (ἀδιαίρετον γὰρ ἐνεργείᾳ), καὶ ἐν χρόνῳ ἀδιαιρέτῳ· ὁμοίως γὰρ ὁ χρόνος διαιρετὸς καὶ ἀδιαίρετος τῷ μήκει. οὔκουν ἔστιν εἰπεῖν ἐν τῷ ἡμίσει τί ἐννοεῖ ἑκατέρῳ· οὐ γὰρ ἔστιν, ἂν μὴ διαιρεθῇ, ἀλλ' ἢ δυνάμει. χωρὶς δ' ἑκάτερον νοῶν τῶν ἡμίσεων διαιρεῖ καὶ τὸν χρόνον ἅμα· τότε δ' οἱονεὶ μήκη. εἰ δ' ὡς ἐξ ἀμφοῖν, καὶ ἐν τῷ χρόνῳ τῷ ἐπ' ἀμφοῖν.

[430^{b}14] τὸ δὲ μὴ κατὰ τὸ ποσὸν ἀδιαίρετον ἀλλὰ τῷ εἴδει νοεῖ ἐν ἀδιαιρέτῳ χρόνῳ καὶ ἀδιαιρέτῳ τῆς ψυχῆς·

430^a **27** *καὶ*$_1$ om W *Si^l*   *καὶ*$_2$ L *Si^l*: *ἤδη καὶ* **b** *cf Th 109,8*   (*σύνεσις* L: *συνθεμένων* W)   **28** (*τις*] *τε τις* V: om W)   *ἤδη τῶν ν.* L W *Si^l A Dexippus^c in categ 9,27*   **29** (*ἢ* LUX) **30** *συντίθεσθαι* **o**: *συντεθεῖσαι* *Si^{c}250,24*   **31** *συντίθεται* LUX: *συντίθεσθαι* CSVWy post *διάμετρος* add *ἢ τὸ σύμμετρον καὶ ἡ διάμετρος* W *Si^{c}250,25* *ἐὰν* W *Si^l ^{c}250,34 Ph^l*   *γενομένων* **o** *Si^{c}250,34 Ph^l Th 109,19*: *γινομένων* *Si^{l}A*

430^b **1** (*τῶν χρόνων* X)   (*πρὸς ἓν νοῶν* L X *Ph^l*)   *καὶ συντιθείς* **o**: *συντίθησι* Torstrik Ross   **2** (*ἀεὶ* om X)   **3** post *λευκὸν*$_1$ ins *φῇ τὸ λευκὸν καὶ* Ross   **4** *τὸ* om L W   **5** (*ἔσται*] *ἐστί* X)   *δὲ* **o**–WX *Si^l*: *δὴ* WX corr U^2 *Ph^l*   **6** (*τούτων* W)   *ποιοῦν τοῦτο ὁ νοῦς ἕκαστον* **o**: *ποιοῦν ἕκαστον τοῦτο ὁ νοῦς* Ross   *ἢ* L CVWy *Si^l*   *(bis) ^{p}251,33 Ph^l*: *ἢ τὸ* SUX **7** post *τὸ* ins *διαιρετὸν ᾗ* Ross   post *ἀδιαίρετον* ins *οἷον* Ross   **9** *καὶ ἀδιαίρετος* **o**–WX *Si^l ^{c}253,22 Ph^l ^{p}549,24 Th 110,9*: om WX, suppl W^2 **10** *ἐννοεῖ* SUVX *Si^l ^{p}253,31 Ph^l*: *ἐνόει* LCWy **12** *τῶν ἡμίσεων* LVW *Si^l Ph^l*: ante *ἑκάτερον* SU: om CXy   (*τόδε* X)   **13** *μήκη* UXy corr L^1 W^x *Si^l ^{c}253,39*: *μήκει* L CSVW [sscr *η* V^1] *Ph^{c}550,12.13*   *ὡς* LCVWy *Si^l*: om SUX [ins X^3] *ἐν* LSUXy *Si^l Ph^{p}550,10*: om CVW   (*τῷ*$_2$] *τὸ* U)   **14** (*τὸ δὲ . . . 15 ψυχῆς* ad l.20 post *μήκει* transp. Bywater Ross)   *ποσὸν* **b**–X *Si^l Ph^l*: *τὸ ποσὸν* L X   **15** (*διαιρετῷ* X)   *ψυχῆς* **o**–V *Si^l ^{c}254,28 cf Ph^{p}550,20*: *ψυχῆς νοήσει* V, ins *νοήσει* C^2 *Th 110,19*

DE ANIMA III 6

Truth and falsity are found in synthetic thinking, not in the thinking of *adiaireta*

Now thinking of objects without division occurs in cases where falsity is not possible. [430a26]
But in those [cases] where both falsity and truth [can be found], [what occurs] is already a certain combination of thoughts as being one—just as Empedocles said "from it [i.e., the earth] many faces sprouted without necks," [30] and [said that] they were then combined by Love, so too these separated [thoughts] are combined; for instance, the incommensurable and the diagonal. And whenever [thinking] is concerned with what has [430b1] been or will be, [one] adds the thought of time and combines it [with the rest]. For falsity is always found in a combination; indeed, even when [one thinks that] a white thing is not white, [one] has combined the not white [with it]. It is also possible, though, to say that all these are instances of division. In any case, false or true is surely not only [the thought] [5] that Cleon is white, but also that he was or will be. And what produces the unity is in each case the capacity for thinking.

Different kinds of *adiaireta*

in quantity

Since there are two ways of being without division—either [without] potential [430b6]
[division] or [without] actual [division]—nothing prevents [one] from thinking an object without division whenever one thinks a length (for it is without actual division), and in a time without division, since the time is divisible and without division in the same way as the [10] length. Accordingly, it is not possible to say what [one] is thinking in each half [of the time], since, as long as the whole has not been divided, there are no parts except in potentiality. And if [one] thinks each of the halves separately, [one] thereby divides the time, too, but then [one thinks] as it were [two] lengths. And if [one thinks the length] as made up of both halves, [one thinks it] also in a time [made up of times] corresponding to both halves.

in form

As for that which is without division not in terms of quantity but of [15] form, [one] [430b14]
thinks it in a time without division and by something without division on the side

κατὰ συμβεβηκὸς δέ, καὶ οὐχ ᾗ ἐκεῖνα, διαιρετὰ ᾧ νοεῖ καὶ ἐν ᾧ χρόνῳ ἀλλ' ᾗ ἀδιαίρετα· ἔνεστι γὰρ κἀν τούτοις τι ἀδιαίρετον, ἀλλ' ἴσως οὐ χωριστόν, ὃ ποιεῖ ἕνα τὸν χρόνον καὶ τὸ μῆκος. καὶ τοῦθ' ὁμοίως ἐν ἅπαντί ἐστι τῷ συνεχεῖ καὶ χρόνῳ καὶ μήκει.

[430^{b}20] *ἡ δὲ στιγμὴ καὶ πᾶσα διαίρεσις, καὶ τὸ οὕτως ἀδιαίρετον, δηλοῦται ὥσπερ ἡ στέρησις. καὶ ὅμοιος ὁ λόγος ἐπὶ τῶν ἄλλων, οἷον πῶς τὸ κακὸν γνωρίζει ἢ τὸ μέλαν. τῷ ἐναντίῳ γάρ πως γνωρίζει. δεῖ δὲ δυνάμει εἶναι τὸ γνωρίζον καὶ ἓν εἶναι ἐν αὐτῷ.*

[430^{b}24] *εἰ δέ τινι μὴ ἐστιν ἐναντίον τῶν αἰτίων, αὐτὸ ἑαυτὸ γινώσκει καὶ ἐνεργείᾳ ἐστὶ καὶ χωριστόν.*

[430^{b}26] *ἔστι δ' ἡ μὲν φάσις τι κατά τινος, ὥσπερ ἡ κατάφασις, καὶ ἀληθὴς ἢ ψευδὴς πᾶσα· ὁ δὲ νοῦς οὐ πᾶς, ἀλλ' ὁ τοῦ τί ἐστι κατὰ τὸ τί ἦν εἶναι ἀληθής, καὶ οὐ τὶ κατά τινος· ἀλλ' ὥσπερ τὸ ὁρᾶν τοῦ ἰδίου ἀληθές, εἰ δ' ἄνθρωπος τὸ λευκὸν ἢ μή, οὐκ ἀληθὲς ἀεί, οὕτως ἔχει ὅσα ἄνευ ὕλης.*

16 *ᾧ*] *ὃ* Vicomercatus Ross **17** *ἀλλ' ᾗ ἀδ.* del Torstrik Förster, legit *Si*^{l} ^{c}*255,34* (*ἢ* X) post *ᾗ* ins *ἐκεῖνα* Ross (*ἔνεστι γὰρ* om X: *ἔστι γὰρ ἐν Si*^{l}) **18** (*ποιεῖ καὶ ἕνα* W) **19** (*ἐν*] *ὂν Si*^{l}*A*) (*παντὶ* W *Si*^{l}*A*) (*τῷ* om *Si*^{l}*A*) **21** (*οὕτως*] *οὔτε* V) **22** (*πῶς καὶ τὸ* W) **24** (*γνωρίζειν* V) *ἓν εἶναι* LX *Ph*^{c}*552,28 Dt*: *ἐνεῖναι* **b**-X *Si*^{lc}*257,26 cf Ph*^{p}*553,4* Förster Ross (*ἐν* om W) *μὴ* **o**: *μηδὲν* Ross **25** *τῶν αἰτίων* **o**-S: *τῶν ἐναντίων* S: *τῶν ὄντων* Torstrik: om Zeller Ross *αὐτὸ ἑαυτὸ* CVXy: *αὐτὸ αὑτὸ* LU: *αὐτὸ αὐτῶ* S: *ὦ τὸ αὐτὸ* W *ἐνεργείᾳ* **o**: *ἐνέργεια* fort *Si*^{p}*258,27.31 Th 112,3* Ross **26** (*ἔτι δ' ἔστιν ἡ* y) (*τις* L) (*ὥσπερ καὶ ἡ* W Torstrik Ross) **27** *κατάφασις* **o**: *ἀπόφασις* Torstrik Ross (*ἢ*] *καὶ* L) **28** (*ἐστιν ἢ κατὰ* X) (*τὶ*$_{3}$ eras X^{2}) **29** (*τοῦ ἰδίου* in *τὸ δί* corr C, *τὸ δὶ* V) **30** *οὕτως* **o** *cf Ph*^{p}*557,9*: *οὕτως δὲ Si*^{l} *A Ph*^{l} *D* (*ὅσα* om W, sscr W^{2}) **31** *ἄνευ τῆς ὕλης* V *Ph*^{l}

of the soul. And that by which one thinks it and the time in which one thinks it are divisible accidentally: not in the way in which the others [i.e., *adiaireta* in quantity are divisible], but in the way in which [the others are] without division. For, in them too there is something without division, but presumably not separable, which makes the time and the length one; and this is similar for every continuous thing, both time and length.

geometrical divisions

A point and every division—that is, all that which is without division in this way— **[430b20]**
is made known just as a privation is. And the same account applies to other cases, such as how one cognizes the bad or the black. For one cognizes it somehow by its opposite. And that which cognizes needs to be in potentiality [with respect to both] and [the two] must be one in it.

causes without opposites

But if any of the causes is such that it has nothing opposite to it, then it cognizes **[430b24]**
itself and is [by itself] in actuality and separate.

Thinking of essences is always true

A statement is [predicating] one thing of another, just as is the case with an affirm- **[430b26]**
ation, and it is in all cases true or false. But this is not so with all thought; rather, the thought of what [something] is in virtue of [its] essence is [always] true, and it is not [predicating] one thing of another. Rather, just as seeing is [always] true with respect to its exclusive object, but it is not always true when it comes to whether the white thing is a human being or not, so it is with whatever is without matter.

DE ANIMA III 7

[431a1] Τὸ δ᾽ αὐτό ἐστιν ἡ κατ᾽ ἐνέργειαν ἐπιστήμη τῷ πράγματι. ἡ δὲ κατὰ δύναμιν χρόνῳ προτέρα ἐν τῷ ἑνί, ὅλως δὲ οὐδὲ χρόνῳ· ἔστι γὰρ ἐξ ἐντελεχείᾳ ὄντος πάντα τὰ γιγνόμενα. φαίνεται δὲ τὸ μὲν αἰσθητὸν ἐκ δυνάμει ὄντος τοῦ αἰσθητικοῦ ἐνεργείᾳ ποιοῦν· οὐ γὰρ πάσχει οὐδ᾽ ἀλλοιοῦται. διὸ ἄλλο εἶδος τοῦτο κινήσεως· ἡ γὰρ κίνησις τοῦ ἀτελοῦς ἐνέργεια, ἡ δ᾽ ἁπλῶς ἐνέργεια ἑτέρα ἡ τοῦ τετελεσμένου.

[431a8] τὸ μὲν οὖν αἰσθάνεσθαι ὅμοιον τῷ φάναι μόνον καὶ νοεῖν· ὅταν δὲ ἡδὺ ἢ λυπηρόν, οἷον καταφᾶσα ἢ ἀποφᾶσα διώκει ἢ φεύγει· καὶ ἔστι τὸ ἥδεσθαι καὶ λυπεῖσθαι τὸ ἐνεργεῖν τῇ αἰσθητικῇ μεσότητι πρὸς τὸ ἀγαθὸν ἢ κακόν, ᾗ τοιαῦτα. καὶ ἡ φυγὴ δὲ καὶ ἡ ὄρεξις ταὐτό ἡ κατ᾽ ἐνέργειαν, καὶ οὐχ ἕτερον τὸ ὀρεκτικὸν καὶ φευκτικόν, οὔτ᾽ ἀλλήλων οὔτε τοῦ αἰσθητικοῦ· ἀλλὰ τὸ εἶναι ἄλλο.

[431a14] τῇ δὲ διανοητικῇ ψυχῇ τὰ φαντάσματα οἷον αἰσθήματα ὑπάρχει, ὅταν δὲ ἀγαθὸν ἢ κακόν, κατάφησιν ἢ ἀπόφησιν καὶ φεύγει ἢ διώκει· διὸ οὐδέποτε νοεῖ ἄνευ φαντάσματος ἡ ψυχή.

[431a17] ὡς δὲ ὁ ἀὴρ τὴν κόρην τοιανδὶ ἐποίησεν, αὕτη δ᾽ ἕτερον, καὶ ἡ ἀκοὴ ὡσαύτως, τὸ δὲ ἔσχατον ἕν, καὶ μία μεσότης, τὸ δ᾽ εἶναι αὐτῇ πλείω. τίνι δ᾽ ἐπικρίνει τί διαφέρει γλυκὺ καὶ θερμόν, εἴρηται μὲν καὶ πρότερον, λεκτέον δὲ καὶ ὧδε. ἔστι γὰρ ἕν

431a **1** δ᾽ *αὐτὸ* LW: *αὐτὸ* δ᾽ CUVXy *Si*^{l} *Ph*^{l}: δ᾽ *αὐτὸ* δ᾽ S **2** (*ποτέρα* U) (*ἔνι ὧ ἔνι* CV) *ὅλως* **o** *Si*^{l} *Ph*^{l} ^{c}*557,27 So 128,34*: *ἁπλῶς Ph*^{v}*557,27* **3** (*ἐντελεχείας* WXy) (*ὄντως* X, [corr in -*ος*] y) **4** *αἰσθητὸν* LCUWy *Ph*^{l} *Th 28,35*: *αἰσθητήριον* SVX *γρ.* mgC^{1}: *αἰσθητικὸν Si*^{l} *A* (*ἐν* X) **6** *εἶδος τοῦτο κινήσεως* L *Si*^{l} *cf* ^{p}*265,6*: *τοῦτο εἶδος κινήσεως* CUVy *Th 28,36*: *τοῦτο κινήσεως* SX [ins *εἶδος* X^{3}] **7** *ἐνέργεια*$_{1}$ LSUX *Si*^{l} ^{c}*265,12 Th 28,37*: *ἐνεργεία* S: *ἐνέργεια ἦν* CVWy (*ἑτέρου Si*^{l} *A*) *ἡ*$_{2}$ **b**–X *Si*^{p}*265,15 Th 29,1*: *ἢ* X: om L *Si*^{l} *A* post *τετελεσμένου* lacunam esse iudicat Susemihl **8** *τῷ* **o**–X *Si*^{l}: *τὸ* X *Ph*^{l} *D* **10** (*ἀποφεύγει* C) *καὶ*$_{2}$ LSX: *ἢ* CUVWy *Si*^{l} ^{c}*266,9* **11** (post *ἀγαθὸν* eras *ᾗ ἀγαθὸν* X) (*ἢ κακὸν* om CS, suppl mg C^{2}) *ᾗ τοιαῦτα* CSUWy *Ph*^{c}*559,10*: *ᾗ τοιαῦται* V: *ᾗ τοιούτου* L: om X: *ἢ τὰ τοιαῦτα Si*^{l} ^{c}*266,10.15* **12** *ἡ*$_{1}$ et *ἡ*$_{2}$ **b**–W: om LW *Si*^{l} *cf Ph*^{l} *D* *δὲ* L W *Ph*^{l}: *δὴ* SUX *Si*^{l}: om CVy *τὸ αὐτὸ* LV, [in ras] X: *ταὐτὸν* C *Si*^{l}: *τοῦτο* SUWy *Ph*^{l} (*ἡ*$_{3}$ om V secl Rodier) **13** (*τὸ*] *τι* V) *φευκτικόν* **b**: *τὸ φ.* L *Si*^{l} ^{p}*266,37 Th 113,27* **14** *δὲ* **o**–S *Si*^{l} *Th 113,14*: *δὴ* S *Ph*^{l} **16** (*κακόν ἐστι* SV) *κατάφησιν ἢ ἀπόφησιν* SUV *Si*^{l}, corr bis in -*φήσειν* S^{2}: *φησὶν ἢ ἀπόφησι* CX: *φήσῃ ἢ ἀποφήσῃ* L: *καταφήσῃ ἢ ἀποφήσῃ* y: *κατάφασις ἢ ἀπόφασις* W *cf Ph*^{p}*559,31 Th 113,18* *καὶ* **b** *Si*^{l}: om L **17** *φαντάσματος* **o** *cf Th 113,20*: *φαντασίας Si*^{l} ^{c}*267,30 cf Ph 560,1* *ὥσπερ* **o** *Si*^{l} ^{c}*269,19.28 Ph*^{l} ^{p}*560,9 So 138,5* *ὡς* scripsit Förster **18** *αὕτη* LSUVXy *Si*^{c} *269,20; 270,17 So 138,6*: *αὐτὴ* CW *Si*^{l} *A* **19** (post *ἓν* add *φεύγει ἢ διώκει* y) *μεσότης* **o**: *ἡ μεσότης* Ross *αὐτῇ* LCWy *Si*^{l}: om SUVX [ins X^{x}] **20** (*τὸ γλυκὺ Si*^{l} *A*) post *πλείω* lacunam esse iudicat Ross **21** (*καὶ*$_{1}$ om W) (*καὶ*$_{2}$ om y) *ὧδε* LSUVX *Si*^{l}: *νῦν* CWy, *cf Si*^{p}*271,2 Ph*^{p}*560,20*

DE ANIMA III 7

The Priority of the Actual: Thought and perception actualized by their objects

Actual knowledge is one and the same with its object, while potential knowledge [431a1] is prior in time in an individual, but generally speaking it is not prior even in time, since it is from something in actuality that everything comes to be. But at least [in the case of the perceptual capacity] it is clear that the object of perception brings the perceptual capacity from being in potentiality to being in actuality, since [the object of perception] is not affected or altered. That is why this is another kind [of actuality] from change: change is actuality of that which is incomplete, whereas unqualified actuality, the actuality of that which is complete, is something else.

Expansion of perception (for action)

Perceiving is similar, then, to mere saying and thinking; and whenever [perception] is pleasant or painful, [the soul] pursues or avoids as if affirming or negating. [431a8] And feeling pleasure or pain is being active with the perceptual mean in relation to the good or bad insofar as they are such. And avoidance and pursuit in actuality are the same thing, and the capacity to pursue and the capacity to avoid do not differ either from one another or from the perceptual capacity, but their being is different.

Ground for the expansion of thought: images

Phantasmata belong to the rational soul like percepts, and whenever [the objects represented by the *phantasmata*] are good or bad, [the soul] affirms or negates, and pursues or avoids. That is why the soul never thinks without an image. [431a14]

Ground for the expansion of perception: a single mean different in being

Just as the air makes the eye-jelly such and such, and this something else, the same [431a17] also hold in the case of hearing. But the end point is one, and [there is] also a single mean, though its being is more than one. That by which [the soul] discriminates upon how sweet and hot differ was established earlier, but it is to be stated

τι, οὕτω δὲ ὡς ὁ ὅρος. καὶ ταῦτα ἓν τῷ ἀνάλογον καὶ τῷ ἀριθμῷ ὄν, ἔχει πρὸς ἑκάτερον, ὡς ἐκεῖνα πρὸς ἄλληλα· τί γὰρ διαφέρει τὸ ἀπορεῖν πῶς τὰ μὴ ὁμογενῆ κρίνει ἢ τὰ ἐναντία, οἷον λευκὸν καὶ μέλαν; ἔστω δὴ ὡς τὸ Α τὸ λευκὸν πρὸς τὸ Β τὸ μέλαν, τὸ Γ πρὸς τὸ Δ [ὡς ἐκεῖνα πρὸς ἄλληλα]· ὥστε καὶ ἐναλλάξ. εἰ δὴ τὰ ΓΔ ἑνὶ εἴη ὑπάρχοντα, οὕτως ἕξει ὥσπερ καὶ τὰ ΑΒ, τὸ αὐτὸ μὲν καὶ ἕν, τὸ δ' εἶναι οὐ τὸ αὐτό, κἀκεῖνο ὁμοίως. ὁ δ' αὐτὸς
[431^{b}1] λόγος καὶ εἰ τὸ μὲν Α τὸ γλυκὺ εἴη, τὸ δὲ Β τὸ λευκόν.

[431^{b}2] τὰ μὲν οὖν εἴδη τὸ νοητικὸν ἐν τοῖς φαντάσμασι νοεῖ, καὶ ὡς ἐν ἐκείνοις ὥρισται αὐτῷ τὸ διωκτὸν καὶ φευκτόν, καὶ ἐκτὸς τῆς αἰσθήσεως, ὅταν ἐπὶ τῶν φαντασμάτων ᾖ, κινεῖται. οἷον αἰσθανόμενος τὸν φρυκτὸν ὅτι πῦρ, τῇ κοινῇ γνωρίζει, ὁρῶν κινούμενον, ὅτι πολέμιος· ὅτε δὲ τοῖς ἐν τῇ ψυχῇ φαντάσμασιν ἢ νοήμασιν, ὥσπερ ὁρῶν, λογίζεται καὶ βουλεύεται τὰ μέλλοντα πρὸς τὰ παρόντα· καὶ ὅταν εἴπῃ ὡς ἐκεῖ τὸ ἡδὺ ἢ λυπηρόν, ἐνταῦθα φεύγει ἢ διώκει, καὶ ὅλως ἐν πράξει. καὶ τὸ ἄνευ δὲ πράξεως, τὸ ἀληθὲς καὶ τὸ ψεῦδος, ἐν τῷ αὐτῷ γένει ἐστὶ τῷ ἀγαθῷ καὶ τῷ κακῷ· ἀλλὰ τῷ γε ἁπλῶς διαφέρει καὶ τινί.

[431^{b}12] τὰ δὲ ἐν ἀφαιρέσει λεγόμενα νοεῖ ὥσπερ ἂν εἰ τὸ σιμόν, ᾗ μὲν σιμόν, οὐ κεχωρισμένως, ᾗ δὲ κοῖλον, εἴ τις ἐνόει ἐνεργείᾳ, ἄνευ

22 ὡς ὁ SUV: καὶ ὁ CXy: ἡ στιγμὴ καὶ ὁ W, ins ἡ στιγμὴ mgC^{2}: καὶ L: «ὥσπερ ὁ» *Ph^{p}560,25*: «ὥσπερ καὶ ὁ» *Si^{p}271,6* ἓν CUWy *Si^{l} ^{p}271,14; 272,7 Ph^{l} ^{p}560,31*: ἐν LSVX καὶ τῷ C *cf Ph^{p}560,26*: ἢ τῶ L y: ἢ UVWX *Si^{l} ^{c}271,14 Ph^{l}*: om S **23** ὄν *Si^{l} ^{c}271,14*: ὄν **o** *Ph^{l}* ὄντα Ross post ἔχει ins ἑκάτερον Ross ἑκάτερον **o**–X *Ph^{l}*: ἑκάτερα X sscr W^{1} *Si^{l} ^{c}271,15.38* ὡς **o** *Ph^{l}*: ᾗ *Si^{l} ^{c}271,15* **24** (διαπορεῖν W *Ph^{l}*) (πῶς om X, ins X^{3}) μὴ LSUVX *Si^{l} Ph^{lp}561,5 So138,25*: om CWy *Si^{p}272,3.7.21* **25** (ὡς ἐν τῶ y) A....B....etc.] πρῶτον...δεύτερον...etc. *Ph^{c}561,9.10* **26** πρὸς LUWXy *Ph^{c}561,9*: καὶ CSV, del et ins πρὸς C^{2} (πρὸς]$_{2}$ ἀέρος X$_{1}$ sscr πρὸς X^{3}) ὡς ... 27 ἄλληλα del Christ qua interpolata ex ^{b}23-24, secl. Rodier Förster Ross **27** (ὥστε] οὕτως W) τὰ LCWy: om SUVX, ins U^{2} ΓΔ **o**: ΓΑ Ross ἑνὶ **o**–Cy: ἐν Cy **28** (οὕτως] καὶ C) (ἕξει ex ἔχει y^{1}) τὰ LW corr U^{2}: τὸ CSUVXy AB **o**: ΔΒ Ross **29** καὶ ἕν LCWy *Ph^{c}561,18*: καὶ S: om UVX δ'$_{1}$ LCVWy *Ph^{c}561,18*: post εἶναι SU: om X (κακεῖνος C, ς eras: κἀκεῖνα Pacius Ross)

431^{b} 1 καὶ LCWy: κἂν SUVX *Si^{c}272,28* τὸ μὲν LCWy: μὲν τὸ SUVX: τὸ *Si^{c}272,28* (τὸ$_{2}$ et τὸ$_{4}$ om W) **3** (ἐν om y) ὥρισται LCWy *Si^{l}*: ὥριστο UVX corr S *Si^{c}273,35* (αὐτῶ C: αὐτὸ y, sscr ω y^{1}) **4** αἰσθήσεως L *Si^{l}*: αἰσθήσεως ὂν CSUVX: αἰσθήσεως ὢν Wy (ἢ X) **5** (κινεῖται corr in κινῆται X^{2}) φρυκτὸν **o** *Si^{l} ^{c}274,15 Ph^{c}561,31 Th 114,1Q^{3}*: φευκτὸν *Th 114,1* vulg (κοινῇ] κόρῃ ut v X, -ει X^{2}) τῇ κοινῇ γνωρίζει ὁρῶν κινούμενον **o**: τῇ κοινῇ ὁρῶν κινούμενον γνωρίζει *Si^{c} 274,15-17* Ross **6** ὅτε LC: ὁτὲ **b**–C *Si^{l} Ph^{l}* τοῖς ἐν **o** *Ph^{l}*: ἐν τοῖς ἐν *Si^{l}* **8** βουλεύεται LCWXy *Si^{l}*: βούλεται SUV **9** ἡδὺ ἢ λυπηρὸν **b**–W *Si^{l}*: ἡδὺ ἢ τὸ λυπηρόν L: λυπηρὸν ἢ ἡδὺ W (καὶ ἐνταῦθα y) **10** ἐν **o**: ἓν Ross τὸ$_{2}$] καὶ τὸ y *Si^{l}A* **11** (τὸ om L) καὶ$_{2}$ CSVy *Si^{l} ^{c}275,22*: καὶ τῷ LUX: ἢ τῷ W **12** τῷ SUVXy *Si^{l}*: τὸ LCW γε L *Si^{l}*: om **b** ἐν LWy *Si^{l} ^{c}276,16 Ph^{l} bis, ^{c}566,10.12*: om CSUVX *Th 114,10* ἐν LWy *Si^{l} ^{c}276,16 Ph^{l} bis, ^{c}566,10.12*: om CSUVX *Th 114,10* **13** ἂν LCWy *Si^{l} Ph^{l} bis*: om SUVX *cf Ph^{p}566,14* (εἰ om y) post εἴ ins τις Ross (σιμόν$_{2}$ om L: σιμότης X) **14** (κεχωρισμένον W) ᾗ δὲ κοῖλον **o**–Xy *Si^{l}A cf Th 114,17*: δὲ ᾗ κοῖλον Ross: ᾗ δὲ κοῖδρη (sic) y: εἰ δὲ καμπύλον X: ᾗ δὲ καμπύλον *Si^{p}278,21 Ph^{l} ^{p}568,27* εἴ τις CSUVW *Si^{p}278,26*: εἴ τι Ly *Si^{c}278,24Aa*: om X Ross: εἴ τι γε *Si^{l} A* ἐνόει **o**–SV *Si^{l}*: ἐννοεῖ SV *Si^{c}278,24Aa* ἐνεργείᾳ om Ross

again in the following way. There is some one thing, and it is so as a boundary; and these [things] too, being one by analogy and in number, stand in relation to each other as those [other things] stand to one another. For what is the difference between puzzling how [the soul] discriminates things not of the same kind and how it discriminates opposites, like white and black? Let A, white, stand in relation to B, black, and C stand in relation to D as those [stand in relation] to each other, with the result that [the relation holds] in alternation too. If, then, CD were to belong to one thing, then it would be the case, just as for AB, that this thing would be one and the same, though its being would not be the same—and likewise for that other thing [CA]. And the same [431b1] relation would hold if A were sweet and B white.

Expansion of thought (for action)

The capacity for thinking, then, thinks the forms in *phantasmata*, and just as the object of pursuit or avoidance is determined for it in those [cases involving perception], so too outside of perception: whenever [one] attends to *phantasmata*, [one] is moved. For instance, perceiving a beacon, that it is fire, seeing with the common [sense] the fire move, one recognizes that it is an alarm sign. And, at times, on the basis of *phantasmata* or thoughts in the soul, just as if seeing, [one] calculates and deliberates about future things with reference to present things; and whenever [one] says that the pleasant or painful is there [in the future], here [in the present] one avoids or pursues—and generally speaking this is the case in action. And what does not involve action, namely the true and the false, is in the same genus as the good and the bad, except that they differ as to whether without qualification and relative to someone. **[431b2]**

Expansion of thought (for theory)

As for things spoken in abstraction, [one] thinks them just as if one [were to think] the snub: insofar as it is snub, [one thinks it] not as something separated, but insofar as it is concave, if [one] were to think it in actuality, one would think it **[431b12]**

τῆς σαρκὸς ἂν ἐνόει, ἐν ᾗ τὸ κοῖλον· οὕτω τὰ μαθηματικά οὐ κεχωρισμένα ὡς κεχωρισμένα νοεῖ, ὅταν νοῇ ἐκεῖνα. ὅλως δὲ ὁ νοῦς ἐστίν ὁ κατ᾽ ἐνέργειαν τὰ πράγματα. ἆρα δ᾽ ἐνδέχεται τῶν κεχωρισμένων τι νοεῖν ὄντα αὐτὸν μὴ κεχωρισμένον μεγέθους, ἢ οὔ, σκεπτέον ὕστερον.

15 (*ἐννοῇ* X) *ἐν ᾗ* LCWXy *Si*^{l} ^{c}*278,28*: om SUV **16** *οὐ κεχωρισμένα* CUVy *Si*^{l} ^{c}*278,32 Ph*^{c}*566,17*: *οὐ κεχωρισμένα τῇ ὑποστάσει* LW, mg C^{2} *cf Th 114,21*: *οὐ κεχωρισμένω* S: *τῶν οὐ κεχωρισμένων* X: *οὐ κεχωρισμένως Si*^{v}*278,33* *ὡς κεχωρισμένα* SUVWXy [sscr *-ω* y^{1}] *Si*^{l} ^{c}*278,33 Ph*^{c}*566,17 cf Th 114,22*: *ὡσεὶ κεχωρισμένω* C [corr in *-α* C^{2}]: om L *Si*^{l}*A*: *ὡς κεχωρισμένως Si*^{v}*278,33* post *οὐ κεχωρισμένα* ins *ὄντα* Ross (*νοεῖ*] *ἐνόει* L) (*ὅτε νοεῖ* W) post *νοῇ* ins *ᾗ* Ross (*ἐκεῖνος* X) **17** *πράγματα* **a** UX *Ph*^{l} ^{p}*566,24; 563,5;* ^{c}*37,27* Ross: *πράγματα νοῶν* CSVWy *Si*^{l} ^{p}*279,9* **18** *ὄντα αὐτὸν* **a**: *αὐτὸν ὄντα* **b** *Si*^{l} *Ph*^{l} **19** (*κεχωρισμεγεθους* E, corr ins *-μένον* E^{2}) (*ὕστερον σκεπτέον* y)

without the flesh in which the concave is present. In this way [one] thinks the mathematical objects, which are not separated [entities] as if separated, whenever [one] thinks them. As a general rule, thinking which is in actuality is [the same as] the objects [it thinks]. The question whether or not it is possible for it to think any of the separated entities, given that it is not itself separate from magnitude, must be investigated later.

DE ANIMA III 8

[431b20] Νῦν δέ, περὶ ψυχῆς τὰ λεχθέντα συγκεφαλαιώσαντες, εἴπωμεν πάλιν ὅτι ἡ ψυχὴ τὰ ὄντα πώς ἐστι πάντα· ἢ γὰρ αἰσθητὰ τὰ ὄντα ἢ νοητά, ἔστι δ' ἡ ἐπιστήμη μὲν τὰ ἐπιστητά πως, ἡ δ' αἴσθησις τὰ αἰσθητά· πῶς δὲ τοῦτο, δεῖ ζητεῖν.

[431b24] τέμνεται οὖν ἡ ἐπιστήμη καὶ ἡ αἴσθησις εἰς τὰ πράγματα, ἡ μὲν δυνάμει εἰς τὰ δυνάμει, ἡ δ' ἐντελεχείᾳ εἰς τὰ ἐντελεχείᾳ. τῆς δὲ ψυχῆς τὸ αἰσθητικὸν καὶ τὸ ἐπιστημονικὸν δυνάμει ταῦτά ἐστι, τὸ μὲν ἐπιστητὸν τὸ δὲ αἰσθητόν. ἀνάγκη δ' ἢ αὐτὰ ἢ τὰ εἴδη εἶναι· αὐτὰ μὲν δὴ οὔ· οὐ γὰρ ὁ λίθος ἐν τῇ ψυχῇ, ἀλλὰ τὸ εἶ-
432a1 δος· ὥστε ἡ ψυχὴ ὥσπερ ἡ χείρ ἐστιν· καὶ γὰρ ἡ χεὶρ ὄργανόν ἐστιν ὀργάνων, καὶ ὁ νοῦς εἶδος εἰδῶν, καὶ ἡ αἴσθησις εἶδος, αἰσθητῶν.

[432a3] ἐπεὶ δὲ οὐδὲ πρᾶγμα οὐθὲν ἔστι παρὰ τὰ μεγέθη, ὡς δοκεῖ, τὰ αἰσθητὰ κεχωρισμένον, ἐν τοῖς εἴδεσι τοῖς αἰσθητοῖς τὰ νοητά ἐστι, τά τε ἐν ἀφαιρέσει λεγόμενα καὶ ὅσα τῶν αἰσθητῶν ἕξεις καὶ πάθη. καὶ διὰ τοῦτο οὔτε μὴ αἰσθανόμενος μηθὲν οὐθὲν ἂν μάθοι οὐδὲ ξυνείη· ὅταν τε θεωρῇ, ἀνάγκη ἅμα φάντασμά τι θεωρεῖν· τὰ γὰρ φαντάσματα ὥσπερ αἰσθήματά ἐστι, πλὴν ἄνευ ὕλης.

431b 20 (νυνὶ *Ph*^{l}) **21** ἐστι πάντα **o**–X *Si*^{l} *Ph*^{c}*567,18*: ἐστιν ἅπαντα [τὰ πάντα X^{2}] X *Th 115,11* **22** ἢ γὰρ **b** *Si*^{l} *Ph*^{c}*567,18 Th 115,12*: γὰρ ἢ **a** *So 138,33 A* [om ἢ *BC*] τὰ **a** UWXy *Si*^{l} *Th 115,12 So 138,33*: om CSV δ' **b** *Th 115,12 So 138,35*: δὴ **a** **24** (ζητεῖν δεῖ U) τέμνεται **b**: τέμνει L *So 138,36*: τεμνε vel τεμνει E, ται add E^{x} εἰς **b**–X: om **a** X *So 138,36*, ins E^{2}X^{2} **25** (ἡ$_{1}$] εἰ E, in ἡ corr E^{3}) τὰ δυνάμει **b** *Si*^{p}*281,6 Ph*^{p}*567,11 Th 115,16*: δυνάμεις [σ eras, τὰ ins E^{2}] **a** *So 138,38* [τὰς δ.] **26** τὰ ἐντελεχείᾳ CWy, corr E^{2}U *Si*^{p}*281,6 Ph*^{p}*567,11 Th 115,16*: τὰς ἐντελεχείας SUX *So 138,38*: ἐντελεχείας **a** (αὐτῆς δὲ τῆς ψ. W) **27** τὸ$_{1}$ CWy *So 138,38*: om **a** SUVX ταῦτά **b** *So 138,38*: ταὐτόν **a**, sscr α E^{x} ταὐτά Ross post μὲν ins τὸ Ross ἐπιστητὸν **a** CWXy *So 138,38*: ἐπιστημονικὸν SUV, corr W^{2} **28** post δὲ ins τὸ Ross αἰσθητὸν **a** CWy *So 138,39*: αἰσθητικὸν SUVX, corr W^{2} (ἢ$_{2}$ om X) (εἶναι] ἐστιν X) **29** μὲν **a** VW *Si*^{l} *Ph*^{c}*567,23 So 139,1B*: μὲν γὰρ CSUXy, ins E^{2}W^{2} *So 139,1AC* ὁ **b** *Si*^{l} *Ph*^{p}*567,19 So 139,1*: om **a** *Th 115,25*
432a 1 (περ om C) ἐστιν **o**–Cy *Si*^{l} *Ph*^{l}: om Cy **2** εἶδος LUWX *Si*$^{l\,c}$*282,27 Ph*^{l} *So 139,2*: om E: ἐστιν εἶδος CSVy mg E^{2} **3** εἶδος αἰσθητῶν delevit Förster (δὲ exp E^{2}, om C, ins C^{x}) οὐδὲ **o**–S *Ph*^{l}: οὐδέν S: οὔτε *Si*^{l}*A*: οὕτω *Si*^{c}*284,14* (ἔστι Ross) **4** (μεγέθει S) **5** (τὸ νοητὸν X) ἐν Wy *Si*$^{l\,c}$*284,1; 285,4*: om **o**–Wy *Ph*$^{l\,c}$*568,22 Th 116,1* **6** ἕξεις **o**–CX *Si*$^{l\,c}$*284,2 Ph*$^{l\,c}$*568,23* ἕξις X, [ι ex η corr] C καὶ$_{2}$ **o** *Si*$^{l\,c}$*284,2 Ph*^{l}: ἢ *Ph*^{c}*568,23* **7** (οὔτε] οὐδὲ y: οὖν ὁ *Ph*^{l} (μὴ ins C: om *Si*^{l}*A*) αἰσθανόμενος **b** *Si*^{l} *Ph*^{l}: αἰσθανόμενον **a** μηθὲν **o**–Cy *Si*^{l}: om Cy *cf Ph*^{l} [sed, quae *568,26.27* leguntur, paraphrasis, non lemma esse videntur] **8** οὐδὲ **o**–W: οὐδ' ἂν W *Ph*^{c}*569,1*: οὔτ' ἂν *Si*^{l}*A* ξυνείη *Ph*^{l}*D*: ξυνίῃ **o**–EW *Ph*^{c}*569,1*: ξυνίοι E [ί in ras, eras vid ει], W *Si*^{l}*A* (δὲ V) ἅμα **a** CWy *Ph*^{l}: ἄρα SUVX: ἆρα *Si*^{l}*A* φάντασμά τι LCU *Si*$^{l\,p}$*284,13 Ph*$^{l\,p}$*569,5*: φαντασματι E [ι in ras], φαντάσματι y corr C^{x} *Th 116,8*: φαντάσματα SVWX (εἰσὶ X)

DE ANIMA III 8

The cognitive soul is somehow all beings

But now, by way of summarizing what we have said about the soul, let us state next that the soul is somehow all beings; for beings are either objects of perception or objects of thinking; and knowledge is somehow the objects of knowledge, and perception the objects of perception. However, it must be investigated in which way this is the case. [431b20]

In which way the cognitive soul is all beings

Knowledge and perception, then, are [each to be] divided according to their [corresponding] objects: [25] the one in potentiality according to those in potentiality and the one in actuality according to those in actuality. The soul's perceptual capacity and its capacity for knowledge are these objects in potentiality, the one [potentially] an object of knowledge and the other [potentially] an object of perception. And it is necessary that they be either these objects [themselves] or their forms. Surely, they are not the things [themselves]: for the stone is not in the soul, but its form. [432a1] And so the soul is just like the hand; for the hand is a tool of tools, and likewise the capacity for thinking is a form of forms, and perception is a form, of perceptible objects. [431b24]

The "empiricist" thesis

And since there is also nothing separate beside perceptible magnitudes, as it seems, [5] the objects of thinking are in the perceptible forms, both those said in abstraction and all those which are states and affections of the objects of perception. And indeed it is also for this reason that one who did not perceive anything could neither learn nor come to understand anything, and that whenever one contemplates, one necessarily at the same time contemplates some *phantasma*; for *phantasmata* are just like sense perceptions are, [10] except that they are without matter. [432a3]

[432ᵃ10] ἔστι δ' ἡ φαντασία ἕτερον φάσεως καὶ ἀποφάσεως· συμπλοκὴ γὰρ νοημάτων ἐστὶ τὸ ἀληθὲς ἢ ψεῦδος. τὰ δὲ πρῶτα νοήματα τί διοίσει τοῦ μὴ φαντάσματα εἶναι; ἢ οὐδὲ τἆλλα φαντάσματα, ἀλλ' οὐκ ἄνευ φαντασμάτων;

10 *καὶ ἀποφάσεως* **a** Cy *Si*[l] *Ph*[l]: om SUVWX, ins X[2]: *ἢ ἀποφάσεως* ins W[2] **11** *νοημάτων ἐστὶ* **a** CWXy *Si*[l]: *ἐστι νοημάτων* SUV (*ἢ τὸ ψ.* W) **12** *νοήματα τί* **b**–X, ins X[2] *Si*[l] *Ph*[p]*569,21* [c]*45,22 Th 116,17 Ammonius in de interpr 6,20*: *νοήματα τίνι* **a**: om X (*φάντασμα* E) **13** *τἆλλα* **o** *Ph*[l] [c]*45,23 Ammonius in de interpr 6,20*: *ταῦτα Si*[l] *Th 116,18* Ross

Phantasmata, assertion, and basic thoughts

Phantasia is unlike affirmation and denial. For that which is true or false is an interweaving of thoughts. But how will the basic thoughts be different from being *phantasmata*? Or is it that not even the others [i.e., those that are part of propositions, if considered in isolation from one another] are not *phantasmata*, but [they are] not without *phantasmata*? [432a10]

Glossary

Actuality (first and second)

To account for the facts of cognition, especially for the status of cognitive capacities, Aristotle resorts to a specific model known since Werner Jaeger as the *Dreistufenlehre* ("the three-stage model"), which may be described as a refinement of his more general doctrine of potentiality and actuality. As such, this model belongs to ontology, but it does not appear explicitly in the ontological treatises except for a few possible allusions. In fact, and although this doctrine is clear and consistent and plays an important role in his philosophy of knowledge and action, Aristotle deals with it in a modest, empirical manner; systematic accounts under the form of a model (including the present entry) derive from commentators. The only, somewhat extended, exposition of this doctrine is to be found in the general introduction to perception in *An.* II 5. We also have significant mentions of it in the discussion of human thinking (*nous*) in *An.* III 4–5, and in *An.* II 1, 412a27–28, where the soul is defined as "the first actuality of a natural body that is potentially alive," the corresponding second actuality being the characteristic life-activities of the relevant creature. It is worth stressing that in this last case the model, which seems to have been elaborated for human activities and capacities implying higher forms of cognition, is used in a salient position to account for the ontology of life taken as a whole.

The most important feature of that model is that it distinguishes a specific intermediate level between the mere potentiality and the full completion consisting in the given activity. Of course, Aristotle thinks that all natural changes are processes that occur by passing through intermediate stages; however, the *Dreistufenlehre* claims that, in some processes, there is a specific level that has a coherence and a permanency of its own, such that one may say that it exists in and of itself. Such is the case of different forms of scientific expertise, and of the soul itself (seen as the principle of life). Aristotle's paradigmatic example is literacy: all human beings, as such, are able to read, because they all possess the required physiological and psychological abilities; but to become an actual reader requires, additionally, a specific training, the outcome of which is the full capacity to read in a given language. The relations between the three levels can be represented as follows:

(1) able to become a reader: *first potentiality*
(2) having learnt to read: *first actuality, second potentiality*
(3) actually reading: *second actuality.*

The ability to read is not spent out or exhausted in one act of reading; on the contrary, it remains intact and available for an unlimited number of subsequent acts. That is why, although it is a *dunamis* and, as such, a potentiality (see *Dunamis*), it may also be described as an actuality.

It might be worth noticing here that Aristotle is flexible in his use of the paradigm of literacy when he applies it to the case of perception. Obviously, our perceptive capacity does not result from teaching or training. However, he claims that it has the character of being a stable permanent capacity (he suggests that the perceptive capacity might then be described as produced by our parents).

That intermediate level divides the generation of an act of cognition into two quite different moments of change. The transition from mere potentiality to first actuality is a complex process that requires some amount of qualitative transformation (i.e., alteration) of the subject and must take some time, whereas Aristotle describes the transition from first to second actuality as an immediate event: as soon as they are in front of a written sentence, skilled readers grasp immediately its contents and meaning. As Aristotle himself remarks, this transition is not, strictly speaking, a change; nevertheless, something must happen then. Aristotle calls it "a preservation (*sôtêria*) of what is in potentiality by the agency of what is in actuality" and "a progress toward itself" (*An.* II 5, 417b3–4, 417b6–7). In this sense, the passage from first to second actuality is also a fulfilment of the relevant potentiality. In the case of cognition, the passage from first to second actuality is also described as a grasping of the form of an object "without its matter" (*An.* II 12, 424a18–19; *An.* III 8, 431b28–29). For Aristotle, this grasping of a form (*eidos*) is the distinctive character of human cognition and, most of all, of human intellectual thinking.

Aisthêma

This is the primary effect of an act of perception. As such, it is causally related to the external object of perception (*to aisthêton*). The *aisthêma* is the perceptual form of the external object; as such, it can only exist in the presence of the external object. An *aisthêma*, along with the external object of perception (*to aisthêton*), constitutes an act of perception. More directly, the *aisthêma* singles out the subjective aspect of an act of perception. We opted to render the Greek *aisthêma* with "percept" to signal its causal dependence on an act of perception.

The *aisthêma* is causally related to a *phantasma* in the sense that the normal operation of perception results in the production not only of an *aisthêma* but also of a *phantasma*. Aristotle illustrates this second causal relation with the help of an analogy. He says the *phantasma* is like the seal (*tupos*) impressed on a letter or some other important document (*Mem.* 1, 450a30–32). This point can be restated by saying that the *phantasma* is the side-effect of an act of perception. The causal dependence of the *phantasma* on an *aisthêma* resurfaces twice in the treatment of the cognitive soul (*An.* III 7–8). Twice Aristotle says that the *phantasma* can perform the role of an *aisthêma* (*An.* III 7, 431a15; *An.* III 8, 432a9). This means that a *phantasma* has the same phenomenal content as an *aisthêma*; the difference is that the *aisthêma* involves the presence of the external object of perception, whereas this is not the case with *phantasma*. (See also PHANTASMA.)

Aisthêsis

Along with *nous*, *aisthêsis* is one of the two basic powers of the cognitive soul (see COGNITIVE SOUL). While rendering *aisthêsis* as perception, we mean by it *sense*-perception: that is, perception which comes through the five sense modalities as explained in *An.* II 7–11. Aristotle defines perception as the capacity to receive the perceptible forms without the matter (*An.* II 12, 424a18–19). Receiving the form without the matter amounts to taking on the perceptual quality of a three-dimensional object (i.e., its perceptible form) without taking on the object itself (i.e., the proximate matter of the perceptual form). Aristotle illustrates his definition with the help of the wax and signet-ring example. The wax takes on the shape of the ring without taking on its matter (the gold or iron out of which the signet-ring is made). Perceiving red is taking on the perceptual quality of redness without the proximate matter (the three-dimensional object).

Aristotle conceives of perception as a discriminative power. Discrimination (*krinein*) is the mechanism by which the perceptible form is separated from its matter. Such a mechanism entails the reproduction of the proportion present in the object in the soul.

Cognitive soul

The cognitive soul is an integrated system of cognitive powers. These powers are always present in an ensouled (i.e., living) body in virtue of the fact that this body possesses a soul. As soon as we reflect on this fact, we see that the study of the cognitive soul amounts to the study of embodied cognition.

The two fundamental modes of cognition present in a living body are perception (*aisthêsis*) and thought (*nous*). For Aristotle, these cognitive powers are separable in definition. By his lights, they can be studied and defined independently from one another as well as from other powers of the soul.

The cognitive soul is the main topic of investigation in *An.* III 7–8. This stretch of text is best understood as a sustained investigation of the cognitive soul conducted from the bottom up. This investigation culminates in the so-called Identity Thesis: the cognitive soul is "all beings"—that is, the cognitive soul cognizes all perceptible and intelligible beings (*An.* III 8, 431b21). Aristotle also provides us with a memorable illustration of the role that the cognitive soul plays in cognition by comparing it to a hand (*An.* III 8, 432a1).

While perception and thought are the two basic powers of the cognitive soul, they are emphatically not its only powers. The cognitive soul has also the powers to feel pleasure and pain, as well as the power to form desire. From *An.* III 7 we learn that these powers are not separate from the basic power of perception. Rather, they are best understood as different applications of the same power (*An.* III 7, 431a12–14). *Phantasia* too (see *Phantasia*) is another important power of the cognitive soul.

We should refrain from thinking of the powers of the cognitive soul as operationally autonomous modules. The cognitive soul is a single cognitive system in which the various powers are operationally fused. This conclusion is already adumbrated in the analogy with rectilinear figures offered in *An.* II 3. There Aristotle is careful to add that "what is prior is always present potentially (*dunamei*) in what follows in a series; for instance, the triangle in the square and the nutritive capacity in the perceptual capacity" (*An.* II 3, 414b29–32).

Dunamis

This is a central concept in Aristotle's philosophical thought well beyond the narrow boundaries of the study of the soul. We render *dunamis* as either "power" or "capacity."

Aristotle offers an elucidation of the concept of *dunamis* and its significance in his philosophical lexicon (*Metaph.* V 12). At the most general level, a *dunamis* is a power that results either in a complete (i.e., non-kinetic) activity or in an incomplete (i.e., kinetic) activity. When understood in this way, a *dunamis* is an explanatory item: namely, the source or cause of an activity or a process. We can restate this point by saying that processes and activities are the *explananda* while the powers (*dunameis*) are among their *explanantia*.

In his *De anima* Aristotle is concerned with the basic powers of the soul. It turns out, in the course of the inquiry into the soul, that the latter is not the sort of thing that *has* powers; rather, it *is* the set of powers that the ensouled (living) bodies possess and in virtue of which they actively do and passively undergo their various life processes. Understood in this way, the powers of the soul are also powers of the ensouled (living) bodies. The only possible exception is *nous*. *Nous* is a power of the soul, but it is in an important sense not a power of the body since it has no bodily organ, and its actuality (*entelecheia*) is not the actuality (*entelecheia*) of any body. (See *Nous* and SEPARATE/SEPARABLE, TO BE SEPARATED, as well as Chapter 6.)

The cognitive powers are among the powers of the soul. Perception (*aisthêsis*) and thought (*nous*) are the two basic cognitive powers. Both are understood as discriminative powers (*An.* III 3, 427a20–21; *An.* III 4, 429b12–13 and 20–21; *An.* III 9, 432a15–16). While perception is the power to discriminate objects of perception (*ta aisthêta*), thought is the power to discriminate objects of thought (*ta noêta*). (See *Noêton* for more on the objects of thought.)

Since they discriminate different kinds of objects, perception and thought are fundamentally different powers. Consequently, their respective activities (*energeiai*) amount to fundamentally different forms of discrimination: namely, *perceptual* discrimination and *intellectual* discrimination.

Explanatory essentialism

Essences play the role of starting points in Aristotle's theory of scientific explanation. They are the basic, necessary, and universal features invoked to explain why certain kinds of things possess the *per se* accidents (i.e., the other necessary and universal features) they do. Essential features so understood are distinguished from merely necessary and universal features by their explanatory role: they are explanatorily primary.

Consider the following zoological example: snakes are a large kind (*megiston genos*) in Aristotle's science of living beings. Certain facts about snakes are to be explained in general for all of them (this follows directly from the methodological insight that explanation ought to be given at the right level of generality to account for the salient features of the kind taken as a whole: see *Posterior Analytics* I 4–5). One fact that surely calls for an explanation is why snakes are footless. The relevant explanation is offered in *Inc. An.* 8 (one of the best-known and most intensely discussed chapters in the whole treatise). Aristotle takes the properties of having an elongated body and of being blooded to be his starting points in the explanation of why snakes are footless. As such these properties are not only necessary but also essential properties. They are employed in the explanation of a non-essential but necessary and universal property (in short, a *per se* property) exhibited by all snakes: being footless. Given these explanatory starting points, there appear to be only two theoretical options: *either* snakes have a foot placed at each of the four points of motion like all other blooded animals do, *or* they have no feet. But having four feet is far from being ideal for bodily displacement in the presence of an extra-long body. A four-footed animal with an extra-long body would move with great difficulty and very slowly. Snakes are clearly better off without feet. Instead of progressing on land (or in water) by using feet, they displace themselves by bending their extra-long body. This turns out to be an extremely effective mode of locomotion for snakes. Although footless, they can displace themselves as efficiently as footed animals.

When we reflect on how Aristotle uses essences in the context of his scientific enterprise, we see that an essence is never a solitary item; rather, it is an item that is always embedded in a larger explanatory system. Aristotle's name for such a system is *epistêmê*.

Noêton

All the capacities of the soul are object-related capacities (*An.* II 4, 415a14–23). The capacity for thinking is no exception to the rule. Like all the other capacities of the soul, this capacity is approached via a discussion of its primary objects. Since Aristotle makes the grasp of an essence—the ultimate cause of why something is what it is (see EXPLANATORY ESSENTIALISM)—the core case of thinking, he approaches the study of human thought via a discussion of the basic types of essences understood as the primary objects of thought. By his lights, there are three basic types of essences: essences of natural substances, essences of mathematical objects, and the separate (immaterial) substances (*An.* III 4, 429b11–12, 430a3–6). These three types of essences are distinguished from one another in virtue of their separability from matter. While the essences of natural and mathematical objects are inseparable from matter in the sense that they can only be thought as a "this-in-this" (*An.* III 4, 429b13–14, 18–20), the essences belonging to the last kind exist and are thought without matter. Moreover, mathematical essences, unlike natural essences, can be thought in separation from perceptible matter, although they cannot exist separately from it (*An.* III 7, 431b12–16).

The first two types of essences (the objects of natural philosophy and mathematics) can only be thought along with something that is not itself an object of thought. Aristotle is very clear on this point when he says that the content of a thought must be thought in a *phantasma* (*An.* III 7, 431a16–17, 431b2), although it is not identical with a *phantasma* (*An.* III 8, 432a10–14). This point can be restated by saying that human beings think of the matter-involving essences only by means of mental representations since those essences are given to them in perceptible forms (*An.* III 8, 432a3–9; cf. *Mem.* 1, 449b32–450a1, where Aristotle offers an independent argument for this claim starting from the case of mathematical objects). This has consequences for separability (see SEPARABLE/SEPARATE, TO BE SEPARATED).

Not all human thinking, of course, amounts to grasping an essence. Indeed, this is a rare achievement. Aristotle, thus, needs to show how the capacity for thinking, defined with respect to essences, can also account for more mundane kinds of thinking, where a predicate is ascribed to a subject in a way that, unlike the grasping of an essence, can turn out to be either true or false. He undertakes this task in *An.* III 6. A propositional thought presupposes that both the subject and the predicate are thought as unitary objects (*adiaireta*). But as long as one thing is predicated of another, the thought falls short of the kind of unity that only the grasp of an essence exhibits (cf. *An.* III 6, 430b26–29) as the exemplary kind of thought. Indeed, the grasp of an essence—which cannot but be true (*An.* III 6, 430b29–31)—alone can provide the ultimate ground of the truth of a propositional thought.

Nous

Aristotle uses the noun *nous* in ways that are not always sharply distinguished. It can refer to: (1) the activity of thinking, being virtually synonymous with *noêsis* or *noein* (see, e.g., *An.* I 4, 408b24–30; *An.* III 6, 430b17–18; *Metaph.* XII 9, 1075a3–5); (2) the capacity to engage in this kind of activity, being virtually synonymous with the thinking part of the soul—namely, *to noêtikon* (see, e.g., *An.* III 4, 429a22–23, 429b4–5; *An.* III 5, 430a24–25); (3) the acquired capacity to think some specific kind of object at one's will (see, e.g., *Posterior Analytics* II 19, 100b5–15; cf. *An.* III 4, 429b5–10).

As a part of the soul, *nous* ("the so-called *nous* of the soul," *An.* III 4, 429a22) is defined very narrowly as the power of grasping essences (*An.* III 4, 429b10–22): the essences of natural and mathematical objects, as well as the separate (immaterial) substances, each of which perfectly coincides with its essence (*An.* III 4, 429b11–12, 430a3–6). As such, *nous* and *noein* (i.e., the activity of thinking) are success terms denoting a very demanding cognitive achievement. For Aristotle, there cannot be any "wrong" *nous* of an essence; there either is or is not the grasp of an essence, which cannot but be true (*An.* III 6, 430b27–31). In this respect, *nous* and *noein* are to be contrasted with *dianoia* and *dianoeisthai.* The latter terms denote discursive thinking, which can be both true and false because it consists in putting things together, *suntithenai* (*An.* III 6, 430a27–b4; see also *Sunthesis*).

It is equally important to stress that this narrowly defined *nous* of the soul is the first explanatory principle of the entire range of human intellectual activities involving discursivity and propositional thought, whether one ever succeeds in grasping an essence or not. It is *nous* that, ultimately, "produces the unity" of each proposition (*An.* III 6, 430b5–6): not, clearly, in the sense that each propositional thought is based on the grasp of an essence, but rather in the sense that in a propositional thought one achieves imperfectly what is only fully achieved in such a grasp.

The human *nous* differs sharply from other powers (*dunameis*) of the soul in that its defining activity—that is, *noein*—is not an activity of the body (*An.* II 1, 413a6–7; cf. *An.* I 4, 408b18–30; *Gener. An.* II 3, 736b28–29). For Aristotle, *nous* has no organ (*An.* III 4, 429a18–b5) and is not a part of human nature (*Part. An.* I 1, 641a32–b10; cf. *An.* I 1, 403a27–28). Nevertheless, as a part of the cognitive soul, human *nous* is operationally fused with other parts (see COGNITIVE SOUL), as manifested in the close interconnection between thinking and *phantasia* (see *An.* III 7, 431a14–15; *An.* III 7, 431b2–3; *An.* III 8, 432a3–10; *Mem.* 1, 449b30–450a7)—an interconnection which, it must be stressed, never amounts to identity (*An.* III 8, 432a10–14). Insofar as thinking is interconnected with *phantasia*, and human *nous* is operationally fused with other parts of the cognitive soul, the human *nous* cannot be *separated* from the soul (see SEPARABLE/SEPARATE, TO BE SEPARATED). This is clearly so for all thinking acts concerned with natural and mathematical objects (*An.* III 8, 432a3–10), for *nous* can think such objects only as an integral part of the cognitive soul.

But *nous* is not limited to "the so-called *nous* of the soul" and its cognitive achievements; it also exists independently from the soul, as suggested by a reflection on separate (immaterial) substances: in the case of such a substance, what is thought perfectly coincides with that which thinks due to the absence of matter (*An.* III 4, 430a3–5); indeed, such a substance thinks itself (*An.* III 6, 430b24–26). While the proof of the existence of separate (immaterial) substances is not on the agenda of *De Anima*, Aristotle's argument here seems to imply that *if* such a substance exists, it is a *nous* in the sense of an eternal self-thinking activity, entirely independent from anything psychic or bodily (*An.* III 5, 430a17–25). Nothing but such a *nous* can be the principle of the motion and order in the universe (*Metaph.* XII 6–10). In this way Aristotle joins the venerable tradition of thinkers starting at least with Anaxagoras who claimed *nous* to be "the principle of everything." But Aristotle also insists that we need to distinguish this kind of *nous* from the *nous* as a part of the soul, and, again, this very specific part of the soul from its natural parts, more sharply than his predecessors did (cf. *An.* I 2, 404a25–b7, 405a8–19).

Phantasia

This is one of the powers of the integrated system that we have called the cognitive soul (see COGNITIVE SOUL). From *An.* III 3 we learn that *phantasia* is a movement or change (i.e., a *kinêsis*) that cannot exist without perception; rather, it exists only in things that are engaged in perception, and in relation to that of which there is perception (*An.* III 3, 428b10–17;

see *Somn.* 1, 459a15–19). Such a characterization of *phantasia* makes it abundantly clear that Aristotle does not consider *phantasia* on a par with the basic cognitive powers of the soul: namely, perception and thought. On the contrary, he makes the presence of *phantasia* contingent on the presence and exercise of perception. In this sense, *phantasia* is something not only different from, but also dependent on, perception. This point can be restated either by emphasizing the functional incompleteness of *phantasia* (see Wedin 1988: 45–57) or by distinguishing the basic powers (i.e., parts) of the soul from the powers that depend for their definition on the basic ones (Corcilius and Gregoric 2010: 81–119).

While functionally incomplete, *phantasia* plays an important role in the explanation of a vast array of phenomena ranging from thinking to animal self-motion, to memory, and to dreaming. Here we limit ourselves to recalling how *phantasia* is involved in the explanation of thinking. Aristotle tells us twice that the cognitive soul cannot think without *phantasmata* (*An.* III 7, 431a15–16, 431b2–3; see PHANTASMA). In both cases Aristotle does not mean to say that thoughts (*noêmata*) are identical with *phantasmata*; rather, he means to say that the content of a thought is always accompanied by a *phantasma*. Aristotle elaborates on this idea in dealing with the phenomenon of memory. There, Aristotle notes that when one proves a geometrical theorem about triangles—for instance, the theorem that the sum of the internal angles of any triangle is equal to two right angles—one always draws a triangle on the blackboard or in the sand. This triangle always has a particular size even if the geometrical proof does not depend on the triangle having any specific size (it depends on the fact that the triangle is a closed figure on a surface bounded by three sides). By reflecting on the relation between mathematical diagrams and *phantasmata*, Aristotle draws the following conclusion: the operation of thinking is always accompanied by *phantasmata*, even though these *phantasmata* are only incidental on thinking (*Mem.* 1, 449b30–450a7 combined with 450a13–14).

Phantasma

A *phantasma* is an affection (*pathos*) of the primary sense organ. (*Mem.* 1, 450a10–11). More directly, and more precisely, it is an affection that is produced by means of an act of perception in the part of the body that contains the [perceptual] soul (*Mem.* 1, 450a27–29). In blooded animals, this part is the heart; in bloodless animals, this part does not have a name, but it is described as something that is functionally analogous to the heart. Aristotle describes the *phantasma* as a movement or change that arises in coincidence with an episode of perception. No temporal space separates the act of perception from the production of a *phantasma*. Rather, the normal operation of perception results in the production of a *phantasma*. In this sense the *phantasma* is best described as a *side-effect* of an act of perception. They are *remnants* (*hupoleimmata*) of the process of perception since they persist in the body after the event of perceiving and preserve the causal powers and presentational qualities of the original acts of perception (*Insomn.* 3, 461b21). Unlike percepts (*aisthêmata*), which are firmly tied to the external objects of perception, the *phantasmata* lose the presentational ties to the external objects that brought them about and become available for new intentional contexts such as memory, anticipation, association, or rational thought. This is possible because *phantasmata* can, as it were, resurface and can be perceived anew (*Insomn.* 2, 460b2–4). Unlike an *aisthêma*, a *phantasma* can be reconfigured and reused in all sorts of ways.

The relation that Aristotle envisions between the *phantasma* and the *aisthêma* is illustrated by means of the analogy with a signatory who uses a signet ring to impress a seal (*tupos*) on a letter or on some other important document (*Mem.* 1, 450a30–32). This analogy is meant to convey the idea of the existence of a causal relation between the *aisthêma* and the *phantasma*. It is not meant to convey the additional idea that there is a privileged connection between the *phantasma* and the *aisthêma*. In other words, the causal story that leads to the imprint of a *phantasma* in the perceptual soul explains the properties of the *phantasma*, but it does not determine what the *phantasma* represents. Whether the *phantasma* represents something, and eventually what, depends on the subsequent *use* that the soul makes of the *phantasma*. We today say that this outcome depends on the *intentional context* in which a *phantasma* (or a sequence of *phantasmata*) occurs. If we are right, a *phantasma* taken by itself is not representational in character. As a matter of fact, a *phantasma* only brings its own qualitative features before the soul. It is a stored and potentially re-activated perceptual stimulus. This is also why we resist translating *phantasma* as either "representation" or "image."

Aristotle employs *phantasmata* to explain not only how memory is possible but also the very possibility of psychological phenomena such as dreams, illusions, and distortions of our sensory experience.

Separable/separate (chôriston), to be separated (chôrizesthai)

Throughout his *De Anima*, Aristotle repeatedly says that *X* is *chôriston*. *Nous* is often the subject of these statements. There are three main questions to be asked in each case:

(1) Does *chôriston* mean "separate" or "separable"? (Both are linguistically possible.)
(2) What is *X* separate/separable *from*?
(3) *In what respect* is *X* separable/separate?

The main candidates for (2) are: (a) the body (matter, magnitude); (b) motion; (c) the other capacities of the soul. The main candidates for (3) are: (a) in place; (b) in definition; (c) in existence. The separability/separateness in existence can be further subdivided into separability/separateness: (c1) in kind (taxonomical); (c2) in number (unqualified or ontological). *X* is *taxonomically* separable from *Y iff* there is a kind of living beings such that *X* is instantiated in them independently from *Y*; *X* is *unqualifiedly* (ontologically) separable from *Y iff* this very *X* can exist independently from *Y*. Aristotle rarely makes these specifications explicit (the usual lack of specification concerning (2) highlights the fact that the separability/separateness relation is not symmetrical). Often various ways of being *chôriston* overlap, so that it would be idle to try to pin down each occurrence exactly. But when it comes to the separateness/separability of *nous*, the way we answer the three questions, especially for some of Aristotle's claims, makes a great difference to his overall position.

Aristotle is very clear about the following: (i) most capacities of the soul are in definition (and *a fortiori* in existence) inseparable from the body and from motion in the sense that their defining activity *is* a bodily activity—that is, a motion (*An*. II 1, 413a4–6); (ii) the nutritive, the perceptive, and the locomotive capacities of the soul of an individual living being are not unqualifiedly separable from each other (*An*. I 5, 411b26; *An*. II 2, 413b16–24; cf. *An*. III 7, 431a13–14 where the capacities of perception and desiring are claimed to be the same in number but different in account); this supports the claims that (iii) these capacities are not separate from each other in place (*An*. II 2, 413b27–29); but (iv) the nutritive capacity is—unlike the perceptive or the motive capacity—taxonomically separable: it exists in plants separately from all other capacities of the soul (*An*. I 5, 411b29–30; *An*. II

2, 413a31–b1). Aristotle is also fairly clear about the following: (v) the nutritive, perceptive, and thinking capacities of the soul are separable in definition both from each other and from the remaining capacities of the soul (cf. Corcilius and Gregoric 2010; Johansen 2012: 53–62); (vi) *nous* is taxonomically separable from all capacities of the soul (as well as from the body and from motion): there is a *nous*—namely, divine *nous*—which exists independently from any soul and, therefore, is unqualifiedly separate (see *An.* III 4, 430a3–5; *An.* III 5, 430a17–25; *Metaph.* XII.7–9; cf. also *An.* II 2, 413a31–32); (vii) the thinking capacity (i.e., the *nous*) of the soul is separable in definition from motion and from the body (*An.* III 4, 429a24–27, 429b5, cf. Chapter 6).

The most difficult question to determine is: (viii) whether the *nous* of the soul is separable from the other capacities of the soul (and so from the body and motion) unqualifiedly (cf. *An.* III 4, 429a11–12). This could only be so if this *nous* were capable of acts which are unqualifiedly separate from the other capacities of the soul and their acts (cf. *An.* I 1, 403a7–12). Aristotle clearly denies that this could be the case for natural and mathematical objects of thought (*An.* III 8, 432a3–10). Indeed, he conceives the level of separateness of the acts of *nous* as, apparently, strictly corresponding to the level of separateness of their objects (*An.* III 4, 429b21–22): since neither natural nor mathematical essences are unqualifiedly separable from matter, neither are the acts of thinking them. The question that Aristotle raises but leaves unaddressed in *De anima* concerns the case of a *nous* of the soul thinking separate substances (*An.* III 7, 431b17–19). Aristotle clearly believes that the human *nous* *can* think separate substances; the difficulty comes from the fact that there are two ways in which the thinking of separate substances may take place: *either* a separate substance can be thought on its own and purely as it is in itself *or* it can be thought in relation to something else—namely, as the unmoved mover *of* the heavenly spheres and the ultimate cause *of* the order of the universe—that is, as a cause and principle of other things and not how it is in itself. Aristotle's treatment of separate substance in *Phys.* VIII 10 and *Metaph.* XII 6–10 is clear evidence for the latter option; it is much more difficult to determine Aristotle's view as to whether the human *nous* can think a separate substance on its own. But, as is clear from the foregoing, the question of unqualified separability of the human *nous* directly depends on this.

If the human *nous* is limited to thinking separate substances, not as they are in themselves, but only in relation to (some of) the things they are causes of, it seems that *all* its thinking acts will depend on *phantasiai*, which represent these things; as a result, the unqualified separability of human *nous* will be excluded. Aristotle's claim at *An.* III 5 430a24–25 that the passive *nous* is perishable suggests that this is, indeed, his view. But that leaves us with the task of interpreting the texts suggesting that human *nous*, or something about it, is imperishable (*An.* I 4, 408b18–30; *An.* II 2, 413b24–27), and that it can be "immortalized" (*EN* X 7, 1077b26–1078a8; cf. *Metaph.* XII 7, 1072b24–28). One upshot of *An.* III 4–8 is that such an imperishability or immortality could only be granted to the human *nous* so far as it can think a separate substance on its own. Aristotle never explicitly discusses this option, and the difficulty of conceiving it comes exactly from the fact that when thinking a separate substance on its own the *nous* in question would have to cease to be a part of the soul: that is, it would be unqualifiedly separated from it—at least for a while, and maybe forever after biological death. It seems that in such a case it could not but coincide with the self-thinking act of the separate substance itself (*An.* III 5, 430a22–23), so that calling it "human" would not make much sense any longer. But this does not mean that the formerly human *nous* has perished; on the contrary, this seems to be the ultimate fulfilment of this capacity. (For more on (viii), see Chapter 6 in this volume.)

Sunthesis

According to Aristotle, neither of the two discriminating activities with respect to which the perceptive and the thinking part of the soul are defined—namely, perceiving (*aisthanesthai*) and thinking (*noein*)—is synthetic. We perceive three-dimensional objects in both their uni-modal and multi-modal aspects without any *synthesis* being involved. And, similarly, no *sunthesis* is involved in the grasp of an essence. That is also why there is nothing like a wrong or incorrect grasp of an essence (see *Nous*). The possibility of error on the level of thinking is explained exactly by the synthetic or compositional nature of propositional thought (*An.* III 6, 430a26–b6). This is also why *An.* III 6 is a non-expendable part of Aristotle's account of *nous* as the principle of human thinking.

The simplicity of the objects of perception and thinking must be sharply distinguished from the simplicity of the material elements. It was, by Aristotle's lights, a fundamental error of the traditional like-is-known-by-like view (in short, the LKL view) to conceive the isomorphism between cognition and the cognized object in terms of material elements constituting both the object and the subject of cognition (for more on this point, see Chapter 1). The very first objection Aristotle raises against this assumption is that isomorphism so understood makes it difficult, if not impossible, to understand how the combinations (*suntheseis*) of the elements can ever be cognized (*An.* I 5, 409b23–410a13). According to Aristotle, what is received in cognition are rather combinations, proportions, or forms themselves without the matter (cf. Chapter 5). In the case of perception, this is primarily the proportion defining each quality. In the case of thinking, it is the essence: that is, what the thing is, as contrasted with what it is made of.

References

Angioni, L. 2013. "Knowledge and Opinion about the Same Thing." In *Dois Pontos* 10: 255–290.

Angioni, L. 2019. "Aristotle's Contrast Between *epistêmê* and *doxa* in its Context (*Posterior Analytics* I.33)." In *Manuscrito* 42: 157–210.

Bäck, A. 2014. *Aristotle's Theory of Abstraction.* Springer, Berlin.

Balme, D. M. 1972. *Aristotle: De Partibus Animalium I and De Generatione Animalium I.* Clarendon Press, Oxford.

Barnes, J. 1993. *Aristotle: Posterior Analytics.* Clarendon Press, Oxford.

Bekker, I. (ed.). 1831. *Aristoteles graece.* 2 vols. Academia Regia Borussica/Reimer, Berlin.

Berti, E. 1978. "The Intellection of 'Indivisibles' according to Aristotle, *De anima* III 6." In G. E. R. Lloyd and G. E. L. Owen (eds.), *Aristotle on Mind and the Senses: Proceedings of the Seventh Symposium Aristotelicum.* Cambridge University Press, Cambridge: 141–163.

Berti, E. 1996. "Encore sur l'intellection des 'indivisibles' selon Aristote, *De anima* III 6." In G. Romeyer Dherbey and C. Viano (eds.), *Corps et âme: Sur le De anima d'Aristote.* Vrin, Paris: 391–404.

Berti, E. 2016. "Aristotle's *nous poiêtikos*: Another Modest Proposal." In G. Sillitti, F. Stella, and F. Fronterotta (eds.), *Il NOÛS di Aristotele.* Academia Verlag, Sankt Augustin: 137–153.

Betegh, G. 2021. "Thinking with Empedocles: Aristotle on the Soul as *harmonia*." In *Oxford Studies in Ancient Philosophy* 59: 1–44.

Betegh, G., and Tsouna, V. 2024. *Conceptualising Concepts in Greek Philosophy.* Cambridge University Press, Cambridge.

Blumenthal, H. 1996. *Aristotle and Neoplatonism in Late Antiquity: Interpretations of the* De anima. Duckworth, London.

Bodéüs, R. 1993. *Aristote: De l'âme.* Traduction et présentation. Flammarion, Paris.

Bonitz, H. 1870. *Index Aristotelicus.* Reimer, Berlin.

Brentano, F. 1867. *Die Psychologie des Aristoteles: insbesondere seine Lehre vom ΝΟΥΣ ΠΟΙΗΤΙΚΟΣ*, Mainz. [Reprinted in 1967 by Wissenschaftliche Buchgesellschaft, Darmstadt. Translated into English by R. George: *The Psychology of Aristotle: In Particular his Doctrine of the Active Intellect.* University of California Press, Berkeley, CA, 1977.]

Broadie, S. 1993. "Aristotle's Perceptual Realism." In *Southern Journal of Philosophy* (Supplement), 31: 137–159.

Broadie, S. 1996. "Νοῦς and Nature in *De anima* III." In *Proceedings of the Boston Area Colloquium in Ancient Philosophy* 12: 163–176.

Broakes, J. 1999. "Aristotle, Objectivity and Perception." In *Oxford Studies in Ancient Philosophy* 17: 57–113.

Bronstein, D. 2016. *Aristotle on Knowledge and Learning: The Posterior Analytics.* Oxford University Press, Oxford.

Bronstein, D. (forthcoming). "Aristotle on the Relation between Definition and Demonstration."

Bruns, I. (ed.). 1886. *Alexandri Aphrodisiensis Scripta minora (De anima liber cum Mantissa).* Academia Regia Borussica/Reimer, Berlin.

Buchheim, T. (ed.). 2016. *Aristoteles De anima: Über die Seele.* Wissenschaftliche Buchgesellschaft, Darmstadt.

Burnyeat, M. F. 1980. "Aristotle on Learning to be Good." In A. Oksenberg Rorty (ed.), *Essays on Aristotle's Ethics.* University of California Press, Berkeley, CA: 69–92. [Reprinted in M. F. Burnyeat, *Explorations in Ancient and Modern Philosophy*, Volume 2. Cambridge University Press, Cambridge, 2012: 259–281.]

Burnyeat, M. F. 2008. *Aristotle's Divine Intellect.* Marquette University Press, Milwaukee, WS.

Busche, H. 2001. *Die Seele als System: Aristoteles' Wissenschaft von der Psyche*. Felix Meiner, Hamburg.

Busche, H., and Perkams, M. (eds.). 2018. *Antike Interpretationen zur aristotelischen Lehre vom Geist*. Felix Meiner, Hamburg.

Butler, T., and Rubenstein, E. 2004. "Aristotle on *Nous* of Simples." In *Canadian Journal of Philosophy* 34: 327–354.

Bywater, I. 1888. "*Aristotelia* III." In *The Journal of Philology* 17: 53–74.

Cagnoli Fiecconi, E. 2019. "Aristotle's Peculiarly Human Psychology." In G. Keil and N. Kreft (eds.), *Aristotle's Anthropology*. Cambridge University Press, Cambridge: 60–76.

Carter, J. 2019. *Aristotle on Earlier Greek Psychology: The Science of the Soul*. Cambridge University Press, Cambridge.

Cassirer, H. 1932. *Aristoteles' Schrift "Von der Seele" und ihre Stellung innerhalb der aristotelischen Philosophie*. Heinrich Mohr, Tübingen 1932. [Reprinted by Wissenschaftliche Buchgesellschaft, Darmstadt, 1968.]

Caston, V. 1993. "Aristotle and Supervenience." In J. Ellis (ed.), *Ancient Minds: Spindel Conference 1992*. Published in *Southern Journal of Philosophy*, Suppl. vol. 31: 49–105.

Caston, V. 1996a. "Why Aristotle Needs Imagination." In *Phronesis* 41: 20–55.

Caston, V. 1996b. "Aristotle on the Relation of the Intellect to the Body: Commentary on Broadie." In *Proceedings of the Boston Area Colloquium in Ancient Philosophy* 12: 177–192.

Caston, V. 1997. "Epiphenomenalisms, Ancient and Modern." In *The Philosophical Review* 106: 309–363.

Caston, V. 1999. "Aristotle's Two Intellects: A Modest Proposal." In *Phronesis* 44: 199–227.

Caston, V. 2002. "Aristotle on Consciousness." In *Mind* 111: 751–815.

Caston, V. 2005. "The Spirit and the Letter." In R. Salles (ed.), *Metaphysics, Soul, and Ethics in Ancient Thought: Themes from the Work of Richard Sorabji*. Oxford University Press, Oxford: 245–320.

Caston, V. 2009. "*Phantasia* and Thought." In G. Anagnostopoulos (ed.), *A Companion to Aristotle*. Blackwell, Oxford: 322–334.

Caston, V. 2013. *Alexander of Aphrodisias*: On the Soul. Part 1: *Soul as Form of the Body, Parts of the Soul, Nourishment, Perception*. Translated by V. Caston. Bristol Classical Press, Bristol.

Charles, D. 2000. *Aristotle on Meaning and Essence*. Oxford University Press, Oxford.

Charles, D. 2021. *The Undivided Self: Aristotle and the 'Mind-Body Problem'*. Oxford University Press, Oxford.

Charlton, W. 1987. "Aristotle on the Place of Mind in Nature." In A. Gotthelf and J. G. Lennox (eds.), *Philosophical Issues in Aristotle's Biology*. Cambridge University Press, Cambridge: 408–423.

Chiba, K. 2010. "Aristotle on Essence and Defining Phrase in his Dialectic." In D. Charles (ed.), *Definition in Greek Philosophy*. Oxford University Press, Oxford: 203–251.

Cohoe, C. 2018. "Why the View of Intellect in *De anima* I 4 is not Aristotle's Own." In *British Journal for the History of Philosophy* 26: 241–254.

Cohoe, C. 2022. "The Separability of *Nous*." In C. Cohoe (ed.), *Aristotle's On the Soul: A Critical Guide*. Cambridge University Press, Cambridge: 229–246.

Connell, S. 2021. "Thinking Bodies: Aristotle on the Biological Basis of the Human Cognition." In J. L. Fink and P. Gregoric (eds.), *Encounters with Aristotelian Philosophy of Mind*. Routledge, London: 223–246.

Cooper, J. 2020. "The Role of Thought in Animal Voluntary Self-Motion." In C. Rapp and O. Primavesi (eds.), *Aristotle's De motu animalium*. Symposium Aristotelicum. Oxford University Press, Oxford: 345–386.

Corcilius, K. 2008a. *Streben und Bewegen: Aristoteles' Theorie der animalischen Ortsbewegung*. Walter de Gruyter, Berlin and New York.

Corcilius, K. 2008b. "Two Jobs for Aristotle's Practical Syllogism?" In C. Rapp and P. Brüllmann (eds.), *The Practical Syllogism*. Special Issue of *Logical Analysis and History of Philosophy* 11: 163–184.

Corcilius, K. 2009. "How are Episodes of Thought Initiated according to Aristotle?" In G. van Riel and P. Destrée (eds.), *Soul and Mind: Ancient Perspectives on the De anima*. Leuven University Press, Leuven: 1–15.

Corcilius, K. 2011a. "Aristotle's Definition of Non-rational Pleasure and Pain and Desire." In J. Miller (ed.), *Aristotle's Nicomachean Ethics: A Critical Guide*. Cambridge University Press, Cambridge: 117–143.

Corcilius, K. 2011b. "Denken." In C. Rapp and K. Corcilius (eds.), *Aristoteles-Handbuch: Leben – Werk – Wirkung*. J.B. Metzler, Stuttgart: 197–206.

Corcilius, K. 2014. "Activity, Passivity and Sensory Discrimination in Aristotle." In J. F. Silva and M. Yrjönsuuri (eds.), *Active Perception in the History of Philosophy: From Plato to Modern Philosophy*. Springer, New York: 31–53.

Corcilius, K. 2015. "Faculties in Ancient Philosophy." In D. Perler (ed.), *The Faculties: A History*. Oxford University Press, Oxford: 19–65.

Corcilius, K. (ed.). 2017. *Aristoteles, Über die Seele / De anima*. Übersetzt, mit einer Einleitung und Anmerkungen. Felix Meiner Verlag, Hamburg.

Corcilius, K. 2019. "Teleology of the Practical in Aristotle: The Meaning of ΠΡΑΞΙΣ." In *Manuscrito* 42: 352–386.

Corcilius, K. 2020a. "*De anima* III 7: The Actuality Principle and the Triggering of Mental Episodes." In G. Guyomarc'h, C. Louget, and C. Murgier (eds.), *Aristote et l'âme humaine: lectures de De anima III offertes à Michel Crubellier*. Peeters, Louvain-la-Neuve: 185–220.

Corcilius, K. 2020b. "Resuming Discussion of the Common Cause of Animal Self-Motion: How Does the Soul Move the Body?" In C. Rapp and O. Primavesi (eds.), *Aristotle's De motu animalium*. Symposium Aristotelicum. Oxford University Press, Oxford: 299–344.

Corcilius, K. 2022. "The Gate to Reality: Aristotle's Account of Perception in *De anima* II 12." In C. Cohoe (ed.), *Aristotle's De anima: A Critical Guide*. Cambridge University Press, Cambridge: 122–154.

Corcilius, K. 2023. "Transformation and Discontinuity: Nature, Rationality, and Self-Motion in Aristotle." In F. Buddensiek (ed.), *Praxis: Handeln und Handelnde in Antiker Philosophie—Akten des VI. Kongresses der Gesellschaft für Antike Philosophie*. Walter De Gruyter, Berlin and New York: 107–137.

Corcilius, K. 2024. "The Soul Itself in Aristotle's Science of Living Things." In D. Lefebvre (ed.), *The Science of Life in Aristotle and the Early Peripatos*. Brill, Leiden.

Corcilius, K., and Gregoric, P. 2010. "Separability vs. Difference: Parts and Capacities of the Soul in Aristotle's *De anima*." In *Oxford Studies in Ancient Philosophy* 39: 81–119.

Corcilius, K., and Gregoric, P. 2013. "Aristotle's Model of Animal Motion." In *Phronesis* 58: 52–97.

Crager, A. (forthcoming). "Aristotle's 'Finest Theorem' and the Project of his *Analytics*."

Crivelli, P. 2004. *Aristotle on Truth*. Cambridge University Press, Cambridge.

Crubellier, M. 2004. "Le 'syllogisme pratique' ou comment la pensée meut le corps." In A. Laks and M. Rashed (eds.), *Aristote et le mouvement des animaux: Dix études sur le De motu animalium*. Septentrion Presses Universitaires, Villeneuve d'Ascq Cédex: 8–15.

Crubellier, M. 2020. "L'âme comme la main: Traduction et commentaire du chapitre III 8." In G. Guyomarc'h, C. Louguet, C. Murgier (eds.), *Aristote et l' âme humaine: lectures de "De anima" III offertes à Michel Crubellier*. Peeters, Louvain-la-Neuve: 221–254.

Crubellier, M. (forthcoming). "The Wax-Tablet in *De anima* III 4, 430a1: The Text and its Philosophical Meaning."

De Koninck, T. 1990. "La *Noêsis* et l'indivisible selon Aristote." In J.-F. Mattéi (ed.), *La naissance de la raison en Grèce. Actes du Congrès de Nice—Mai 1987*. Presses Universitaires de France, Paris: 215–228.

De Koninck, T. 2008. "L'intelligence et l'indivisible." In *L´intelligence et dieu*. Presses Universitaires de France, Paris: 95–123.

Delcomminette, S. 2020. "*De anima* III 6." In C. Murgier, C. Louguet, and G. Guyomarc'h (eds.), *Aristote et l' âme humaine: lectures de "De anima" III offertes à Michel Crubellier*. Peeters, Leuven: 157–184.

Denniston, J. D. 1954. *The Greek Particles*. Clarendon Press, Oxford.

Esfeld, M. 2000. "Aristotle's Direct Realism in *De anima*." In *The Review of Metaphysics* 54: 321–336.

Everson, S. 1999. *Aristotle on Perception*. Oxford University Press, Oxford.

Falcon, A. 2021. "Eternalism in Aristotle and After." In J. Verheyden, G. Roskam, and G. van Riel (eds.), *From Protology to Eschatology: Competing Views on the Origin and the End of the World in Platonism and Christian Thought.* Mohr Siebeck, Tübingen: 7–22.

Falcon, A. 2024. *The Architecture of the Science of Living Beings: Aristotle and Theophrastus on Animals and Plants.* Cambridge University Press, Cambridge.

Falcon, A., and Corcilius, K. 2022. "Aristotle on Memory and Remembering." In *Medicina nei secoli* 34: 12–30.

Falcon, A., and Lefebvre, D. 2017. "Introduction: Aristotle's Philosophy and the *Generation of Animals.*" In A. Falcon and D. Lefebvre (eds.), *Aristotle's Generation of Animals.* Cambridge University Press, Cambridge: 1–12.

Finamore, J. F. 1989. "Intellect and Common Sense in Aristotle's *De anima* III.7." In *Syllecta classica* 1: 27–41.

Förster, A. 1912. *Aristoteles: De anima.* Accademia Litterarum Hungarica, Budapest.

Frede, D. 1992. "The Cognitive Role of *Phantasia.*" In M. C. Nussbaum and A. Oksenberg (eds.), *Essays on Aristotle's De anima.* Oxford University Press, Oxford: 279–295.

Frede, D. 2020. "The Two Meanings of *Phantasia* in *De anima* III 3." In G. Guyomarc'h, C. Louget, and C. Murgier (eds.), *Aristote et l'âme humaine: lectures de De anima III offertes à Michel Crubellier.* Peeters, Louvain-la-Neuve: 53–74.

Frede, M. 1992. "On Aristotle's Conception of Soul." In M. C. Nussbaum and A. Oksenberg Rorty (eds.), *Essays on Aristotle's De anima.* Clarendon Press, Oxford: 93–107.

Frede, M. 1996a. "Aristotle's Rationalism." In M. Frede and G. Striker (eds), *Rationality in Greek Thought.* Oxford University Press, Oxford: 157–174.

Frede, M. 1996b. "La théorie aristotelicienne de l'intellect agent." In G. Romeyer Dherbey and C. Viano (eds), *Corps et âme: Sur le De anima d'Aristote.* Vrin, Paris: 377–390.

Frey, C. 2018. "Aristotle on the Intellect and Limits of Natural Science." In J. Sisko (ed.), *Philosophy of Mind in Antiquity.* Routledge, London: 160–174.

Fronterotta, F. 2007. "*OU MNHMONEUOMEN DE . . .* Aristotele. *De anima* Γ 5. 430 a 23–25." In *Elenchos* 27: 79–104.

Gasser-Wingate, M. 2021. *Aristotle's Empiricism.* Oxford University Press, New York.

Geach, P. 1957. *Mental Acts: Their Content and Their Objects.* Routledge, London.

Gerson, L. P. 2004. "The Unity of Intellect in Aristotle's *De anima.*" In *Phronesis* 49/4, 348–373.

Gregoric, P. 2007. *Aristotle on the Common Sense.* Oxford University Press, Oxford.

Gregoric, P. 2019. "Aristotle's Perceptual Optimism." In *Croatian Journal of Philosophy* 17: 543–560.

Gregoric, P., and Fink, J. L. 2021. *Encounters with Aristotelian Philosophy of Mind.* Routledge, Abingdon and New York.

Gregoric, P., and Pfeiffer, C. 2015. "Grasping Aristotle's Intellect." In *Documenti e studi sulla tradizione filosofica medievale* XXVI: 13–31.

Guthrie, W. K. C. 1981. *A History of Greek Philosophy.* Volume 6: *Aristotle: An Encounter.* Cambridge University Press, Cambridge.

Hahmann, A. 2016. *Aristoteles' "Über die Seele": Ein systematischer Kommentar.* Reclam, Leipzig.

Hamlyn, D. W. 1993^2. *Aristotle: De anima,* Books II and III (with passages from Book I). Clarendon Press, Oxford.

Harvey, J. 1978. "Aristotle on Truth and Falsity in *De anima* III 6." In *Journal of the History of Philosophy* 16: 219–220.

Hasper, P. S. 2002. *The Metaphysics of Continuity: Zeno, Democritus and Aristotle.* PhD Dissertation, University of Groningen.

Hayduck, M. (ed.). 1883. *Sophoniae In Aristotelis De anima libros paraphrasis.* Academia Regia Borussica/Reimer, Berlin.

Hayduck, M. (ed.). 1992. *Simplicii In Aristotelis De anima libros commentaria.* Academia Regia Borussica/Reimer, Berlin.

Hayduck, M. (ed.). 1997. *Ioannis Philoponi In Aristotelis De anima libros commentaria.* Academia Regia Borussica/Reimer, Berlin.

Heinze, R. (ed.). 1899. *Themistii In Aristotelis De anima libros paraphrasis.* Academia Regia Borussica/Reimer, Berlin.

Hicks, R. D. 1907. *Aristotle: De anima*. Translation, Introduction, and Notes by R. D. Hicks. Cambridge University Press, Cambridge. [Facsimile reprint: Georg Olms Velag, Hidesheim, Zürich, and New York, 1990.]

Horn, H.-J. 1994. *Studien zum dritten Buch der aristotelischen Schrift De anima*. Vandenhoeck and Ruprecht, Göttingen.

Inwood, B. 2001. *The Poem of Empedocles: A Text and Translation with an Introduction*. University of Toronto Press, Toronto.

Jannone, A., and Barbotin, E. 1966. *Aristote: De l'âme*. Texte établi par A. Jannone. Traduction et notes de E. Barbotin. Les Belles Lettres, Paris.

Jiménez, E. R. 2017. *Aristotle's Concept of Mind*. Cambridge University Press, Cambridge.

Johansen, T. K. 2006. "What Is New in Aristotle's *De sensu*? The Place of the *De sensu* in Aristotle's Psychology." In R. A. H. King (ed.), *Common to Body and Soul: Philosophical Approaches to Explaining Living Behavior in Greco-Roman Antiquity*. Walter de Gruyter, Berlin and New York: 140–164.

Johansen, T. K. 2012. *The Powers of Aristotle's Soul*. Oxford University Press, Oxford.

Johansen, T. K. 2020. "The Principle that 'Like Perceives Like' in Theophrastus' *De sensibus*." In *Rhizomata* 7: 226–248.

Judson, L. 2020. *Aristotle: Metaphysics. Book Λ*, Clarendon Press. Oxford.

Jung, C. 2011. *Die doppelte Natur des menschlichen Intellekts bei Aristoteles*. Königshausen and Neumann, Würzburg.

Kahn, Charles H. 1992. "Aristotle on Thinking." In M. C. Nussbaum and A. Oksenbert Rorty (eds.), *Essays on Aristotle's De anima*. Oxford University Press, Oxford: 359–379.

Kampe, F. 1870. *Die Erkenntnistheorie des Aristoteles*. Fues, Leipzig.

Kamtekar, R. 2009. "Knowing by Likeness in Empedocles." In *Phronesis* 54: 215–238.

Kelsey, S. 2022. *Mind and World in Aristotle's De anima*. Cambridge University Press, Cambridge.

Kietzmann, C. 2019. "Aristotle on the Definition of What It Is to Be Human." In G. Keil and N. Kreft (eds.), *Aristotle's Anthropology*. Cambridge University Press, Cambridge: 25–43.

Kosman, A. 1992. "What Does the Maker Mind Make?" In M. C. Nussbaum and A. Oksenberg Rorty (eds.), *Essays on Aristotle's De anima*. Oxford University Press, Oxford: 343–358.

Krämer, H. J. 1967. *Der Ursprung der Geistmetaphysik*. Zweite unveränderte Auflage. B. R. Grüner, Amsterdam.

Kühner, R., and Gerth, B. 1898. *Ausführliche Grammatik der Griechischen Sprache*. Dritte Auflage. 2 Bände. Zweiter Teil: *Satzlehre*. Hahnsche Buchhandlung, Hannover.

Kullmann, W. 1974. *Wissenschaft und Methode: Interpretationen zur aristotelischen Theorie der Naturwissenschaft*. Walter de Gruyter, Berlin and New York.

Kurfess, H. 1911. *Zur Geschichte der Erklärung der aristotelischen Lehre vom sog. ΝΟΥΣ ΠΟΙΗΤΙΚΟΣ und ΠΑΘΗΤΙΚΟΣ*. G. Schnürlen, Tübingen.

Labarrière, J.-L. 1993. "Aristote et la question du langage animal." In *Mètis: Anthropologie des mondes grecs anciens* 8: 247–260.

Labarrière, J.-L. 2004. *Langage, vie politique et mouvement des animaux*. Vrin, Paris.

Laks, A. 2020. "The Lever, or How to Act at a Distance: A Backdrop to Theophrastus' *De sensibus*." In *Rhizomata* 7: 168–187.

Le Blond, J.-M. 1997^2. *Aristote: Parties des animaux. Livre I*. Flammarion, Paris.

Lefebvre, D. 2002. "L'argument du sectionnement des vivants dans les *Parva naturalia*: le cas des insectes." In *Revue de philosophie ancienne* 20: 5–28.

Lennox, J. G. 1999. "The Place of Mankind in Aristotle's Zoology." In *Philosophical Topics* 27: 1–16.

Lennox, J. G. 2001. *Aristotle: On the Parts of Animals I–IV*. Clarendon Press, Oxford.

Lennox, J. G. 2008. "'As If We Were Investigating Snubness': Aristotle on the Prospects for a Single Science of Nature." In *Oxford Studies in Ancient Philosophy* 35: 149–186.

Lennox, J. G. 2009. "Aristotle on Mind and the Science of Nature." In M. Rossetto et al. (eds.), *Greek Research in Australia: Proceedings of the Eighth Biennial International Conference of Greek Studies, Flinders University June 2009*. Flinders University Department of Languages—Modern Greek, Adelaide: 1–18.

Lennox, J. G. 2019. "Is Reason Natural? Aristotle's Zoology of Rational Animals." In G. Keil and N. Kreft (eds.), *Aristotle's Anthropology*. Cambridge University Press, Cambridge: 99–117.

Lennox, J. G. 2021. *Aristotle on Inquiry: Erotetic Framework and Domain-Specific Norms*. Cambridge University Press. Cambridge.

Lewis, F. A. 1996. "Self-Knowledge in Aristotle." In *Topoi* 15: 39–58.

Lloyd, A. C. 1970. "Non-discursive Thought: An Enigma of Greek Philosophy." In *Proceedings of the Aristotelian Society* 70: 261–274.

Loening, R. 1903. *Die Zurechnungslehre des Aristoteles*. Verlag Gustav Fischer, Jena. [Facsimile reprint: Georg Olms, Hildesheim, Zürich, and New York, 1967].

McCready-Flora, I. 2014. "Aristotle's Cognitive Science: Belief, Affect and Rationality." In *Philosophy and Phenomenological Research* 89: 394–435.

McCready-Flora, I. 2019. "Speech and Rational Soul." In G. Keil and N. Kreft (eds.), *Aristotle's Anthropology*. Cambridge University Press, Cambridge: 44–59.

Malink, M. 2017. "Aristotle on Principles as Elements." In *Oxford Studies in Ancient Philosophy* 53: 163–214.

Maurus, S. 1668. *Aristotelis Opera quae extant omnia*. Paris (repr. 1885–1886).

Mendell, H. 2004. "Aristotle and Mathematics." In *Stanford Encyclopedia of Philosophy* (https://plato.stanford.edu/entries/aristotle-mathematics/)

Menn, S. 1994. "The Origins of Aristotle's Concept of *energeia*: *energeia* and *dunamis*." In *Ancient Philosophy* 14: 73–114.

Menn, S. 2012. "Aristotle's Theology." In C. Shields (ed.), *The Oxford Handbook of Aristotle*. Oxford University Press, Oxford: 211–265.

Menn, S. 2020. "From *De anima* III 4 to *De anima* III 5." In G. Guyomarc'h, C. Louguet, and C. Murgier (eds.), *Aristote et l'âme humaine: lectures de De anima offertes à Michel Crubellier*. Peeters, Louvain-la-Neuve: 95–156.

Menn, S. (forthcoming). *The Aim and the Argument of Aristotle's Metaphysics*. https://www.philosophie.hu-berlin.de/de/lehrbereiche/antike/mitarbeiter/menn/contents

Mignucci, M. 1996. "Vérité et pensée dans le *De anima*." In G. Romeyer Dherbey and C. Viano (eds.), *Corps et Âme: Sur le De anima d'Aristote*. Vrin, Paris: 405–422.

Miller, F. D. 2012. "Aristotle on the Separability of Mind." In C. Shields (ed.), *The Oxford Handbook of Aristotle*. Oxford University Press, Oxford: 306–339.

Miller, F. D. 2018. *Aristotle: On the Soul and Other Psychological Works*. Oxford University Press, Oxford.

Mingucci, G. 2015. *Fisiologia del pensiero in Aristotele*. Il Mulino, Bologna.

Moraux, P., Harlfinger, D., Reinsch, D., and Wiesner, J. 1976. *Aristoteles Graecus: Die griechischen Manuskripte des Aristoteles*. Volume 1: *Alexandrien—London*. Walter De Gruyter, Berlin and New York.

Morel, P.-M. 2006. "Common to the Body and the Soul in the *Parva naturalia*." In R. A. H. King (ed.), *Common to Body and Soul: Philosophical Approaches to Explaining Living Behavior in Greco-Roman Antiquity*. Walter de Gruyter, Berlin and New York: 121–139.

Morel, P.-M. 2008. "The Practical Syllogism in Context: *De motu* 7 and Zoology." In C. Rapp and P. Brüllmann (eds.), *The Practical Syllogism*. Special Issue of *Logical Analysis and History of Philosophy* 11: 185–196.

Morison, B. 2002. *On Location: Aristotle's Concept of Place*. Oxford University Press, Oxford.

Morison, B. 2019. "Theoretical *Nous* in the *Posterior Analytics*." In *Manuscrito* 42: 1–43.

Moss, J. 2012. *Aristotle on the Apparent Good, Perception, Phantasia, Thought and Desire*. Oxford University Press, Oxford.

Nussbaum, M. 1985[2]. Aristotle's *De motu animalium: Text with Translation, Commentary and Interpretive Essays*. University of Princeton Press, Princeton, NJ.

Oehler, K. 1962. *Die Lehre vom noetischen und dianoetischen Denken bei Platon und Aristoteles*. Verlag C. H. Beck, München.

Osborne, C. 1998. "Perceiving White and Sweet (again): Aristotle's *De anima* 3.7, 431a20–b2." In *Classical Quarterly* 48: 433–446.

Perfetti, S. 1998. "'*An anima nostra sit mortalis*': Una *quaestio* inedita discussa da Pietro Pomponazzi nel 1521." In *Rinascimento* 38: 205–226.

Perkams, M. 2008. *Selbstbewusstsein in der Spätantike: Die neuplatonischen Kommentare zu Aristoteles' De anima*. De Gruyter, Berlin and New York.
Pfeiffer, C. 2018. *Aristotle's Theory of Bodies*. Oxford University Press, Oxford.
Polansky, R. 2007. *Aristotle's De anima*. Cambridge University Press, Cambridge.
Politis, V. 2001. "Aristotle's Account of the Intellect as Pure Capacity." In *Ancient Philosophy* 21: 375–401.
Primavesi, O., and Corcilius, K. 2018. *Aristoteles: Über die Bewegung der Lebewesen / De motu animalium*. Philologische Einführung, neuer griechischer Text von Oliver Primavesi, philosophische Einführung, Übersetzung und Kommentar von Klaus Corcilius. Meiner, Hamburg.
Pritzl, K. 1984. "The Cognition of Indivisibles and the Argument of *De anima* 3.4–8." In *Proceedings of the American Catholic Philosophical Association* 58: 140–150.
Rapp, C. 2020a. "Joints and Movers in the Cliffhanger Passage at the end of Aristotle, *De anima* III 10." In G. Guyomarc'h, C. Louget, and C. Murgier (eds.), *Aristote et l'âme humaine: lectures de De anima III offertes à Michel Crubellier*. Peeters, Louvain-la-Neuve: 273–302.
Rapp, C. 2020b. "Introduction: The Argument of the *De motu animalium*." In C. Rapp and O. Primavesi (eds.), *Aristotle's De motu animalium*. Oxford University Press, Oxford: 1–66.
Rapp, C. 2021. "Whose State? Whose Nature? How Aristotle's *Polis* is 'Natural.'" In P. Adamson and C. Rapp (eds.), *State and Nature: Studies in Ancient and Medieval Philosophy*. De Gruyter: Berlin and New York: 81–118.
Rashed, M. 2007. *Essentialisme: Alexandre d'Aphrodise entre logique, physique et cosmologie*. Walter de Gruyter, Berlin and New York.
Reeve, C. D. C. 2017. *Aristotle: De anima*. Hackett, Indianapolis, IN.
Rodier, G. 1900. *Commentaire du "Traité de l'âme" d'Aristote*. Leroux, Paris.
Roreitner, R. 2020. "Blood, *Pneuma*, or Something More Solid? Aristotle on the Material Structure of Perceptual Apparatus." In H. Bartoš and C. King (eds.), *Heat,* Pneuma, *and Soul in Ancient Greek Philosophy and Science*. Cambridge University Press, Cambridge: 288–309.
Roreitner, R. 2021a. "The *Nous*-Body Relationship in Aristotle's *De anima*." In P. Gregoric and J. L. Fink (eds.), *Encounters with Aristotelian Philosophy of Mind*. Routledge, Abingdon and New York: 249–280.
Roreitner, R. 2021b. "Themistius Against Porphyry (?) on 'Why We Don't Remember.'" In *Classical Quarterly* 71: 379–385.
Roreitner, R. 2024. "Human Ontogeny in Aristotle and Theophrastus." In *Apeiron*.
Roreitner 2025. *Aristotle on the Nature and Causes of Perception*. Cambridge University Press, Cambridge.
Roreitner, R. (forthcoming a). "The *prooimion* to the *De sensu*: The Primacy of Perception and the Usefulness of the Senses (*Sens.* 1 436b1–437a17)." In K. Corcilius (ed.), *Text and Idea of Aristotle's* De Sensu. Mohr Siebeck, Tübingen.
Roreitner (forthcoming b). *Aristotle on Receptive Reason*.
Ross, W. D. 1956. *Aristotelis De anima recognovit brevique adnotatione instruxit*. Oxford Classical Text. Oxford University Press, Oxford. [Ross, *editio minor*]
Ross, W. D. 1961. Aristotle's *De anima*. Edited, with Introduction and Commentary by D. W. Ross. Clarendon Press, Oxford [Ross, *editio maior*].
Schmitz, H. 1985. *Die Ideenlehre des Aristoteles. Band 1/2. Ontologie, Noologie, Theologie*. Bouvier, Bonn.
Segev, M. 2017. "Aristotle on Nature, Human Nature and Human Understanding." In *Rhizomata* 5: 177–209.
Shields, C. 2016. *Aristotle: De anima*. Translated with an Introduction and Commentary by C. Shields. Clarendon Aristotle Series. Oxford University Press, Oxford.
Siwek, P. 1965. *Aristotelis tractatus de anima*. Edidit, versione latina auxit, commentario illustravit. Desclée & Co., Rome.
Sorabji, R. 1980. *Necessity, Cause and Blame: Perspectives on Aristotle's Theory*. Cornell University Press, Ithaca, NY.
Sorabji, R. 1981. "Definitions: Why Necessary, and in What Way?" In E. Berti (ed.), *Aristotle on Science: The "Posterior Analytics."* Proceedings of the Eighth Symposium Aristotelicum Held in Padua from September 7 to 15, 1978. Editrice Antenore, Padua: 205–244.

Sorabji, R. 1982. "Myths about Non-propositional Thought." In M. Schofield and M. C. Nussbaum (eds.), *Language and Logos: Studies in Ancient Greek Philosophy Presented to G. E. L. Owen*. Cambridge University Press, Cambridge: 295–314.

Sorabji, R. 1983. *Time, Creation, and the Continuum: Theories in Antiquity and the Early Middle Ages*. Duckworth, London.

Szlezák, T. A. 1979. *Platon und Aristoteles in der Nuslehre Plotins*. Schwabe, Basel.

Teichmüller, G. 1873. *Geschichte des Begriffs der Parusie*. Verlag von G. Emil Barthel, Halle.

Theiler, W. 1979[3]. *Aristoteles: Über die Seele*. Akademie Verlag, Berlin.

Thillet, P. 2005. *Aristote: De l'âme*. Traduction, présentation et notes. Gallimard, Paris.

Torstrik, A. 1862. *Aristoteles: De anima libri III recensuit A. Torstrik*. Weidemann, Berlin. [Facsimile reprint: Georg Olms, Hildesheim, Zürich, and New York, 1970.]

Trendelenburg, F. A. 1877. *Aristotelis De anima libri tres: Interpretum graecorum auctoritatem et codicum fidem recognivit commentariis illustravit—Editio altera emendata et aucta*. [Facsimile reprint: Akademische Druck- U. Verlagsanstalt, Graz, 1957.]

Trentini, S. 2016. "The Internal Coherence of *De anima* III 6." In G. Sillitti, F. Stella, and F. Fronterotta (eds.), *Il NOÛS di Aristotele*. Academia Verlag, Sankt Augustin: 175–213.

Tricot, J. 1934. *Aristote: De l'âme*. Vrin, Paris.

Van der Eijk, P. 1997. "The Matter of Mind: Aristotle on the Biology of 'Psychic' Processes and the Bodily Aspects of Thinking." In W. Kullmann and S. Föllinger (eds.), *Aristotelische Biologie: Intentionen, Methoden, Ergebnisse*. Steiner, Stuttgart: 231–258.

Verbeke, G. 1966. *Commentaire sur le de anima d'Aristote, traduction de Guillaume de Moerbeke*. Editions Béatrice-Nauwelaerts, Paris.

Wedin, M. V. 1988. *Mind and Imagination in Aristotle*. Yale University Press, New Haven, CT and London.

Wedin, M. V. 1993. "Content and Cause in the Aristotelian Mind." In *The Southern Journal of Philosophy* 31: 49–105.

Wedin, M. V. 1994. "Aristotle on the Mind's Self-Motion." In M.-L. Gill and J. G. Lennox (eds.), *Self-Motion from Aristotle to Newton*. Princeton University Press, Princeton, NJ: 86–116.

Zeller, E. 1921. *Die Philosophie der Griechen in ihrer geschichtlichen Entwicklung*. Zweiter Teil, zweite Abteilung. *Aristoteles und die alten Peripatetiker*. Vierte Auflage. O. R. Reisland, Leipzig.

Zucca, D. 2015. *L'anima del vivente: Vita, cognizione e azione nella psicologia aristotelica*. Morcelliana, Brescia.

Zucca, D. 2019. "What is Aristotle's Active Intellect?" In D. Zucca and R. Medda (eds.), *The Soul/Body Problem in Plato and Aristotle*. Academia Verlag, Baden Baden: 133–157.

Index of Passages

For the benefit of digital users, indexed terms that span two pages (e.g., 52–53) may, on occasion, appear on only one of those pages.

General Index

For the benefit of digital users, indexed terms that span two pages (e.g., 52–53) may, on occasion, appear on only one of those pages.

Tables and figures are indicated by an italic *t* and *f* following the page number.

The manufacturer's authorised representative in the EU for product safety is Oxford University Press España S.A. of el Parque Empresarial San Fernando de Henares, Avenida de Castilla, 2 – 28830 Madrid (www.oup.es/en or product.safety@oup.com). OUP España S.A. also acts as importer into Spain of products made by the manufacturer.

www.ingramcontent.com/pod-product-compliance
Lightning Source LLC
Chambersburg PA
CBHW050926070726
47757CB00003B/31
* 9 7 8 0 1 9 8 9 2 1 7 9 0 *